Self-regulation in Health Behavior

Self-regulation in Health Behavior

Edited by

Denise T.D. de Ridder and John B.F. de Wit

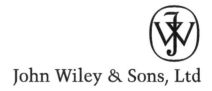

John Wiley & Sons, Ltd

Other Wiley Editorial Offices

John Wiley & Sons Inc., 111 River Street, Hoboken, NJ 07030, USA

Jossey-Bass, 989 Market Street, San Francisco, CA 94103-1741, USA

Wiley-VCH Verlag GmbH, Boschstr. 12, D-69469 Weinheim, Germany

John Wiley & Sons Australia Ltd, 42 McDougall Street, Milton, Queensland 4064, Australia

John Wiley & Sons (Asia) Pte Ltd, 2 Clementi Loop #02-01, Jin Xing Distripark, Singapore 129809

John Wiley & Sons Canada Ltd, 22 Worcester Road, Etobicoke, Ontario, Canada M9W 1L1

Wiley also publishes its books in a variety of electronic formats. Some content that appears in print may not
be available in electronic books.

Library of Congress Cataloging-in-Publication Data

Self-regulation in health behavior/edited by Denise T.D. de Ridder
and John B.F. de Wit.
    p. cm.
    Includes bibliographical references and index.
    ISBN-13: 978-0-470-02407-2 (cloth : alk. paper)
    ISBN-10: 0-470-02407-0 (cloth : alk. paper)
    ISBN-13: 978-0-470-02408-9 (pbk. : alk. paper)
    ISBN-10: 0-470-02408-9 (pbk. : alk. paper)
1. Health behavior.   2. Self-control.   3. Self-management (Psychology)
4. Control (Psychology)   5. Behaviorism (Psychology)
6. Health–Decision making. I. Ridder, Denise T. D. de. II. Wit, John Bertha Franciscus de, 1965-
    RA776.9.S45 2006
    613′.0433–dc22   2006000889

British Library Cataloguing in Publication Data

A catalogue record for this book is available from the British Library

ISBN-13 978-0-470-02407-2 (hbk)   978-0-470-02408-9 (pbk)
ISBN-10 0-470-02407-0 (hbk)   0-470-02408-9 (pbk)

Typeset in 10/12 pt Times by Thomson Press (India) Limited, New Delhi

This book is printed on acid-free paper responsibly manufactured from sustainable forestry
in which at least two trees are planted for each one used for paper production.

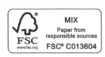

To Paul, Daniel, and Charlotte Leseman
DdR
To Philippe Adam, for everything
JdW

Contents

About the Editors

Denise T.D. de Ridder, Ph.D. is professor of Health Psychology at Utrecht University (The Netherlands) and scientific director of the Dutch Research Institute for Psychology and Health. Her research focuses on topics at the interface of coping and self-regulation with an emphasis on self-care behavior and adherence in chronic illness and eating and overweight in healthy individuals. She is co-editor of *Psychology and Health* and associate editor of *Health Psychology Review.*

John B.F. de Wit, Ph.D. is associate professor of Social Psychology of Health at Utrecht University (The Netherlands), and executive director of the master program in psychology at Utrecht University. His research interests encompass determinants of health behavior and strategies of change, and combine cognitive, motivational and volitional approaches to self-regulation. He has a longstanding involvement in the domains of sexuality and health, emphasizing the promotion as well as the maintenance of protective behaviors in vulnerable populations. Other work is concerned with motivational processes in risk perception and persuasion.

Contributors

Hugo J.E.M. Alberts is Ph.D. student at Maastricht University, Maastricht, The Netherlands.

Sander M. Bot is Ph.D. student at the Institute of Family and Child Care, University of Nijmegen, Nijmegen, The Netherlands.

Denise T.D. de Ridder is professor of health psychology at Utrecht University, Utrecht, The Netherlands.

John B.F. de Wit is associate professor of social psychology of health at Utrecht University, Utrecht, The Netherlands.

Jennifer L. Dykstra is graduate assistant at the Department of Psychology, Iowa State University, Ames, USA.

Rutger C.M.E. Engels is professor of psychology at the Institute of Family and Child Care, University of Nijmegen, Nijmegen, The Netherlands.

Winifred A. Gebhardt is assistant professor in clinical and health psychology at Leiden University, Leiden, The Netherlands.

Meg Gerrard is professor of psychology at Iowa State University, Ames, USA.

Frederick X. Gibbons is professor of psychology at Iowa State University, Ames, USA.

Peter M. Gollwitzer is professor of psychology at New York University, New York, USA.

Amy E. Houlihan is graduate assistant at the Department of Psychology, Iowa State University, Ames, USA.

Roeline G. Kuijer is assistant professor of health psychology at Utrecht University, Utrecht, The Netherlands.

Carolien Martijn is assistant professor of experimental psychology at Maastricht University, Maastricht, The Netherlands.

Elizabeth A. Pomery is graduate assistant at the Department of Psychology, Iowa State University, Ames, USA.

Rachel A. Reimer is graduate assistant at the Department of Psychology, Iowa State University, Ames, USA.

Klaus Rothermund is professor of psychology at Friedrich-Schiller Universität, Jena, Germany.

Paschal Sheeran is professor of psychology at the University of Sheffield, Sheffield, UK.

Michelle L. Stock is graduate assistant at the Department of Psychology, Iowa State University, Ames, USA.

Nanne K. de Vries is professor of health education and health promotion at Maastricht University, The Netherlands.

Thomas L. Webb is a lecturer in social psychology at the School of Psychological Sciences, University of Manchester, Manchester, UK.

Foreword

The psychology of health and illness has come a very long way since its inception. In the course of its evolution, the field has developed a fairly elaborate substructure of specializations. Some areas of health psychology focus on how the body responds to stressful experiences by setting into motion a cascade of cardiovascular, neuroendocrine, and immune changes—changes that adaptively prepare the body for the demands of high levels of activity but which can have longer-term residual effects that are problematic. Other areas of the field focus on how people with health problems go about regaining pre-illness levels of social and emotional functioning, or alternatively how they adapt to the restrictions their diseases place on them. Yet other areas of this field focus on the health-damaging behaviors that people sometimes engage in, in an effort to understand better what processes promote and maintain those behaviors and how those processes can be harnessed to make those behaviors less likely.

Different people find appeal in various aspects of this growing field. To me, the appeal of health psychology has always been less about the health than about the psychology. For example, I have long believed that what we sometimes treat as a special topic called "stress and coping" is simply human behavior under conditions of greater than typical adversity. As such, it displays essentially the same properties as human behavior in other contexts where obstacles exist. I think of adversity as any condition that represents a threat to, or interference with, attainment of goals the person values as important. Interestingly enough, it is not always outside forces that create such obstacles. It often turns out that the various goals a given person holds are not always fully compatible with one another. Sometimes attaining one goal interferes with the attainment of another. Thus even a success can be an obstacle to a different success. When the attainment of a goal is threatened, the person has to decide (and often must do so over and over again) whether to keep pursuing the goal or give it up. Because the negative emotions that come when goal attainment is threatened are unpleasant and undesired, people will often take steps to reduce them, even if only temporarily. They will often do this without regard to longer-term effects of the emotion-soothing actions, which in some cases can be deleterious. Increasingly, social and personality psychologists are also interested in the idea that behavior sometimes is managed from the top down (intentions leading to actions), but sometimes is triggered from the bottom up (via self-organization or reflexive triggering without the formation of an intention).

All the elements of this portrayal of stress and coping are represented in mainstream psychology. The idea that human behavior is about approaching (and maintaining proximity to) desired conditions (whether these conditions are thought of as goals, values, desires, or pathways to the future) is a common element of psychological theory today. We also understand, though, that people do not always (or even often) have completely smooth sailing to those goals. Reality throws a wide variety of obstacles in people's way (obstacles ranging in severity from closed doors to hurricanes). The idea that people's values are often less than fully compatible with each other is part of many approaches to understanding behavior. Thus, the same person may want to be healthy and also want to pursue other interests that take time and attention away from the goal of health. Many theories also posit that how people respond to difficulty, whether created by obstacles or conflicts, depends partly on their confidence of prevailing. The fact that people's goal-directed actions can be automatic or effortful—well thought out or impulsive—is of increasing interest today. Determinants of whether people choose to do things that feel good in the short run or instead make choices that are better in the long run have been studied for years under such labels as self-control and delay of gratification. All these ideas are embedded in contemporary psychology. All of them are also represented in this volume on health behavior.

These ideas interweave with one another (some perhaps more easily than others). The picture they form has an intrinsic dynamic. It fits the idea that living systems are composed of simple processes that draw them forward to desired ends, while keeping key parameters within certain comfortable ranges. Some such processes are labeled homeostatic, others are sometimes called homeodynamic. The processes are simple, but simple processes can be linked into arrays of great complexity. Many desired ends are pursued at once, sometimes in competition with each other and sometimes just concurrently. There are systems within systems, natural forces acting to regulate movement and control of many values simultaneously within plausible orbits. Humans are not linear strings of causal paths. Humans are self-regulating systems.

The idea that health-related behavior represents self-regulating systems is given clear expression in this excellent volume. As a group, the contributors take seriously the idea that people have consciously held goals and also goals that are implicit; the idea that goal pursuit can be effortful but can also be automatic; the idea that people often choose between short-term gratification and deeper longer-term well-being. The contributors to this volume understand that people confront conflict not just between impulse and restraint, but also between incompatible desires. They understand that whether people stay on track depends in part on their confidence, and that staying on track is a long-term proposition. In short, as a group they apply diverse aspects of a broadly grounded view of behavior-in-general to the specific problem of health behavior. The view is that of a self-regulating system. Many of the ideas represented in these discussions are present in more general statements on self-regulation (e.g., Carver & Scheier, 1998). However, the authors of these chapters extend such ideas more directly into the domain of health-related behavior.

The Chapters and Their Themes

The notion that health-promoting behavior is goal-directed (in some ways the core of self-regulatory models) is implicit in many of these chapters and a core feature of some of them. Gebhardt (Chapter 2) focuses closely on the personal goals that underlie health-promoting behavior. De Wit (Chapter 10) makes the point that change in behavior can be viewed as a process of goal setting and effortful action toward attaining the goal. Sheeran, Webb and Gollwitzer (Chapter 6) focus on the fact that having broad, general goals is typically not enough; people also benefit from having concrete if-then connections in mind, to help them start acting when appropriate circumstances arise and to help them continue acting when the going gets difficult.

The idea that desires to behave in health-promoting ways can conflict with other desires is one that is important in many of these chapters. It forms a main focus for Gebhardt (Chapter 2), for de Ridder and Kuijer (Chapter 7), and for Rothermund (Chapter 10). Gebhardt focuses on organizations of goals within the self that can make health behaviors more likely or less likely to be adopted. De Ridder and Kuijer consider the frustrations and distractions that often emerge in the course of efforts toward the desired goal of behavior change, and argue that it is important to attend to those frustrations, because they signal other important goals. By satisfying those short-term goals periodically, the person may be able to facilitate the more difficult longer-term goals. Similarly, Rothermund uses the idea of conflict among goals as a basis for stressing the importance of sometimes accommodating to the reality of goals besides those directed at better health. The notion of conflict among goals also plays a more minor role in several other chapters.

The role of expectancies is taken up by several of these authors, in several forms. Rothermund (Chapter 10) stresses the fact that the decision whether to continue making efforts toward health goals depends in part on confidence about ultimate outcomes of the efforts. De Wit (Chapter 9) notes as well that confidence is a key determinant of continued efforts to maintain health behavior changes, once such changes are initiated. Martijn, Alberts and De Vries (Chapter 8) address a different sort of expectancy. They argue that people's self-control efforts are guided by their expectations: in particular, expectations about whether continued efforts at self-control exhaust resources. Their very intriguing findings raise serious questions about whether the capacity for self-control is limited in the way that Baumeister and colleagues have argued.

The proposition that behavior is sometimes guided top-down by intentions and sometimes guided bottom-up by impulses suggested by the social environment plays a role in the Engels and Bot chapter (Chapter 4) and takes center stage in the interrelated chapters by Gibbons et al. (Chapter 3) and Gerrard et al. (Chapter 5). Engels and Bot review a variety of literature indicating that neither parents nor peers exert strong influence on adolescent risk behavior, but then turn to another source of evidence—direct behavioral observation—which shows strong situational modeling effects. These effects are relatively spontaneous, in contrast to the self-reports that form the bulk of the other literatures. As such, they suggest that the behavior itself is relatively spontaneous. Gibbons et al. go a step further, arguing that health-promoting behavior tends to be deliberative and derived from planful intentions, but that health-risk behavior tends to be more spontaneous and impulsive. The Gerrard et al. chapter delves more deeply into the conceptual basis of this difference. Based on a review of ideas from the developmental literature, they propose that one important source of risk behavior is poor self-control, the relative inability to override impulses. This is quite different from the active tendency to seek out risks as a source of excitement. Instead, it is about the spontaneous nature of many acts of behavior, particularly in childhood and adolescence.

It is very satisfying to me to see health behavior approached from this conceptual framework. I think it is a general framework that offers great promise to future research efforts on these topics. I hope other readers will find it as interesting and valuable a perspective on health behavior as I do.

Charles S. Carver
Coral Gables, Florida

CHAPTER 1

Self-regulation in Health Behavior: Concepts, Theories, and Central Issues

Denise T.D. de Ridder and John B.F. de Wit

Good health is of critical importance to many people while they are generally aware that their behavior plays an important role in achieving and maintaining physical well-being. In Western societies, it is difficult *not* knowing that one is, to some extent, responsible for one's own health as people are continuously reminded of the importance of their behavior for staying healthy by both public health campaigns and medical care professionals (Brownell, 1991). Yet, even though good health is generally considered important, and many people have good intentions for health behavior, the vast majority report difficulties in consistently performing those behaviors. They may find it hard, for instance, to maintain a healthy diet or a pattern of regular exercise in the face of temptations of modern life (e.g., Rothman, Baldwin & Hertel, 2004). Changing a bad health habit seems even more difficult than maintaining a good one (Polivy & Herman, 2002; cf. Norcross, Ratzin & Payne, 1989).

The proverbial road to hell does indeed seem to be paved with good intentions (cf. Powers, Koestner & Topciu, 2005). The question is: Why is it so difficult to act upon intentions or maintain attempts for changing health behavior, even for people who seem to be motivated? Only recently has the so-called "intention-behavior gap" started to attract substantial attention, and currently this is one of the most researched aspects of health behavior (e.g., Sheeran, 2002; Sheeran, Milne, Webb & Gollwitzer, 2005; also see Sheeran, Webb & Gollwitzer, this volume), and a crucial aspect of self-regulation. Self-regulation broadly refers to the processes of goal setting and goal striving, and includes dealing with a range of challenges that individuals may face when trying to achieve something that is important but, almost by definition, difficult to attain (Mischel, Cantor & Feldman, 1996). Important new questions arise from a self-regulation approach to health behavior, such as the following: How do people set health goals, and do they in fact

Self-regulation in Health Behavior. Edited by Denise T.D. de Ridder and John B.F. de Wit.

have health goals? Are these goals authentic or merely a response to persuasive health messages or other social influences that are not well considered and therefore prone to failure? Which types of health goals motivate behavior, and what happens when health goals are in conflict with other goals? What are the conditions that promote or hinder the successful pursuit of health goals? And how do people deal with distractions and temptations when striving for health goals?

Self-regulation theories have not been designed uniquely to explain and understand health behavior and they are relevant in other important contexts as well, such as learning or organizational behavior (cf. Karoly, Boekaerts & Maes, 2005; for an overview, see Boekaerts, Pintrich & Zeidner, 2000). However, the health domain poses special challenges for self-regulation theories because of the substantial discrepancy that has been noted between the importance of individuals' health goals (or at least, what they report to be important health goals) and their frequent failure to act upon these goals. In fact, self-regulation failure in the health domain is a prototypical case to illustrate the relevance of a self-regulation approach to behavior (Baumeister, Heatherton & Tice, 1994). In turn, health behavior research can benefit from a self-regulation approach as this explicitly frames health behavior as a process of investing in long-term goals that require the control of immediate needs, which is one of the most important and difficult self-regulatory tasks (Brandtstädter & Renner, 1990; Mischel et al., 1996).

We feel that the self-regulation approach opens new perspectives for the study of complex health-related behaviors, and we are convinced that applying a self-regulation approach to critical issues in health behavior will result in a better understanding of why and when people effectively invest in their long term health than traditional approaches so far have done. In our overview of self-regulation approaches to health behavior we will not limit ourselves to one or two particular perspectives, as others have done (e.g., Cameron & Leventhal, 2003), but instead adopt a broad view that highlights important basic processes of self-regulation of health behavior, notably those involved in flexible goal setting and tenacious goal striving (Mischel et al., 1996). In the remainder of this chapter, we will first discuss what generally is meant by self-regulation, and briefly trace the historical roots of this approach. Next, we elaborate on different theoretical approaches to self-regulation, highlighting the cybernetic control approach (e.g., Carver & Scheier, 1998), a strength perspective of self-control (e.g., Muraven & Baumeister, 2000), and behavioral enaction strategy (e.g., Gollwitzer, 1999), respectively. We then proceed with highlighting critical issues related to the self-regulation of health behavior. In the last section we will give an overview of the book.

WHAT IS SELF-REGULATION?

Compared to other living creatures, human beings are noted for having an extensive ability to exert control over their inner states, processes, and responses (Baumeister et al., 1994). People are able to resist their own impulses, adapt their behavior to a range of standards, and change their current behaviors in the service of attaining distal goals (Baumeister, 1999). The term self-regulation is often used to refer broadly to efforts by humans to alter their thoughts, feelings, desires, and actions in the perspective of such higher goals (Carver & Scheier, 1998; Vohs & Baumeister, 2004). Hence, self-regulation refers to the person as an active agent and decision-maker, and is a vital aspect of human adaptation to life without which the individual would be a helpless spectator of events (Baumeister, 2005).

Psychologists' interest in self-regulation has burgeoned in recent years, and as an illustration Leventhal, Brisette and Leventhal (2003) found that two thirds of more than 2,700 publications containing the keyword "self-regulation" were published after 1990. This growing popularity promoted a range of views that differ in the various principles of self-regulation they emphasize and the specific mechanism they propose, but nevertheless share two basic properties (Cameron & Leventhal, 2003). A first common feature is to construe self-regulation as a dynamic motivational system of setting goals, developing and enacting strategies to achieve those goals, appraising progress, and revising goals and strategies accordingly. A second common characteristic is that self-regulation is also concerned with the management of emotional responses, which are seen as crucial elements of the motivational system, and that are conceived of as intricately linked with cognitive processes.

An issue of particular relevance in self-regulation concerns the processes involved in effective goal-pursuit that often extends over long periods of time and is frequently confronted with obstacles and temptations. How do individuals manage to successfully quit smoking, for instance, even though from time to time they may experience urges and cravings, and encounter numerous situations in which a cigarette is on offer? More generally, how do people manage the trade-offs and choices between distal goals and immediate urges? And how do they stay on track in cycles of waxing and waning commitment to their goals (cf. Klinger, 1977)? Some of these "preliminaries of willing" (cf. James, 1890), are related to the process of goal setting, and effective self-regulation is more likely when a goal is construed as personally meaningful, supported by favorable expectations about one's ability to execute the necessary actions, and the choice of appropriate standards for performance (Mischel et al., 1996). Several other processes contribute to the successful enaction of intentions, such as effective planning and adequate self-instruction to implement plans. Detailed overviews of "goal-guidance processes" (Maes & Karoly, 2005) are presented by other authors (e.g., Gollwitzer & Moskowitz, 1996; Kuhl, 2000; Maes & Karoly, 2005; Mischel et al., 1996).

Successful self-regulation requires the strategic mobilization of thought, feeling, and action (Cantor, 1990; Gollwitzer, 1996; Kuhl, 2000), in particular when facing obstacles and conflicts between goals, and self-regulation generally is construed as a systematic process that involves conscious effort to influence thoughts, feelings, and behaviors in order to achieve a goal in the context of a changing environment (cf. Zeidner, Boekaerts & Pintrich, 2000). Phrased differently, self-regulation entails individuals' involvement in the management of their own change processes (Abraham, Norman & Conner, 2000), including the conscious consideration of the relative importance of potentially competing goals, and goal prioritization in particular (Abraham & Sheeran, 2000). The unique contributions of the psychological self-regulation perspective to an explanation of (health) behavior can best be understood when considered in the historic context of other perspectives on behavior, especially insofar as they relate to the role of motivation (Bandura, 1986; Mischel et al., 1996).

The Emergence of a Self-regulation Perspective

Since the emergence of psychological science in the late 19th century, psychologists have proposed a range of substantially different views on the nature of motivational processes that underlie human behavior. However, be it the trait-disposition view, the biological perspective, psychoanalytic thinking or learning theory, to name but the most important perspectives, the approaches that have dominated thinking about motivation and behavior for most of the 20th century shared one critical assumption. All considered behavior to mostly result from non-reasoned processes. The precise processes that have been proposed differed between these perspectives, but none included reasoning. Indeed, for much of the history of psychological thought, motivational processes have been considered as substantially different from and independent of cognitive processes. Only more recently have scholars started to invoke human agency and systematically address the ways in which motivation and cognition are intricately linked (cf. Mischel et al., 1996). A major change in thinking about how motivation and cognition are related is evident in Bandura's view that cognitive processes play a central role in human learning as well as motivation (Bandura, 1977). An important cognitive process underlying motivation is that reinforcements create expectations of future outcomes, which guide behavior through the processes of goal setting and self-evaluation against these standards, a notion that has become central to the self-regulation perspective of behavior. Indeed, it has been noted that the concept of self-regulation originates with attempts to make learning theory more sophisticated and flexible to encompass a larger portion of behavior (Baumeister, 1998).

Bandura's writings (e.g., 1977, 1986) have proven particularly seminal for the emergence of a self-regulation perspective, highlighting central issues such as the symbolic representations of goals and self-reflective monitoring of behavior in the pursuit of goals. Bandura's Social Cognitive Theory posits that individuals engage in behavior because of the outcomes they hope to achieve, and these action expectations reflect the motivational function of reinforcement (Bandura, 1977, 1986). People strive to gain anticipated positive outcomes and to forestall potential negative outcomes, and this goal striving is further governed by individuals' self-efficacy beliefs. As a general rule, people undertake those tasks for which they judge themselves efficacious. Self-efficacy is particularly important to self-regulation because it influences a host of variables that come into play as people strive to regulate their behavior (Cervone, Mor, Orom, Shadel & Scott, 2004). Self-efficacy beliefs affect the level and type of goal individuals adopt, which in turn influences performance. Explicit, challenging goals raise motivation and goal attainment (Locke & Latham, 2002), and individuals with high self-efficacy are more likely to adopt and remain committed to highly challenging goals.

The major contribution of Social Cognitive Theory arguably lies in the proposition that self-efficacy beliefs affect standards of performance (i.e., goal setting), a suggestion that has rapidly been included in other motivational theories of behavior. Only recently increasing attention is being devoted to explicating the ways in which self-efficacy beliefs also affect strategies for achieving goals (Bandura, 1991; Cervone et al., 2004; Luszczynska & Schwarzer, 2005; Schwarzer, 1992), but the proposed mechanisms substantially overlap with processes that are central to other accounts of self-regulation. Also, according to Carver and Scheier (1998), Bandura has been somewhat reluctant to adopt the vocabulary of feedback control, which constitutes another important feature of self-regulation (Miller, Gallanter & Pribam, 1960; Carver & Scheier, 1982), and one that we will discuss in the next section.

MODELS OF SELF-REGULATION

Cameron and Leventhal (2003) note that the term self-regulation has been so widely used in recent years that one cannot but wonder whether all theories of (health) behavior are self-regulation models. Obviously, the answer should be no. Following other authors in the field of self-regulation (Carver & Scheier, 1998; Mischel et al., 1996), we apply three criteria for including models of behavior as self-regulatory models: (a) The explicit consideration of goals, (b) a view of the person as an active agent in shaping his or her own behavior, and (c) an emphasis on volitional processes in goal striving.

Central to all self-regulation models of behavior is the concept of goals. Different type of goal constructs have been proposed, including personal strivings (Emmons, 1986), life tasks (Cantor & Kihlstrom, 1987), personal projects (Little, 1983) or self-guides (Higgins, 1987), each emphasizing different aspects of goals but having in common the idea that goals energize and direct activities as they give meaning to people's lives (Baumeister, 1989). Indeed, understanding the person means understanding the person's goals (Carver & Scheier, 1999). By definition, goals are future-oriented as they relate to how people think of their unrealized potential and the kind of things they might want to achieve. Most theoretical accounts of self-regulation cast goals as guiding principles that people consciously and intentionally set to effectively steer their behavior (e.g., Austin & Vancouver, 1996; Elliott & Dweck, 1988; Pervin, 1989). We consider a theory to be a self-regulation model when it starts from the assumption that individuals are agents that somehow are involved in shaping their own destiny. This can be as active decision-makers, but also includes instances in which individuals act to achieve goals of which they are not consciously aware (e.g., Bargh & Chartrand, 1999; Fitzsimons & Bargh, 2004; Strack & Deutsch, 2004).

In addition to acknowledging the importance of goals and goal setting as motivational underpinnings of human action, a self-regulation theory of human behavior also should make explicit the processes that are involved in striving to attain the specified goal. That is, self-regulation theories are not only concerned with motivation but also with volition, and the processes of goal setting and goal striving are construed as intricately linked in a recursive process, which dynamically adapts to changes in the context in which the self-regulation occurs. We next introduce major theoretical approaches to self-regulation that differ in the extent in which they incorporate these different features. We distinguish among cybernetic control theory (e.g., Carver & Scheier, 1998), models of willpower and self-control resources (e.g., Baumeister et al., 1994; Mischel et al., 1996), and behavioral enaction theories (e.g., Gollwitzer, Fujita & Oettingen, 2004; Schwarzer, 2001).

Cybernetic Control Theory

For a long time, the cybernetic view of self-regulation developed by Carver and Scheier (Carver, 2004; Carver & Scheier, 1998; Scheier & Carver, 2003) has more or less been equated with the self-regulation perspective, not in the least because it was one of the first self-identified self-regulation theories. Central to Carver and Scheier's approach to self-regulation, which continues to be "the bedrock of self-regulation science" (Vohs & Baumeister, 2004, p. 4), is the notion that "individuals live life by identifying goals and behaving in ways aimed at attaining those goals" (Scheier & Carver, 2003, p. 17). Behavioral self-regulation hence entails that individuals hold a goal, monitor progress towards the attainment of this goal, and act in ways to reduce any discrepancy between the current state and a standard as specified by the goal, and they do this in ways that fit the situation and their personalities (Carver, 2004).

This dynamic process of feedback control is summarized by the Test-Operate-Test-Exit cycle (TOTE; Miller et al., 1960; Powers, 1973), in which stimulus input is evaluated through a comparison with a reference value or standard (Test), acted upon to bring the person's situation in line with the standard (Operate), which constitutes the systems output function, and tested again to evaluate whether the standard has been reached (Test). If so, the control process is ended (Exit). Feedback loops are discrepancy reducing (or "negative") when behavior decreases any discrepancy between the person's current state and the goal. This process is seen when someone attempts to attain a valued goal or conform to a standard, such as exercising more or eating more fruits, and refers to approach behaviors. A discrepancy enlarging ("positive") feedback loop is involved in acts of avoidance, as in not eating high caloric foods or reducing alcohol intake. It is in particular the consequences of behavior that constitute useful feedback, and self-regulation in essence refers to an internal guidance system that operates on the short-term effects of actions (Carver & Scheier, 1998), and can override normal response tendencies.

A central idea in Carver and Scheier's theorizing of self-regulation is that goals differ in abstraction, and are organized hierarchically. They similarly propose a hierarchy of feedback loops in which lower order goals are controlled by higher order goals (Carver & Scheier, 1982; cf. Powers, 1973). In this hierarchical system of self-regulation, a lower level represents the means towards the ends specified at the next higher level, and what results is a "cascade of control" (Scheier & Carver, 2003, p. 20), which extends from the most abstract top level at which system concepts (or "be" goals) are represented, such as being a healthy person, down to motor control goals at the lowest level, such as walk to work instead of driving by car (Carver & Scheier, 1982). An implication of the notion of hierarchy is that goals vary in importance. The higher in the organization, the more goals are tied to the sense of self and the more an individual is committed to this goal. In turn, high goal commitment is often associated with affect, and affect in particular is thought to be involved in priority management (Carver, 2004). Carver and Scheier (1998) have suggested that the feelings a person experiences reflect how well the behavior regulation process is doing. This self-awareness or self-monitoring of affect is crucial for the understanding of self-regulation processes as the affect resulting from either slower or faster than expected progress to the standard is believed to determine further action.

Given that the function of feedback systems is to reduce discrepancies, positive affect is suggested to promote slowing down or *coasting*, as a result of which the positive affect gradually fades (Carver, 2004). While people are generally thought to strive for continued pleasure, this makes functional sense because it can explain why someone would ever stop a pleasurable activity and attend to other important issues and concerns. Negative affect is proposed to promote that a person tries harder, but an impulse to withdraw or disengage may also occur when the person's expectancy of being able to reduce the discrepancy is unfavorable (cf. Carver, 1979). Sometimes this disengagement involves scaling back to the pursuit of a less demanding goal, which adaptively keeps the person in specific domain of goal pursuit. An import issue concerns when it is adaptive to give up, and Scheier and Carver (2003) suggest that this is the case when it leads to taking up of other goals, which can be substitutes for the abandoned goal (Wrosch, Scheier, Miller, Schulz & Carver, 2003; see also Rothermund, this volume).

Theories of Willpower and Self-control Resources

Whereas the Carver and Scheier approach to self-regulation highlights the process of self-monitoring as crucial in acting upon the experience of discrepancy between a current state and a desired goal, Baumeister's self-control strength theory emphasizes the resources involved in making changes and adjustments in one's behavior to achieve a goal (Baumeister, Bratslavsky, Muraven & Tice, 1998). In cybernetic terms this self-regulation resource approach focuses on the operate phase of the TOTE loop, and much less on performance standards or monitoring progress (Baumeister & Heatherton, 1996). As such, both approaches are believed to be complementary, and to address different aspects of self-regulation (Vohs & Baumeister, 2004). The approach advocated by Baumeister and colleagues entails that self-control or willpower plays an essential role in self-regulation, as self-control is required to resist urges and temptations that would otherwise interfere with the individual's long-term interests. This emphasis on the importance of self-control and willpower is shared with earlier theories concerning postponing the fulfillment of immediate needs, such as Mischel's delay of gratification paradigm (Mischel, Shoda & Rodriguez, 1989).

The Baumeister model holds three central assumptions. First, it states that there is a limited capacity for self-regulation because self-regulation is an effortful process. Second, the theory holds that all self-regulation tasks draw on the same (limited) resource, making it difficult to engage in continued self-control once the resource has been employed for an initial task. The third and probably most important assumption is that successful self-regulation entirely depends on the availability of the resource. A series of experimental studies have provided evidence for the first two assumptions, demonstrating that the capacity for controlling the self draws on a resource that resembles a strength, more than a skill or a knowledge structure and is hence vulnerable to depletion (Baumeister et al., 1998; Muraven, Tice & Baumeister, 1998). That is, the resource for self-regulation is limited in such a way that expending it is followed by a period of reduced capacity until it builds up again, much like a muscle works (Muraven & Baumeister, 2000). However, it has been suggested that depletion effects may also be related to decreased motivation (Martijn, Alberts & De Vries, this volume; Muraven & Slessareva, 2003).

Regarding the third assumption of the model, evidence is mixed. To date, most studies applying self-control resource theory have been concerned with explaining self-regulation failure, which seems reasonable because of its emphasis on the limited availability of self-control (Baumeister & Heatherton, 1996; Baumeister et al., 1994; Muraven et al., 1998). Indeed, the scarce capacity for self-regulation may provide a good account of why so many people fail in acting upon their intentions or do not maintain initial attempts to change their behavior. That is, they may be able to withstand the temptations of cigarettes, alcohol or fattening foods for a short while but, as the theory predicts, sooner or later they will give in because of self-control depletion. Often they do so for the hedonistic motive of feeling good in the short term or because they fail to recognize the long-term benefits of self-control (Leith & Baumeister, 1996; Tice, Bratslavsky & Baumeister, 2001).

Despite its relevance for understanding self-regulation failure, which seems especially important in the field of health behavior, the resource approach has some trouble in explaining why and how people may achieve successful self-regulation. There is some evidence that self-control may improve as a result of exercise (Muraven, Baumeister & Tice, 1999), but overall the theory is more concerned with explaining the conditions that hinder self-regulation than those that may promote it. Because of its emphasis on self-control as the essential feature of self-regulation the theory also tends to neglect other important aspects of self-regulation, most notably how people determine their strategies for goal achievement in the face of distractions and frustrations (an issue we will discuss later in this chapter). Thus, although self-control may be a powerful device in withstanding immediate urges that may interfere with striving for long-term goals, the resource approach remains rather implicit about how people engage in successful goal pursuit once they have effectively inhibited their impulses. In addition, the resource approach also is somewhat vague about the way goals regulate behavior, and implicitly seems to hold that people are driven by immediate interests only. These issues are addressed by a third type of self-regulation models, which we will discuss in the next section.

Behavioral Enaction Theories

In contrast to classic social-cognitive models that focus on the role of motivation in behavior (for a discussion of social-cognitive models of health behavior, see later this chapter), more recent models in this tradition have become increasingly concerned with the volitional processes involved in the initiation and maintenance of actions to achieve one's goals (Abraham & Sheeran, 2000). These models have been termed behavioral enaction models, and we consider them models of self-regulation because they not only address processes involved in goal setting but also distinguish important aspects of goal striving.

In recent years a number of theories have been proposed that have in common the assumption that the process of behavior change can be best described as a passing through a number of distinct stages, and that suggest factors that might influence the transition from one stage to another. Stage models hold that individuals in different stages will behave in qualitatively different ways, and propose that interventions needed to move individuals further in the process of change should vary from stage to stage (Weinstein, Rothman & Sutton, 1998). These models differ in the number of stages they propose and, more importantly, in how specific they are with respect to the psychological mechanisms and strategies that are involved at different points in the process of behavior change.

Well-known stage models of behavior change, notably the Transtheoretical Model (Prochaska & DiClemente, 1984), but also Weinstein's Precaution Adoption Process model (Weinstein, 1988), propose five to six distinct stages of change. These refer to the transitions a person experiences from initially unaware of a problem to undecided about taking action, considering action, initiating effective action, and through to successful maintenance and avoidance of relapse. While these models have intuitive appeal and hold substantial heuristical value for large scale prevention as well as change attempts in therapeutic settings, the mechanisms of change that are involved in stage transitions remain rather unspecified (Weinstein et al., 1998). Armitage and Conner (2000) note that in both these models the description of what occurs in terms of social-cognitive processes is rather imprecise, and it remains unclear whether they truly describe the change process, or strategies for goal pursuit at all. In addition, these models are rather implicit about the role of personal goals, which is probably related to their development in the context of behavioral interventions that may often serve to convince individuals of the need to adopt a particular health goal.

Other important stage models distinguish between a motivational and a volitional phase to behavior change, as implied by the classic distinction between goal setting and goal striving (Lewin, Dembo, Festinger & Sears, 1944). A model that has proven particularly influential is the model of action phases (Heckhausen & Gollwitzer, 1987; Gollwitzer, 1993). This model argues that an individual selects a particular behavior because of expected consequences, and then sets out to implement it in a specific way. The entire behavior change process is thought to consist of four stages: 1) a predecisional phase in which potential goals are deliberated, and a decision to pursue one of them is made; 2) a post-decisional phase in which ways of implementing goals are considered, and some means of goal attainment are selected; 3) an actional phase in which functional behaviors to attain the goal are initiated; and 4) a postactional phase in which attained outcomes are evaluated.

While no empirical work has directly assessed the propositions of the model (Armitage & Conner, 2000), it has proven an important conceptual basis for contemporary work on the implementation of intentions (cf. Gollwitzer, 1996). Gollwitzer, Heckhausen and Steller (1990) propose that each phase involves a distinct mindset that tailors a person's cognitive processing to meet the task demands of that phase (i.e., cognitive tuning). Gollwitzer and colleagues reported a number of studies examining the deliberative mindset of the predecisional phase and the implemental mindset of the post-decisional phase, and made clear that goal setting and goal striving differ in nature. They further noted that researchers interested in goal-oriented behavior did not develop distinct theories to account for goal striving, but rather stretched expectancy-value theories to make them account for goal setting as well as goal striving (Gollwitzer et al., 1990).

Gollwitzer (1996) advances the view that planning promotes the willful implementation of a person's goal and thus provides volitional benefits. In particular, it is proposed that planning helps to alleviate crucial volitional problems of goal achievement, such as being too easily distracted or giving up in the face of difficulties when instead increased effort and persistence are needed. These beneficial effects of planning are achieved by the formation of implementation intentions (if-then plans that specify when, where and how an instrumental goal-directed response is to be initiated) that should be particularly facilitative when faced with implemental problems (for overviews, see Gollwitzer, 1999;

Gollwitzer et al., 2004; Sheeran, 2002; Sheeran et al., this volume). It is proposed that, in short, the formation of implementation intentions delegates control over goal-directed action to the situation, similar to the operation of habits. However, the automatic control implied in implementation intentions is created at once through a willful act, rather than established over time via repeated pairings of stimulus and response.

Applying Self-regulation Theories to Health Behavior

Our previous discussion of major theoretical approaches to self-regulation illustrated that each of these theories emphasize different aspects of the self-regulation process. However, regardless of the specific processes of self-regulation that are highlighted in these approaches, none of them were specifically designed for understanding and explaining self-regulation processes in health behavior. In that respect these models differ from, for example, the self-regulation approach to health behavior developed by Howard Leventhal and his co-workers (e.g., Leventhal et al., 2003), which will be discussed in a later section. Important issues, therefore, are to what extent these three generic approaches to self-regulation are relevant for the health behavior domain, and whether some approaches are more suited to promote understanding of self-regulation of health behavior than others. This entails the question whether health behaviors represent a special category of behavior or are more or less equivalent to other types of behavior.

Health behaviors may be governed by the same principles as other behaviors that are subject to self-regulation because they involve the person as an active agent and draw on volitional processes of goal striving. However, there is some debate about the extent to which goals are true guides of health behavior. For instance, are we really self-regulating (choosing our own goals) or are we being regulated (following doctors orders) when we decide to quit smoking or eat a healthy diet (cf. Brownlee, Leventhal & Leventhal, 2000)? If the latter would be the case, then a self-regulation perspective would not add much to our understanding of why people either succeed or fail in that behavior. In a similar vein, we may wonder whether people who consume plenty of fruit and vegetables or who exercise a lot, do this for the sake of their long-term health or simply because they enjoy the taste of fresh fruit or love being physically active.

In a way, then, one of the important questions for self-regulation theories of health behavior is to what extent people have adopted health goals that direct their behavior (see also Gebhardt, this volume; Rothermund, this volume). Nevertheless, it seems reasonable to assume that when people are practicing health behaviors, that is, when they do things that bear relevance for their health, they mostly engage in acts that require substantial effort, and need an active self to resist impulses that may threaten involvement in the behavior. These are the types of actions self-regulation theories generally are concerned with, and the next issue is to determine the relevance of each of the genereric self-regulation approaches described earlier for the domain of health behaviors.

All three theoretical perspectives on self-regulation have been successfully employed in examining issues related to striving for health goals, albeit with different emphases. The framework offered by cybernetic control theory, for example, has been used to explain self-regulation processes in patients dealing with chronic illness and has drawn special attention to the way positive outcome expectancies (optimism) may affect these processes (Carver, Scheier & Pozo, 1992; Carver et al., 1993; Scheier & Carver, 1992). Unfortunately, no studies have directly tested the full TOTE cycle in the context of health behavior, or any other types of behavior for that matter. However, this approach proposes a series of assumptions that seem relevant for health behavior and require further examination. For instance, is it really true that people will try harder to attain their goals when they are confronted with difficulties in goal attainment, and is it equally true that negative affect that may result from the less than optimal pursuit of a particular health goal can motivate people to put more effort in their strivings? These propositions are central in Carver and Scheier's theory but seem at odds with most observations of striving for health goals that suggest that people give up rather easily in the face of obstacles.

Further issues that are central to the Carver and Scheier theory, but have not yet been examined empirically relate to the proposed hierarchical structure of goals: At what level do people conceive of their health goals? Are health goals "be" goals or more instrumental types of goals? And when do people pay attention to health goals? It may be that in particular people who experience positive affect related to other, non-health goals can afford to pay attention to goals in need of repair, and people may hence attend to health goals only when other things are going well (Carver, 2003). The Carver and Scheier approach thus raises a myriad of important issues that require further examination in the health behavior domain. In fact, health behaviors may provide excellent cases to examine these issues because at first glance findings in this domain seem at odds with essential propositions of the theory.

The self-control strength approach advocated by Baumeister and colleagues highlights the importance of resources to regulate the self and has intuitive appeal when attempting to explain why so many people fail in their striving for health goals. Indeed, health behaviors provide a host of good examples of unsuccessful goal striving, such as that many people eventually fail when trying to control their appetites and cravings for fatty foods and nicotine, as exemplified in Baumeister's seminal work on self-regulation failure (Baumeister et al., 1994). Unlike cybernetic control theory, the limited resource approach has been applied to a range of health problems, including overeating (Kahan, Polivy & Herman, 2003; Vohs & Heatherton, 2000), smoking (Sayette, 2004), alcohol abuse (Muraven, Collins & Nienhaus, 2002), and condom use (Bryan, Schinkeldecker & Aiken, 2001).

In a series of studies Vohs and Heatherton (2000), for example, found that a depletion of resources as a result of overriding the temptation of chocolate candies, led to more ice-cream eating among chronic dieters (but not among nondieters who were not actively trying to inhibit caloric intake). These findings support the resource model of self-regulation as an explanation for dieting failure: Exertions of self-control, whether or not related to inhibiting an impulse to eat, may make it more difficult to inhibit eating immediately thereafter. The model thus bears relevance for an understanding of health behavior, especially those that involve the restraint of impulses. The model does not, however, offer a full understanding of the conditions under which people will successfully control their impulses and maintain their striving for health goals. That is, having enough resources may be an essential but not sufficient ingredient of self-regulation, especially insofar as complex behavior is involved.

As outlined above, this is addressed in behavioral enaction models, which represent an approach to self-regulation that probably has been most extensively tested in the domain of health behavior (e.g., Gollwitzer & Oettingen, 2000; Sheeran et al., 2005; Sheeran & Orbell, 2000; also see Sheeran et al., this volume). Indeed, a fair amount of studies have shown that implementation intentions are useful devices to promote acting upon good intentions to perform a wide range of health behaviors, including exercise (Milne, Orbell & Sheeran, 2002), testicular self-examination (Steadman & Quine, 2004), and cervical cancer screening (Sheeran & Orbell, 2000). Recent findings, however, seem to suggest that effects of implementation intentions in the domain of health behavior are partly influenced by the extent to which people are intrinsically motivated to perform that behavior (Sheeran, Webb & Gollwitzer, 2005) Again, the nature of health goals seems to be crucial for understanding self-regulatory processes in health behavior. There is some evidence that suggests that implementation intentions arouse negative affect in those who have adopted high standards, and consequently make these individuals actually perform worse (Powers et al., 2005).

In sum, it appears that each of the three theoretical approaches to self-regulation bears relevance for understanding the self-regulation of health behavior. Depending on what part of the self-regulation process is under study—how health goals guide behavior, why people fail in maintaining the pursuit of health goal, or how they may increase the likelihood of acting upon their good intentions—specific approaches can provide a useful framework for explaining health behaviors. Nevertheless, a number of issues that are particularly relevant to understand how self regulation of health behavior works, remain hitherto unaddressed. We will address some of these in the next section.

CRITICAL ISSUES IN SELF-REGULATION OF HEALTH BEHAVIOR

Despite the relevance of the self-regulation approach for a better understanding of the processes involved in striving for health goals, the lack of an encompassing theoretical framework to examine the processes involved in self-regulation remains a particularly important issue, as exemplified in our discussion of theoretical models of self-regulation in the previous section. Even though all approaches more or less share an emphasis on difficulties associated with goal pursuit, each approach seems to highlight different aspects of self-regulation. This state of affairs has brought some authors to wonder whether the field of self-regulation is mature enough to be discussed in a handbook (Royer, 2003) or to complain that self-regulation theory may be "too good to be true" (McKeachie, 2000, p. xxii).

However, notwithstanding these critical notes we believe that a self-regulation approach to health behavior has some unique features that have surplus value as compared to more traditional approaches to health behavior, in particular social-cognitive models. In this section we discuss views derived from other theoretical approaches to health behavior to delineate the unique contribution of a self-regulation perspective on goal-related processes involved in health behavior. By doing so, we will address critical issues that merit further attention, and that in part will be addressed in this volume.

Social Cognition and Self-regulation

Social-cognitive models have been the predominant approach to understanding and explaining health behavior since the 1950s (for overviews, see Armitage & Conner, 2000; Conner & Norman, 1996; De Wit & Stroebe, 2004). Models like the Health Belief Model (Rosenstock, 1974), Protection-Motivation theory (Rogers, 1983), and Theory of Planned Behavior (Ajzen, 1991) have in fact dominated theorizing of health behavior for decades. The common ground of this type of model of behavior is that they specify a limited set of beliefs that are proposed as proximal determinants of motivation, often represented as an intention to act. The different models are loosely derived from a predominantly economic expectancy-value or subjective expected utility view that suggests that individuals are motivated to strive for those goals and enact those behaviors that are most likely to result in highly valued outcomes. By far the most popular model in this category, the Theory of Planned Behavior (Ajzen, 1991), is exemplary of the kind of reasoning adopted in many motivational models that view motivation as sufficient for successful action: If a person holds a positive attitude about the behavior, thinks others would approve of the behavior, and the behavior is under personal control, he or she forms an intention and subsequently acts upon it.

Social-cognitive models of health behavior can be regarded as rudimentary self-regulation models, as they are somewhat concerned with the way people engage in future action. Most of these models also incorporate concepts of volitional control. In a way, then, social-cognitive models include the processes of goal setting and goal striving that are central to self-regulation (cf. Bagozzi, 1992; Maes & Gebhardt, 2000). However, intention formation is not necessarily identical to goal setting, because intentions often tend to involve rather specific acts whereas goals tend to be of a higher-order, abstract nature (Austin & Vancouver, 1996; see also Gebhardt, this volume). In a similar vein, perceived personal control is not equivalent to goal striving, as people will not always engage in behavior they consider under their personal control (Armitage & Conner, 1999; cf. Abraham, Sheeran & Johnston, 1998).

In a more general sense, the Theory of Planned Behavior and other motivational models that highlight behaviors as resulting from weighting the pros and cons, may be criticized because of their "consequentionalist" nature (Loewenstein, Weber, Hsee & Welch, 2001). By focusing on the role of future outcomes of behavior as leading factors in behavioral decision-making these models tend to underestimate the role of the here and now in whether or not individuals act on intentions. Deliberate intentions are often overruled by reactions to compromising situations, as is for example demonstrated in research on behavioral willingness to act against one's intentions (e.g., Gibbons, Gerrard, Blanton & Russell, 1998; also see Gibbons et al., this volume). For this reason, some authors consider models like the Theory of Planned Behavior more as theories of intentions than of behavior (Greve, 2001). It can be argued that because of their emphasis on intention formation, and because the relation between intention and behavior is considered as unproblematic, motivational models of health behavior provide only a limited account of how people may strive to attain health goals.

Coping and Self-regulation

One of the most challenging self-regulatory tasks is tenacity in goal pursuit when difficult or frustrating situations are encountered (Brandtstädter & Renner, 1990; Mischel et al., 1996). Indeed, distractions and temptations are often regarded as the main causes of self-regulatory failure (Baumeister & Heatherton, 1996). However, compared with processes of goal setting and goal striving relatively little is known about how people deal with adversity during goal pursuit and how ways of coping may affect goal attainment. The way people respond to frustration and distress has been highlighted in the stress and coping literature. Unfortunately, however, the literatures on self-regulation and coping have largely developed independently, even though they share a concern with what people do when they anticipate or encounter adversity (Carver & Scheier, 1999; Lazarus & Folkman, 1984).

Only few authors have attempted to integrate concepts derived from stress-coping theory in the theoretical framework of self-regulation, and Leventhal's self-regulation model is one of the exceptions that explicitly pay attention to the role of coping (Leventhal, Meyer & Nerenz, 1980). The model holds that mental representations of actual or future health threats elicit coping "procedures" for dealing with these threats, and that dimensions of these representations in terms of timeline, causes, or consequences determine the selection of coping strategies. However, as the concept of health goals is rather implicit in Leventhal's model, or at least not more specified than a general assumption that people are motivated to act in response to a health threat, this approach provides little information about the role of coping in staying on track during goal pursuit. Moreover, the role of coping has not been a point of great interest in the model as most research has been focused on the dimensions of mental representations of illness (Leventhal et al., 2003; Hagger & Orbell, 2003). Extending self-regulation models with concepts derived from stress-coping theory seems to be important, however (Aspinwall, 2004; De Ridder & Kuijer, this volume).

Self-regulation theories emphasize long-term goal pursuit without explicitly considering the short-time regulation of goal frustrations, and theories of stress and coping may be helpful in explaining how effective dealing with such frustrations might benefit continued goal striving. In addition, the coping literature may provide more insight in how conditions of high distress create major shifts in goal priorities (Emmons, Colby & Kaiser, 1998). Research at the interface of coping and self-regulation is scarce, however. One particularly interesting attempt to consider the role of coping in the context of goal striving is the proactive coping model developed by Aspinwall and Taylor (1997). This model explicitly deals with coping processes in the service of long-term goals and highlights how people may employ coping efforts to prevent potential future stressors that may pose a threat to their goals. It is important to note that the coping literature may not only be informative for a better understanding of self-regulation processes. In a similar vein, the coping literature might benefit from the extended self-regulation framework. In recent years, critical reviews of the coping concept have been published pointing to such problems as a failure to understand how stressful situations may shape coping responses (Aspinwall, 2004; De Ridder & Kerssens, 2003). Explaining stressful situations in terms of interruptions of goal striving or in terms of threats to goals (Lazarus, 1990), therefore seems a promising area of future research.

Self-control and Self-regulation

Many authors emphasize the role of willpower or self-control in self-regulation (Mischel et al., 1996), as exemplified in the limited resource approach to self-regulation discussed previously. The general idea is that when faced with the temptation of immediate rewards people need to exert some control over their impulses to continue striving for long-term goals. Yet, the extent to which self-control is sufficient for successful self-regulation is the subject of recent debate. Whereas some authors tend to consider self-control as synonymous with self-regulation (Muraven & Slessareva, 2003; Vohs & Baumeister, 2004), others question the central role of self-control and find positive outcome expectancies more important for explaining self-regulatory behavior (Scheier & Carver, 1992). Some authors even argue that self-control may compromise self-regulation as the stoic denial of immediate needs may affect efforts to engage in future-directed behavior, implying that attention to immediate needs is more adaptive for long-term goal striving (Fishbach, Friedman & Kruglanski, 2003).

These diverging opinions on the role of self-control may be explained by different views on the nature of self-control: Is self-control an individual "strength" that people may or may not have? Or is self-control related to the situational circumstances that may or may not allow the individual to exert control? While trait explanations emphasizing self-control as a strength can predict stable individual differences in self-control, they do not resolve one of the most important questions for a theory of self regulation that should specify what makes self-control possible (Mischel et al., 1996). Several studies have shown that conditions of uncertainty are highly relevant for self-control in terms of inhibiting impulses. For instance, in the typical delay of gratification task the motivation to exhibit self-control is strongly affected by the certainty of the delayed reward (Mischel & Ayduk, 2004). It has been argued that the decreased motivation for engaging in self-control under conditions of uncertainty is adaptive. If it is highly uncertain whether one will be able to collect the long-term reward, it may be wiser to choose the immediate reward even when it is smaller or one would have no reward at all: "The future is uncertain, eat dessert first," like the proverb states. Uncertainty of long-term gains while confronted with big immediate rewards is typical for many health goals: Even if one refrains from highly rewarding but unhealthy habits like smoking or eating fattening foods, it is uncertain whether one will remain healthy in the long run. As we are not prepared by evolution to recognize the dangers of hamburgers, cigarettes or unsafe sex but still experience their rewarding value, inhibiting these impulses may be a difficult task (Loewenstein et al., 2001).

In the domain of health behavior then, self-control in terms of the capacity to override impulses seems to be a necessary but not sufficient factor in successful self-regulation. Recently, it has been argued that there may be actually two distinct systems of self-regulation with two sorts of operating characteristics; one system dealing with the restraint of unwanted or unplanned impulses and the other system dealing with acting upon premeditated and planful actions, labeled as the hot system and cool system respectively (Metcalfe & Mischel, 1999). This distinction may have important implications for the psychology of health behavior as it might explain why the effortful, planful system is functioning less when the individual is confronted with impulses that require immediate control, leaving in charge impulsive, hot system with only short-term goals (see also De Ridder & Kuijer, this volume).

Initiating and Maintaining Goal Pursuit

Most social-cognitive models of health behavior hitherto have approached health behavior change as a static event: Once people have made a commitment to behavior change they will engage in attempts for actually changing their behavior. This is even true for most applications of stage models as they tend to focus on the early stages of behavioral change, describing the transition from considering change to initiating change. One of the potentially interesting contributions of a self-regulation perspective to health behavior derives from its emphasis on behavior in a more extended time framework. The prominent role of goals in self-regulation models dictates that behavior should be viewed in the context of the long-term goals that people have adopted. As health goals are almost by definition distal goals, pursuit should be maintained over a long period of time while the outcome is uncertain. Indeed, one may successfully stop smoking or lose some pounds, but there is no guarantee that one will not die from cancer or heart disease. In other words, even if one manages to change behavior, the reward for these efforts may only be manifest many years afterwards, and the issue of behavioral maintenance is thus particularly relevant for health behavior.

Maintenance of health behavior change has only infrequently been studied from the perspective of self-regulation approaches (cf. Maes & Karoly, 2005; also see De Wit, this volume), but research hitherto suggests that the initiation and maintenance of health behavior are affected by different factors (cf. Rothman et al., 2004). Rothman and colleagues argue that whereas the initiation of behavior change is related to the health goals people cherish, continuation of their goal-related efforts may be more related to their satisfaction with perceived progress to this goal (cf. Carver & Scheier, 1998). In a more general sense, a self-regulation perspective on behavioral maintenance is interesting because effortful attempts for self-regulation seem to alter perception of time (Vohs & Schmeichel, 2003), which may be one reason why continued attempts for behavioral change are prone to failure, if they do not become a routine or habit.

OVERVIEW OF THIS VOLUME

This volume brings together overviews of theorizing and research on self-regulation processes that are involved in health behavior and health behavior change. We have divided the chapters into two sections, one dealing primarily with processes involved in goal setting, the other related to processes of goal striving. In the first part, four chapters address topics related to the adoption of health goals and initial attempts for goal striving in the perspective of competing interests. Gebhardt (Chapter 2) discusses issues related to the role of health goals in personal goal structures. She specifically calls attention to the way health goals may interfere with other cherished goals. The next three chapters all deal with health goals of adolescents and the way these goals, if present at all, affect health behavior.

The health behavior of adolescents poses some interesting questions for those who study self-regulation processes, as many adolescents seem not very keen on spending a lot of effort in attaining these goals, despite a sincere interest in health. As a result, many studies on adolescent health behavior focus on what determines whether or not adolescents engage in risky health behaviors, such as smoking, excessive alcohol use, or unprotected sex. In Chapter 3, Gibbons, Gerrard, Reimer, and Pomery challenge the central assumption of many theories of health behavior as a reasoned and intentional activity. More specifically, they argue that health behavior, and especially behavior involving health risks, in adolescents is not premeditated but a reaction to social circumstances. As social goals seem more salient than health goals in adolescents, engagement in health risk behavior is explained as behavioral willingness to adapt to the social situation.

In Chapter 4, Engels and Bot provide a detailed analysis of how parents and peers affect adolescents, smoking and drinking behavior, which reveals that parents have a significant role in adolescent health risk behavior, although the social processes amongst peers have not yet been examined in detail. Chapter 5 by Gerrard, Gibbons, Stock, Houlihan and Dykstra also discusses the role of parents in the way adolescents react to health risk situations, with a focus on the development of temperament-based self-regulatory processes. The authors argue that these individual differences in self-regulatory competence determine how adolescents react to potentially risky social situations, but that parents can play an important role in helping their children to develop more self-control.

The second part of this volume addresses processes related to goal striving and goal persistence in the face of difficulties. Sheeran, Webb and Gollwitzer (Chapter 6) discuss the role of implementation intentions in the pursuit of health goals. They argue that forming so-called if-then plans is an essential self-regulatory tool when confronted with common problems in the pursuit of health goals, such as overcoming initial reluctance to act upon a health goal or maintaining initial strivings over a prolonged period of time. The formation of if-then plans may help to identify opportunities to act upon health goals. In Chapter 7, De Ridder and Kuijer address the role of coping and emotion regulation in the self-regulation of health behavior. They argue that in order to maintain striving for health goals, individuals need to take care of their short term frustrations and distraction that otherwise might interfere with goal directed behavior.

In Chapter 8, Martijn, Alberts, and De Vries discuss the role of self-control in self-regulation. They specifically argue that depletion of self-control is related to the beliefs people hold about the nature of self-control, and that depletion may be prevented when people are encouraged to persist. De Wit (Chapter 9) also addresses issues related to the persistence of initial efforts, and reviews the multitude of factors that seem involved. The prolonged maintenance of behavior change is rarely addressed in theory-based research, and understanding sustained change poses novel challenges to self-regulation theory and research. Finally, in Chapter 10 Rothermund addresses the important issue to what extent it is adaptive to continue striving for health goals when personal control is limited and resources are scarce. He raises the possibility that it is better to give up on health goals when striving is doomed to fail. Coming to terms with goals that might be pursued only with substantial costs allows a shift in attention to more promising goals and thus eventually benefits well-being.

Together, these chapters demonstrate the potential of a self-regulation approach to health behavior. They point to new areas for future research that may help us to understand and explain why and how people engage in behavior that is relevant for their health, although they often fail to take advantage of opportunities to perform that behavior and have difficulties in sustaining change.

REFERENCES

Abraham, C., Norman, P. & Conner, M. (2000). Towards a psychology of health-related behaviour change. In P. Norman, C. Abraham & M. Conner (Eds), *Understanding and Changing Health Behaviour: From health beliefs to self-regulation* (pp. 343–369). Amsterdam: Harwood.

Abraham, C. & Sheeran, P. (2000). Understanding and changing health behaviour: From health beliefs to self-regulation. In P. Norman, C. Abraham & M. Conner (Eds), *Understanding and Changing Health Behaviour: From health beliefs to self-regulation* (pp. 3–24). Amsterdam: Harwood.

Abraham, C., Sheeran, P. & Johnston, M. (1998). From health beliefs to self-regulation: Theoretical advances in the psychology of action control. *Psychology and Health, 13*, 569–591.

Ajzen, I. (1991). The theory of planned behavior. *Organizational Behavior and Human Decision Processes, 50*, 179–211.

Armitage, C.J. & Conner, M. (1999). The theory of planned behavior: Assessment of predictive validity and 'perceived control'. *British Journal of Social Psychology, 38*, 35–54.

Armitage, C.J. & Conner, M. (2000). Social cognition models and health behaviour: A structured review. *Psychology and Health, 15*, 173–189.

Aspinwall, L.G. (2004). Dealing with adversity: Self-regulation, coping, adaptation, and health. In M. Hewstone & M.B. Brewer (Eds), *Applied Social Psychology* (pp. 3–27). Malden, MA: Blackwell.

Aspinwall, L.G. & Taylor, S.E. (1997). A stitch in time: Self-regulation and proactive coping. *Psychological Bulletin, 121*, 417–436.

Austin, J.T. & Vancouver, J.B. (1996). Goal constructs in psychology: Structure, process, and content. *Psychological Bulletin, 120*, 338–375.

Bagozzi, R.P. (1992). The self-regulation of attitudes, intentions, and behaviour. *Social Psychology Quarterly, 55*, 178–204.

Bandura, A. (1977). Self-efficacy: Toward a unifying theory of behavioral change. *Psychological Review, 84*, 191–215.

Bandura, A. (1986). *Social Foundations of Thought and Action: A social cognitive theory.* Englewood Cliffs, NJ: Prentice Hall.

Bandura, A. (1991). Social cognitive theory of self-regulation. *Organizational Behavior and Human Decision Processes, 50*, 248–287.

Bargh, J.A. & Chartrand, T.L. (1999). The unbearable automaticity of being. *American Psychologist, 54*, 462–479.

Baumeister, R.F. (1989). The problem of life's meaning. In D.M. Buss & N. Cantor (Eds), *Personality Psychology: Recent trends and emerging directions* (pp. 138–148). New York: Springer.

Baumeister, R.F. (1998). The self. In D.T. Gilbert, S.T. Fiske & G. Lindzey (Eds), *Handbook of Social Psychology*, (4th edn, pp. 680–740). New York: McGraw-Hill.

Baumeister, R.F. (1999). The nature and structure of the self: An overview. In R.F. Baumeister (Ed.), *The Self in Social Psychology* (pp. 1–24). Philadelphia, PA: Psychology Press.

Baumeister, R.F. (2005). *The Cultural Animal: Human nature, meaning, and social life.* New York: Oxford University Press.

Baumeister, R.F., Bratslavsky, E., Muraven, M. & Tice, D.M. (1998). Ego-depletion: Is the active self a limited resource? *Journal of Personality and Social Psychology, 74*, 1252–1265.

Baumeister, R.F. & Heatherton, T.F. (1996). Self-regulation failure: An overview. *Psychological Inquiry, 7*, 1–15.

Baumeister, R.F., Heatherton, T.F. & Tice, D.M. (1994). *Losing Control: How and why people fail at self-regulation*. San Diego, CA: Academic Press.

Boekaerts, M., Pintrich, P.R. & Zeidner, M. (Eds) (2000). *Handbook of Self-regulation*. San Diego, CA: Academic Press.

Brandstädter, J. & Renner, G. (1990). Tenacious goal pursuit and flexible goal adjustment: Explication and age-related analysis of assimilative and accommodative strategies of coping. *Psychology and Aging, 5*, 58–67.

Brownell, K.D. (1991). Personal responsibility and control over our bodies: When expectation exceeds reality. *Health Psychology, 10*, 303–310.

Brownlee, S., Leventhal, H. & Leventhal, E.A. (2000). Regulation, self-regulation, and construction of the self in the maintenance of physical health. In M. Boekaerts, P.R. Pintrich & M. Zeidner (Eds), *Handbook of Self-regulation*, (pp. 369–416). San Diego, CA: Academic Press.

Bryan, A., Schindeldecker, M.S. & Aiken, L.S. (2001). Sexual self-control and male condom-use outcome beliefs: Predicting heterosexual men's condom use intentions and behaviours. *Journal of Applied Social Psychology, 31*, 1911–1939.

Cameron, L.D. & Leventhal, H. (2003): Self-regulation, health and illness: An overview. In L.D. Cameron and H. Leventhal (Eds), *The Self-regulation of Health and Illness Behaviour* (pp. 1–13). London: Routledge.

Cantor, N. (1990). From thought to behavior: "Having" and "doing" in the study of personality and cognition. *American Psychologist, 45*, 735–750.

Cantor, N., & Kihlstrom, J.F. (1987). *Personality and Social Intelligence*. Englewood Cliffs, NJ: Prentice-Hall.

Carver, C.S. (1979). A cybernetic model of self-attention processes. *Journal of Personality and Social Psychology, 37*, 1251–1281.

Carver, C.S. (2003). Pleasure as a sign that you can attend to something else: Placing positive feelings within a general model of affect. *Cognition and Emotion, 17*, 241–261.

Carver, C.S. (2004). Self-regulation of action and affect. In R.F. Baumeister & K.D. Vohs (Eds), *Handbook of Self-regulation. Research, Theory, and Applications* (pp. 13–39). New York: Guilford.

Carver, C.S. & Scheier, M.F. (1982). Control theory: A useful conceptual framework for personality—social, clinical, and health psychology. *Psychological Bulletin, 92*, 111–135.

Carver, C.S. & Scheier, M.F. (1998). *On the Self-regulation of Behavior*. New York: Cambridge University Press.

Carver, C.S. & Scheier, M.F. (1999). Stress, coping, and self-regulatory processes. In L.A. Pervin & J.P. Oliver (Eds), *Handbook of Personality Theory and Research*, (pp. 553–575). New York: Guilford.

Carver, C.S., Scheier, M.F. & Pozo, C. (1992). Conceptualizing the process of coping with health problems. In H.S. Friedman (Ed), *Hostility, Coping, and Health* (pp. 167–199). Washington, DC: American Psychological Association.

Carver, C.S., Pozo, C., Harris, S.D., Noriega, V., Scheier, M.F., Robinson, D.S., Ketcham, A.S., Moffat, F.L. Jr. & Clark, K.C. (1993). How coping mediates the effects of optimism on distress: A study of women with early stage breast cancer. *Journal of Personality and Social Psychology, 65*, 375–390.

Cervone, D., Mor, N., Orom, H., Shadel, W.G. & Scott, W.D. (2004). Self-efficacy beliefs and the architecture of personality. In R.F. Baumeister & K.D. Vohs (Eds), *Handbook of Self-regulation. Research, Theory, and Applications* (pp. 188–210). New York: Guilford.

Conner, M. & Norman, P. (1996). *Predicting Health Behavior.* Buckingham, UK: Open University Press.

De Ridder, D. & Kerssens, J. (2003). Owing to the force of circumstances? The impact of situational features and personal characteristics on coping patterns across situations. *Psychology and Health, 18,* 217–236.

De Wit, J. & Stroebe, W. (2004). Social cognition models of health behaviour. In A. Kaptein & J. Weinman (Eds), *Health Psychology,* (pp. 52–83). Oxford, UK: Blackwell.

Elliott, E.S. & Dweck, C.S. (1988). Goals: An approach to motivation and achievement. *Journal of Personality & Social Psychology, 54,* 5–12.

Emmons, R.A. (1986). Personal strivings: An approach to personality and subjective well-being. *Journal of Personality & Social Psychology, 51,* 1058–1068.

Emmons, R.A., Colby, P.M. & Kaiser, H.A. (1998). When losses lead to gains: Personal goals and the recovery of meaning. In P.T. Wong & P.S. Fry (Eds), *The Human Quest for Meaning: A handbook of psychological research and clinical applications* (pp. 163–178). Mahwah, NJ: Erlbaum.

Fishbach, A., Friedman, R.S. & Kruglanski, A.W. (2003). Leading us not unto temptation: Momentary allurements elicit overriding goal activation. *Journal of Personality & Social Psychology, 84,* 296–309.

Fitzsimons, G.M. & Bargh, J.A. (2004). Automatic self-regulation. In R.F. Baumeister & K.D. Vohs (Eds), *Handbook of Self-regulation. Research, Theory, and Applications* (pp. 151–170). New York: Guilford.

Gibbons, F.X., Gerrard, M., Blanton, H. & Russell, D.W. (1998). Reasoned action and social reaction: Willingness and intention as independent predictors of health risk. *Journal of Personality and Social Psychology, 74,* 1164–1181.

Gollwitzer, P.M. (1993). Goal achievement: The role of intentions. In W. Stroebe & M. Hewstone (Eds), *European Review of Social Psychology* (Vol. 4, pp. 141–185). Chichester, UK: John Wiley & Sons, Ltd.

Gollwitzer, P.M. (1996). The volitional benefits of planning. In P.M. Gollwitzer & J.A. Bargh (Eds), *The Psychology of Action: Linking cognition and motivation to behavior* (pp. 287–312). New York: Guilford.

Gollwitzer, P.M. (1999). Implementation intentions: Strong effects of simple plans. *American Psychologist, 54,* 493–503.

Gollwitzer, P.M., Fujita, K. Oettingen, G. (2004). Planning and the implementation of goals. In R.F. Baumeister & K.D. Vohs (Eds), *Handbook of Self-regulation. Research, Theory, and Applications* (pp. 211–228). New York: Guilford.

Gollwitzer, P.M., Heckhausen, H. & Steller, B. (1990). Deliberative versus implemental mindsets: Cognitive tuning towards congruous thoughts and information. *Journal of Personality and Social Psychology, 59,* 1119–1127.

Gollwitzer, P.M. & Moskowitz, G.B. (1996). Goal effects on action and cognition. In E.T. Higgins & A.W. Kruglanski (Eds), *Social Psychology: Handbook of basic principles* (pp. 361–399). New York: Guilford.

Gollwitzer, P.M. & Oettingen, G. (2000). The emergence and implementation of health goals. In P. Norman, C. Abraham & M. Conner (Eds), *Understanding and Changing Health Behaviour: From health beliefs to self-regulation,* (pp. 229–260). Amsterdam: Harwood.

Greve, W. (2001). Traps and gaps in action explanation: Theoretical problems of a psychology of human action. *Psychological Review, 108,* 435–451.

Hagger, M.S. & Orbell, S. (2003). A meta-analytic review of the common-sense model of illness representations. *Psychology and Health, 18,* 141–184.

Heckhausen, H. & Gollwitzer, P.M. (1987). Thought contents and cognitive functioning in motivational versus volitional states of mind. *Motivation and Emotion, 11,* 101–120.

Higgins, E. T. (1987). Self-discrepancy: A theory relating self and affect. *Psychological Review, 94,* 319–340.

James, W. (1890). *The Principles of Psychology* (Vol. 2). Retrieved December 20, 2005, from York University, Classics in the History of Psychology web site: http://psychclassics.yorku.ca/index.htm.

Kahan, D., Polivy, J. & Herman, P.C. (2003). Conformity and dietary disinhibition: A test of the ego-strength model of self-regulation. *International Journal of Eating Disorders, 33,* 165–171.

Karoly, P., Boekaerts, M. & Maes, S. (2005). Toward consensus in the psychology of self-regulation: How far have we come? How far do we have yet to travel? *Applied Psychology: An International Review, 54,* 300–311.

Klinger, E. (1977). *Meaning and Void: Inner experience and the incentives in people's lives.* Minneapolis: University of Minnesota Press.

Kuhl, J. (2000). A functional-design approach to motivation and self-regulation: The dynamics of personality systems interactions. In M. Boekaerts, P.R. Pintrich & M. Zeidner (Eds), *Handbook of Self-regulation* (pp. 111–169). San Diego, CA: Academic Press.

Lazarus, R.L. (1990). Theory-based stress measurement. *Psychological Inquiry, 1,* 3–13.

Lazarus, R.L. & Folkman, S. (1984). *Stress, Appraisal, and Coping.* New York: Springer.

Leith, K.P.M. & Baumeister, R.F. (1996). Why do bad moods increase self-defeating behavior? Emotion, risk-taking, and self-regulation. *Journal of Personality and Social Psychology, 71,* 1250–1267.

Leventhal, H., Brisette, I. & Leventhal, E. (2003). The common-sense model of self-regulation of health and illness. In L.D. Cameron & H. Leventhal (Eds), *The Self-regulation of Health and Illness Behavior* (pp. 42–65). London: Routledge.

Leventhal, H., Meyer, D. & Nerenz, D. (1980). The common sense representation of illness danger. In S. Rachman (Ed), *Medical Psychology* (Vol. 2, pp. 7–30). New York: Pergamon.

Lewin, K., Dembo, T., Festinger, L. & Sears, P.S. (1944). Level of aspiration. In J. McHunt (Ed.), *Personality and the Behavior Disorders* (pp. 333–378). New York: Ronald.

Little, B.R. (1983). Personal projects: A rationale and methods for investigation. *Environment and Behavior, 15,* 273–309.

Locke, E.A. & Latham, G.P. (2002). Building a practically useful theory of goal setting and task motivation. *American Psychologist, 57,* 705–717.

Loewenstein, G., Weber, E.U., Hsee, C.K. & Welch, N. (2001). Risk as feelings. *Psychological Bulletin, 127,* 267–287.

Luszczynska, A. & Schwarzer, R. (2005). Social cognitive theory. In M. Conner & P. Norman (Eds), *Predicting Health Behaviour* (pp. 127–169). Maidenhead, UK: Open University Press.

Maes, S. & Gebhardt, W. (2000). Self-regulation and health behaviour: The health behaviour goal model. In M. Boekaerts, P.R. Pintrich and M. Zeidner (Eds), *Handbook of Self-regulation* (pp. 343–368). San Diego, CA: Academic Press.

Maes, S. & Karoly, P. (2005). Self-regulation assessment and intervention in physical health and illness: A review. *Applied Psychology: An International Review, 54,* 267–299.

McKeachie, W.J. (2000). Foreword. In M. Boekaerts, P.R. Pintrich & M. Zeidner (Eds), *Handbook of Self-regulation,* (pp. xxi–xxiii). San Diego, CA: Academic Press.

Metcalfe, J. & Mischel, W. (1999). A hot/cool-system analysis of delay of gratification: Dynamics of willpower. *Psychological Review, 106,* 3–19.

Miller, G.A. Galanter, E. & Pribam, K.H. (1960). *Plans and the Structure of Behavior.* New York: Holt, Rinehart & Winston.

Milne, S., Orbell, S. & Sheeran, P. (2002). Combining motivational and volitional interventions to promote exercise participation: Protection motivation theory and implementation intentions. *British Journal of Health Psychology, 7,* 163–184.

Mischel, W. & Ayduk, O. (2004). Willpower in a cognitive-affective processing system: The dynamics of delay of gratification. In R.F. Baumeister & K.D. Vohs (Eds), *Handbook of Self-regulation. Research, Theory, and Applications* (pp. 99–129). New York: Guilford.

Mischel, W., Cantor, N. & Feldman, S. (1996). Principles of self-regulation: The nature of willpower and self-control. In E.T. Higgins & A.W. Kruglanski (Eds), *Social Psychology. Handbook of Principles* (pp. 329–360). New York: Guilford.

Mischel, W., Shoda, Y. & Rodriguez, M.L. (1989). Delay of gratification in children. *Science, 244,* 933–938.

Muraven, M & Baumeister, R.F. (2000). Self-regulation and depletion of limited resources: does self-control resemble a muscle? *Psychological Bulletin, 126,* 247–259.

Muraven, M., Baumeister, R.F. & Tice, D.M. (1999). Longitudinal improvement of self-regulation through practice: Building self-control strength through repeated exercise. The *Journal of Social Psychology, 139,* 446–457.

Muraven, M., Collins, R.L. & Nienhaus, K. (2002). Self-control and alcohol restraint: An initial application of the self-control strength model. *Psychology of Addictive Behaviors, 16,* 113–120.

Muraven, M. & Slessareva, E. (2003). Mechanisms of self-control failure. Motivation and limited resources. *Personality and Social Psychology Bulletin, 29,* 894–906.

Muraven, M., Tice, D.M. & Baumeister, R.F. (1998). Self-control as a limited resource: Regulatory depletion patterns. *Journal of Personality and Social Psychology, 74,* 774–789.

Norcross, J.C., Ratzin, A.C. & Payne, D. (1989). Ringing in the New Year: The change processes and reported outcomes of resolutions. *Addictive Behaviors, 14,* 205–212.

Pervin, L.A. (Ed) (1989). *Goal Concepts in Personality and Social Psychology.* Hillsdale, NJ: Erlbaum.

Polivy, J. & Herman, C.P. (2002). If at first you don't succeed. False hopes of self-change. *American Psychologist, 57,* 677–689.

Powers, W.T. (1973). *Behavior: The control of perception.* Chicago: Aldine.

Powers, T.A., Koestner, R. & Topciu, R.A. (2005). Implementation intentions, perfectionism, and goal progress: Perhaps the road to hell *is* paved with good intentions. *Personality and Social Psychological Bulletin, 31,* 902–912.

Prochaska, J.O. & DiClemente, C.C. (1984). *The Transtheoretical Approach: Crossing the traditional boundaries of change.* Homewood, IL: Irwin.

Rogers, R.W. (1983). Cognitive and physiological processes in fear appeals and attitude change: A revised theory of protection motivation. In T.T. Cacioppo & R.E. Petty (Eds), *Social Psycho-physiology* (pp. 153–176). New York: Guilford.

Rosenstock, I.M. (1974). Historical origins of the Health Belief Model. *Health Education Monographs, 2,* 1–8.

Rothman, A.J., Baldwin, A.S. & Hertel, A.W. (2004). Self-regulation and behavior change. In R.F. Baumeister & K.D. Vohs (Eds), *Handbook of Self-regulation. Research, Theory, and Applications* (pp. 130–148). New York: Guilford.

Royer, J.M. (2003). Almost everything you would want to know about self-regulation. *Contemporary Psychology. APA Review of Books, 48,* 56–58.

Sayette, M.A. (2004). Self-regulatory failure and addiction. In R.F. Baumeister & K.D. Vohs (Eds), *Handbook of Self-regulation. Research, Theory, and Applications* (pp. 447–465). New York: Guilford.

Schwarzer, R. (1992). Self-efficacy in the adoption and maintenance of health behaviors: Theoretical approaches and a new model. In R. Schwarzer (Ed), *Self-efficacy: Thought control of action* (pp. 217–243). London: Hemisphere.

Schwarzer, R. (2001). Social-cognitive factors in changing health-related behavior. *Current Directions in Psychological Science, 10,* 47–51.

Steadman, L. & Quine, L. (2004). Encouraging young males to perform testicular self-examination: A simple, but effective, implementation intentions intervention. *British Journal of Health Psychology, 9,* 479–487.

Sheeran, P. (2002). Intention-behavior relations: A conceptual and empirical review. In W. Stroebe & M. Hewstone (Eds), *European Review of Social Psychology* (Vol. 12, pp. 1–30). Chichester, UK: John Wiley & Sons, Ltd.

Sheeran, P., Milne, S.E., Webb, T.L. & Gollwitzer, P.M. (2005). Implementation intentions. In M. Conner & P. Norman (Eds), *Predicting Health Behaviour* (pp. 276–323). Maidenhead, UK: Open University Press.

Sheeran, P., & Orbell, S. (2000). Using implementation intentions to increase attendance for cervical cancer screening. *Health Psychology, 19*, 283–289.

Sheeran, P., Webb, T.L. & Gollwitzer, P. M. (2005). The interplay between goal intentions and implementation intentions. *Personality and Social Psychology Bulletin, 31*, 87–98.

Scheier, M.F. & Carver, C.S. (1992). Effects of optimism on psychological and physical well-being: Theoretical overview and empirical update. *Cognitive Therapy and Research, 16*, 201–228.

Scheier, M.F. & Carver, C.S. (2003). Goals and confidence as self-regulatory elements underlying health and illness behaviour. In L.D. Cameron & H. Leventhal (Eds), *The Self-regulation of Health and Illness Behaviour* (pp. 17–41). London: Routledge.

Strack, F. & Deutsch, R. (2004). Reflective and impulsive determinants of social behavior. *Personality and Social Psychology Review, 8*, 220–247.

Tice, D.M., Bratslavsky, E. & Baumeister, R.F. (2001). Emotional distress regulation takes precedence over impulse control: If you feel bad, do it! *Journal of Personality and Social Psychology, 80*, 53–67.

Vohs, K.D. & Baumeister, R.F. (2004). Understanding self-regulation: An introduction. In R.F. Baumeister and K.D. Vohs (Eds), *Handbook of Self-regulation. Research, Theory, and Applications* (pp. 1–9). New York: Guilford.

Vohs, K.D. & Heatherton, T.F. (2000). Self-regulatory failure: A resource-depletion approach. *Psychological Science, 11*, 249–254.

Vohs, K.D. & Schmeichel, B.J. (2003). Self-regulation and the extended now: Controlling the self alters the subjective experience of time. *Journal of Personality and Social Psychology, 85*, 217–230.

Weinstein, N.D. (1988). The precaution adoption process. *Health Psychology, 7*, 355–386.

Weinstein, N.D., Rothman, A.J. & Sutton, S.R. (1998). Stage theories of health behavior. *Health Psychology, 17*, 290–299.

Wrosch, C., Scheier, M.F., Miller, G.E., Schulz, R. & Carver, C.S. (2003). Adaptive self-regulation of unattainable goals: Goal disengagement, goal reengagement, and subjective well-being. *Personality and Social Psychology Bulletin, 29*, 1494–1508.

Zeidner, M., Boekaerts, M. & Pintrich, P.R. (2000). Self-regulation: Directions and challenges for future research. In M. Boekaerts, P.R. Pintrich, & M. Zeidner (Eds), *Handbook of Self-regulation* (pp. 750–768). San Diego, CA: Academic Press.

Goal Setting in Health Behavior: Conflicting Desires and Social Influences

CHAPTER 2

Contextualizing Health Behaviors: The Role of Personal Goals

Winifred A. Gebhardt

Humans pursue multiple goals simultaneously: They wish to feel good, look good, be successful, socially embedded, healthy, and experience pleasure all at the same time (e.g., Karoly, 1998; Riediger & Freund, 2004). Although such goals may sometimes be aligned, they are likely to be in conflict at other times. Conflict occurs when various incompatible goals are equally desirable (Miller, 1944). Humans have to choose which goal to pursue and which actions to undertake to achieve it. They have to balance their strivings, taking into account the goals they wish to accomplish, both in the short term and the long term. Thus, in order to understand the behavior of humans, it is crucial to capture their personal goals, and to comprehend how these may influence behavioral decisions. Personal goals are likely to have an effect on all phases of behavioral change. This chapter, however, will be limited to the influence of personal goals on the first phase of behavioral change when the individual is deciding whether or not to engage in a certain health behavior.

HEALTH GOALS AND THE SOCIAL-COGNITIVE PERSPECTIVE

In general, humans wish to remain healthy and to prolong their lives. Yet, while it is widely known that most serious health problems in our society, including coronary heart disease, cancer, and diabetes, are to a considerable extent caused by unhealthy lifestyles, many individuals continue to perform health-compromising behaviors. The predominant theories that have been applied to the study of health behaviors involve a social cognitive perspective on behavioral change. They consider individuals to be rational and "economic", maximizing the utility of behavior in terms of positive outcomes. This perspective finds its origin in the Subjective Expected Utility Theory (Edwards, 1954), in which choices

Self-regulation in Health Behavior.   Edited by Denise T.D. de Ridder and John B.F. de Wit.
© 2006 John Wiley & Sons Ltd.

are assumed to be based on the estimated probability that a certain goal will be reached, as well as on the subjective value attached to this goal.

The Subjective Expected Utility Theory has had a vast influence on theories explaining health behaviors that were developed in the early fifties and the following decades, such as the Health Belief Model (Becker, 1974; Rosenstock, 1974) and Protection Motivation Theory (Rogers, 1975, 1983). These and other more general theories of social behavior, including Bandura's Social Cognitive Theory (Bandura, 1986), the Theory of Reasoned Action (Fishbein & Ajzen, 1975) and the Theory of Planned Behavior (Ajzen, 1985) have been frequently applied in health behavior research. Expectations of future events and outcomes are considered to be the main determinants of the intention or motivation to change behavior.

In both the Health Belief Model and Protection Motivation Theory, the cognitive representations of emotions, in particular fear, have been given a major role. It is assumed that the perceived likelihood ("perceived vulnerability") and seriousness ("perceived severity") of a health threat as well as the estimated effectiveness of the health behavior to reduce this threat ("response efficacy") determine whether people may wish to change their behavior. In the more general theories of social behavior the perceived outcomes are not limited to fear-related expectancies. For example, in social learning theories, such as Bandura's theory, the social component of behavioral change receives more attention. The effects of expected reinforcement from the social environment are assumed to be crucial in the development of the expectancies, which precede the decision to act. Furthermore, the role of the social environment on the formation of specific expectancies is extended to include learning through observation and modelling. In the Theory of Reasoned Action and the Theory of Planned Behavior, the social component is specified in the form of subjective norms. That is, the individual is expected to be influenced by perceptions related to whether or not others will approve of the behavior. Finally, most of the social cognitive theories suggest that expectancies regarding one's capabilities of performing the behavior, either in the form of self-efficacy (Bandura, 1977) or "perceived behavioral control" (Ajzen, 1985) play a key role in the decisional process.

The social cognitive perspective has generated a substantial amount of research (e.g., Ogden, 2003). However, though popular, empirical tests of the models indicate that a large amount of the variance in behavior is left unexplained (e.g., Armitage & Conner, 2000; see also De Ridder & De Wit, this volume). One of the main criticisms is that health behavior is regarded in isolation, and other, non-health related goals are not taken into account (Abraham & Sheeran, 2003; Gebhardt & Maes, 2001). Within social-cognitive theories the decision whether a health behavior is adopted depends on the expectancies related to this particular behavior. If performance of the behavior is expected to lead to many positive outcomes (e.g., "high response efficacy" or "approval of others") and if it is perceived as relatively easy to perform, the behavior is likely to be conducted. However, this perspective does not incorporate the notion that individuals are engaged in many different tasks and roles concurrently. They must divide their resources among multiple life pursuits and these strivings may at times be irreconcilable. Focusing on the outcomes of a health behavior in isolation is therefore a too limited approach and, as Weinstein (1988, p. 357) stated, ignores "... other life responsibilities that compete for time, energy, and material resources". For a more accurate prediction of behavioral change, then, there is a definite need to consider the health behavior within the context of other goals a person is pursuing: To understand a human's actions "... means to understand the person's goals" (Carver & Scheier, 1999, p. 554). The other pursuits of the individual may simply not leave enough time, attention, or energy to perform the health behavior, or even to seriously consider doing so. In such instances a person may choose not to adopt a certain health behavior, even if he or she may be convinced that the outcomes would be highly beneficial and that practicing the behavior would be easy. A completely unrelated goal may just appear to be far more important at that specific moment in time.

GOALS AND SELF-REGULATION

Self-regulation theories provide a useful framework for personal goals as a determining factor of behavioral change. Self-regulation refers to the processes that enable humans to guide their behavior over time (Karoly, 1993), and is based on the capacity of humans to influence, modify, and control their own behavior (Baumeister & Heatherton, 1996). It enables one to bring the environment in line with one's wishes, or to bring one's wishes in line with realistic situational limitations (Rothbaum, Weisz & Snyder, 1982). Self-regulation involves the "mental and behavioral processes by which people enact their self-conceptions, revise their behavior, or alter the environment so as to bring about outcomes in line with their self-perceptions and personal goals" (Fiske & Taylor, 1991, p. 181). Consequently, self-regulation removes behavior from the direct effects of immediate situational stimuli. Most of the responses to the environment depend less on the cues available within that specific situation than on how these cues relate to the goals that are currently being pursued. Although these goals are not necessarily represented in consciousness, they are generally accessible to active awareness (Bargh & Chartrand, 1999).

The primary underlying tenet of self-regulation theories is that humans are by nature goal-oriented organisms (e.g., Ford, 1992). Behavior is primarily instigated to achieve one's previously set goals. Furthermore, the array of personal goals is unique to the individual and is defined by the individual's developmental history and idiosyncratic interpretation of desired consequences (e.g., Ford, 1992; Higgins, 1996; Little, 1983; Winell, 1987).

People select and pursue the goals that support their definition of the self, based on the general need to create a coherent, stable, and positive sense of the self (Shahar, Henrich, Blatt, Ryan & Little, 2003). The ultimate aim of self-regulatory endeavors, therefore, is to affirm, sustain or enhance the self (Stets & Burke, 2000). People act to bring evaluations of the self in line with their identity standards, which leads to consistent self-conceptions across situations and over time. It generates positive feelings reinforcing the process of self-regulation itself (Sedikides, Gaertner & Toguchi, 2003).

Goals guide actions and give meaning to life (Kruglanski, 1996). Individuals actively select the goals they wish to pursue as well as the environments in which they believe that they are likely to achieve these goals (Cantor, 1994). They always hold some sort of conception of their actions in terms of what they are doing and why (Vallacher & Wegner, 1989). Thus, action is accompanied by the mental representations of its purpose. Naturally, these representations may be incomplete and changeable, but they allow behaviors to be known and planned in advance of their occurrence (Wegner, Vallacher & Dizadji, 1989). As such, these mental representations, or goals, organize and direct behavior over time. Furthermore, the effects of actions, or perceived outcomes of behavior, form a source of input for future goal setting and consequently for future action.

What Is a Goal?

Goals have been defined as desired future states that people seek to obtain, maintain or avoid (e.g., Austin & Vancouver, 1996) through action (e.g., Kruglanski, 1996). Humans are inclined to engage in behaviors that move the current self closer to a desired value ("approach goals") or further away from an undesired value ("avoidance goals"; also referred to as "anti-goals," Carver & Scheier, 1999).

According to Carver and Scheier (1982) the desired end-states are contrasted with the person's perception of his or her present condition. In the case of a discrepancy between desired and actual states, behavior will be initiated to reduce the difference. The main purpose of this negative feedback loop is, thus, to restore homeostasis. The perceived discrepancy leads to self-referent processes that motivate the person to deliberate on how to reduce the gap between states and to choose the most suitable behavior accordingly (Gollwitzer & Oettingen, 1998). Behavior, as an output of the negative feedback loop, has an impact on the environment. Subsequently, the outcomes of the behavior are assessed in terms of the extent to which they have led to the desired state. During this so-called assessment loop, the relative progress rather than the absolute effect of the behavior is considered. The rate of discrepancy reduction between actual and desired states, relative to an expected reduction rate, is believed to determine the valence and intensity of the emotions that accompany the process of self-regulation (Boldero & Francis, 2002).

Since goals are derived from anticipated desired states, they can be conceptualized as knowledge structures (Kruglanski, 1996), or stored expectations of the outcomes of their attainment. These expectations are based on the personal history of experiences with goal pursuit as well as on the observation of goal pursuit as carried out by others (Bandura, 1977). Humans have a unique personal history with regard to behaviors and the extent to which they lead to desired outcomes. The experiences of the past define what individuals believe they should possess or attain, how they wish to be, and how they wish others to view them. Clearly, not all desired states or goals are of equal importance to the individual. In this regard it is important to note that the primary motive for a behavior (e.g., "studying hard") is often not so much the achievement of a directly corresponding goal in itself ("passing an exam"), but rather what it represents for the individual ("admiration by others on graduation day"). The more the goal is related to the central concept of the self, the more salient it is.

Goal Hierarchies

Goals are structured and organized in a hierarchical manner. The goals that are the highest in the hierarchy, for example "to become successful" or "to develop one's talents", are the most abstract and distal, and they are imbedded in many meaningful cognitive networks

(Baumeister, Heatherton & Tice, 1994). Thus, these goals are associated with many other goals which are relevant to the individual, because they represent an important part of the self. They involve the representation of how individuals would like to regard themselves as well as how they would like others to perceive them. Thus, every human possesses, and actively (re)creates a cognitive representation of the self. The goals on this highest level of abstraction are frequently referred to in the literature as "possible selves" or future representations of the self (Markus & Nurius, 1986). Possible selves include both the "ideal selves" that refer to hopes, wishes, and desires, and their opposites, namely "feared selves" that refer to a concept of self someone does not want to be and that reflect fears and anxieties (Carver, Lawrence & Scheier, 1999). Possible selves may also refer to "ought selves" (a person one is morally required to be) that relate to perceived duties, obligations, and responsibilities (Higgins, 1987, 1996).

At the middle level of the goal hierarchy are "program goals," roles or scripts, which involve a set of behaviors that together may lead to a positive reinforcement of related elements of the self concept and as such facilitate a higher order goal. By taking on role identities, humans give meaning to their behaviors within specific contexts. Which set of roles are activated within a specific situation varies across persons, as each person has a unique combination of identities (Stets & Burke, 2000). Humans regard themselves to be distinct from each other by having their own aims, duties, and resources, which are derived from their perception of the self, and the accompanying roles they have chosen to embrace. These goals have been investigated under the name of "personal projects" that involve self-generated accounts of what an individual is doing or is planning to do (Little, 1983), "current concerns" that refer to the things that matter to a person at a particular time in life (Klinger, 1977), "personal strivings" or the things individuals are trying to do in their life (Emmons, 1986), and "life tasks" that comprise what a person is working on during a specified period in life related to socially and culturally prescribed age-graded tasks (Cantor & Kihlstrom, 1987).

At the lower level of the goal hierarchy, individuals have behavioral aims related to specific actions or so-called behavioral episodes (Ford, 1992). A behavioral episode consists of a distinct behavior, which is performed within a specific, limited time frame. Health behaviors (e.g., quitting smoking or exercising) are specific actions and fall in this category of lower level goals which are pursued to obtain higher order goals (e.g., to be healthy or to be attractive).

To illustrate the concept of goal hierarchy consider the following example: A young mother may wish to regard herself as a loving, fun, and responsible person. Being a wife, mother, daughter, employee, and friend, she fulfills many different roles and tries to accomplish the many accompanying life tasks. Feedback from others is evaluated along the relevant dimensions of her concept of the self. One day, after she has heard a friend make a remark that she would never ever want to wear a size 16, the size she currently wears, she may feel that she would like to reduce her weight. She may believe that she is already very sensible about her food choices for the main daily meals, and decides that she should quit eating unhealthy snacks in between. In doing so she would also set a good example to her children, which is in line with her self-perception of being a responsible person. However, at the same time she realizes that she loves eating chocolate and associates it with rewarding herself after a hard day's work. Also, in her youth, her mother used to bake cakes, and she connects the smell of a cake in the oven with being at home in a warm atmosphere. This is something she wishes to create for her children as well. Therefore, on a behavioral level she may well continue to buy sweets and bake cakes, while this conflicts with her wish to lose weight.

The various levels of goals are interconnected. Goals at the higher levels generate input for goal setting at lower levels of the hierarchy (Carver & Scheier, 1999). Thus, higher level goals activate the means or strategies to attain them through top-down mechanisms. For example, if one strives to be a loving mother, this may define some goals at a middle level, such as "providing my children with a warm and cozy atmosphere at home," which may lead to several goals at the behavioral level, including "bake a cake together." Goals at a higher level may also be elicited by goals at a lower level through bottom-up mechanisms. For example, one day the young mother may be forced to cycle to work because the car broke down. She may find the experience very pleasant. This could elicit the goal of "promoting fitness" as a feasible and desirable aim for her to pursue, and would be in line with her self-image of being a responsible person. Simultaneously her new health goal may facilitate her goal of reducing weight.

Goal Conflict

Some goals within a hierarchy may be in alignment with each other, while others may be incompatible. In this regard, Sheldon and Kasser (1995) distinguish between a horizontal and vertical degree of coherence. Horizontal coherence represents the degree to which a goal leads to the attainment of another goal at the same hierarchical level, rather than to hindrance of that goal. A high level of horizontal coherence leads to relatively low demands on personal resources. However, if two or more goals at the same hierarchical level are in conflict then the individual is confronted with an incompatibility between goals. Vertical coherence refers to the degree to which a proximal or subordinate goal serves one or more distal or superordinate goals at a higher hierarchical level. For example, participating in sports activities may serve one's health goals, such as becoming more fit, as well as one's social goals, such as meeting other persons in a nice atmosphere. When a goal at a certain level serves multiple purposes at a higher level, this increases the motivation to perform this action. Alternatively, if a goal is in conflict with another, this leads to a reduction in positive affect and to goal avoidance.

Two different sources of incompatibility between goals have been identified (Riediger, 2001). First, goals may be irreconcilable because they are drawn from the same limited resources, such as time, money, or energy. If exercising three times a week entails that a father is not able to spend time with his son, the two goals of being fit and being a good father are competing with each other for time. If, on the other hand, the father could participate in a sport together with his son, the two goals could be aligned and no conflict would exist. If an employee is frequently too tired after work to prepare a meal and therefore decides to eat fast food, the two goals of pursuing a career and healthy diet are at odds because the limited amount of energy available to the person does not allow the fulfillment of both goals. Again, if for example the cooking of the meal were to be experienced as a method of relaxation, conflict would not occur or would be reduced.

Second, goals may be logically incompatible: This situation occurs when a goal may require a certain behavior while another equally valued goal may call for an opposite behavior. For example, the goal to "behave healthily" may necessitate declining a high-calorie piece of birthday cake while the goal of "being polite" may require one to consume it. Obviously, these goals cannot be achieved simultaneously in this situation. This type of conflict also includes the conflict between short term goals, such as experiencing direct pleasure, and desired long term states, such as being healthy—which has proven to be a prototypical conflict in striving for health goals (see also De Ridder & Kuijer, this volume).

The personal goal structure and goal conflict in particular are the core constructs of the Health Behavior Goal Model (Gebhardt, 1997; Gebhardt & Maes, 2001; Maes & Gebhardt, 2000). It is based on the notion that at every stage of behavioral change personal goals may conflict with each other. The likelihood that a certain type of behavior will occur, as a means to reach a specific goal, depends on the strength of the underlying goal in relation to the strength of other goals. The next section will elaborate on the role of competing personal goals in the process of adopting a health goal.

ADOPTING HEALTH BEHAVIOR AS A PERSONAL GOAL

As discussed previously, social cognition theories emphasize the importance of outcome expectancies, which refer to the desirability of the behavior, and of self-efficacy expectancies, which refer to the feasibility of the behavior. Theories of self-regulation incorporate this insight with the notion that these expectancies are generated within the context of the pursuit of many other personal goals.

In order to change one's health behavior a health goal has to become personally salient—that is, more salient than other, competing goals. The more the behavior is expected to serve other goals, and the higher these goals are in the hierarchy, the more likely it is to be adopted. In addition, low expected conflict between the health behavior and other valued goals will increase the chances of its acceptance. Alternatively, a lack of goal relevance and high levels of expected conflict will decrease the chances of goal adoption. For instance, a smoker may become motivated to quit if she frequently experiences a sense of addiction when she runs out of cigarettes and has to rush to the store to buy them. This may be at odds with her wish to be independent and to function autonomously. Yet, if she does not care about a desire to be independent and experiences positive consequences of her behavior, it is not likely that her motivation will change. Change is the least likely to occur if the positive consequences of the unhealthy behavior are related to highly valued parts of the self concept such as "smoking with others is pleasurable and sociable," and "I am a social person." A health behavior will become a goal in itself only when it is linked to many other goals, including goals that are unrelated to health.

Knowledge and beliefs about behavioral outcomes are accumulated and stored in memory over time (cf., Anderson, 1983). Knowledge and beliefs are also connected with other available concepts within complex associative networks. These concepts and relationships are applied to generate inferences about future states within the corresponding domain. Moreover, the individual is capable of moving beyond the existing connections by making new associations through constructive reasoning. However, time constraints and motivational deficiencies may limit the number of concepts and relations within the networks used for any given decision (Fazio, 1990). Therefore, the decision whether or not to adopt a health behavior is not only dependent on expectancies related to the behavior itself. Frequently, other considerations related to different personal goals will be given priority.

Activation of cognitive networks containing outcome beliefs in situations in which decisions have to be made concerning behavior (e.g., whether to light a cigarette), depends on how the knowledge on the outcomes of the behavior is organized in memory, the strength of the connections between the concepts, and the salience in terms of vividness and its relevance to the decision-maker's personal goals. Certain knowledge (e.g., on the negative effects of smoking) may not be accessible to the working memory of an individual, simply because other networks that are unrelated to health (e.g., boosting self-image) are more important. In certain situations such as being under pressure to make an on-the-spot decision (e.g., social pressure to smoke at a party) only the strongest, most easily accessible networks will be activated. This explains why frequently accurate information on the detrimental effects of certain behaviors, even when it is well comprehended and processed, does not lead to a corresponding change in behavior.

However, knowledge of the outcomes of behavior may be processed and stored in one or more of the individual's cognitive networks. It may, therefore, be retrieved at any other moment. The more frequent the information that is in conflict with the current behavior is elicited, the more likely it is that the individual becomes more ambivalent towards his or her current unhealthy behavior—a postulate that is addressed in the literature on attitudinal ambivalence (e.g., Thomson, Zanna & Griffin, 1995). From this ambivalence an action tendency or a need for behavioral change is formed, in which the likelihood that the new course of action will lead to the new desired state is taken into account. The negative emotional state related to ambivalence functions as a signal to take action (Schwarz & Bohner, 1996).

The decision to change behavior can, thus, be preceded by ambivalence and by the recognition that the current behavior is incongruent with important long-standing personal goals. This awareness is in most instances not brought about by the direct consequences of the behavior itself, but by the effects it has on other valued life-goals. For example, not being able to fit into one's summer clothing may make one become aware of the fact that one feels highly uncomfortable with the weight one has gained over the past winter months. The "turning point" (Kearny & O'Sullivan, 2003), then, is not so much a specific event, but rather the critical self-evaluation that follows it, and the awareness that if one were to continue to perform the current behavior, negative emotions would re-occur repeatedly in the future. Thus, internal or external cues including critical life events (Rosenstock, 1974; Weinstein, 1988), such as not being able to climb stairs without panting, receiving a flyer from new sports facilities in the neighborhood, or becoming ill, may give rise to a reorganization of the goal structure. Through this reorganization, the health behavior may become (one of) the most important goals within the personal goal hierarchy. However, the exact manner in which the reorganization will be expressed in terms of behavior depends on the idiosyncratic content and organization of goals within the personal goal structure.

For example, a middle-aged man who suffers from a blood vessel disease may have been repeatedly and urgently advised by his doctors to quit smoking. Over time he has experienced more difficulties with walking due to his condition. However, several years after the diagnosis, although having tried to quit, he is still a regular, heavy smoker. He may frequently hear about the detrimental consequences of his behavior, but he actively distorts or denies this threatening information in order to cope with the health threat (i.e., "disengage"; Bandura, 1996). Perhaps he fears the day that he will be dependent on a wheel chair, but at the same time he claims that smoking is a part of his life. Smoking as such for him symbolizes some of the central parts of his identity. One day, after hearing about the prolonged life expectancy of dog owners, he may, however, decide to change some other aspect of his lifestyle. He may buy himself a puppy and take it out for a walk several times a day—while simultaneously enjoying his cigar.

Problems in Goal Adoption

Several problems may interfere with the decision to select a new health behavior as a personal goal that needs to be pursued. First of all, a health goal may not be considered, simply because a person is unaware that his or her current behavior may have serious negative consequences (Weinstein, 1988), or because he or she does not believe that these consequences are relevant to the personal situation ("unrealistic optimism"; Weinstein, 1988; Weinstein & Klein, 1996). The current unhealthy behavior may also be accommodated by personal norms, which sustain it. That is to say, the current unhealthy behavior may be defined as part of the self (e.g., "it suits me just the way I am"), and this may lead individuals to discount their negative feelings about the long-term negative consequences. People may even lack the motivation to perceive the discrepancy between the actual and the desired states as such motivation requires a certain degree of action-orientation (Kuhl, 1981). In addition, in many situations the number of choices and conflicting wishes and desires may overwhelm individuals, and they may therefore be inclined to choose maintenance of their current behavior rather then to accept a new behavioral alternative (Mischel, Cantor & Feldman, 1996).

The foregoing shows that often the consideration of a new health behavior may not turn into health goals. At other times, the health behavior may be conceived as important, but other goals that are incompatible with the health goal may be of higher relevance to the self. The health behavior, then, simply does not sufficiently connect to important parts of self-concept in comparison with other behaviors, and does not get prioritized. Sometimes a behavior is in line with several, but not all important personal goals at a higher level. In such instances of goal incongruence, the individual holds at least to some extent an ambivalent attitude towards the health behavior (see for attitudinal ambivalence in health behavior Broemer, 2002; Lipkus et al., 2005; Sparks, Harris & Lockwood, 2004). For example, if using a condom is associated with low levels of mutual trust and intimacy, this behavior is less desirable for someone who has a strong need for bonding with a romantic partner, even if he or she is convinced that condoms are effective in minimizing the risks of contracting a sexually transmitted infection. In addition, goal importance may fluctuate, depending on the circumstances that are encountered. Distractions and temptations and the way they are processed, may change the strength of any action tendency (Klinger, 1996). As a result, other behaviors may be given priority.

To summarize, people may be unaware of the need to change behavior, or may be unmotivated to seriously consider it. Even if they are convinced that they should adopt a health behavior, the reality is that they may not be able to fulfill all of their wishes at once. The organism is filled with action tendencies, which compete with each other for expression (Atkinson & Birch, 1970). We have to select which goals we will pursue and how, and the outcome of the decisional process depends on a large variety of factors.

It should be mentioned that a conflict between goals is not always experienced at a conscious level. In fact, any existing tension between the goals is often first noticed through the negative emotions that accompany it. From a natural tendency to reduce tension, the individual responds by changing cognition and behavior almost automatically. Sorrentino (1996) has argued that, although the "battle" between action tendencies, or goals may at times occur at a non-conscious level, conscious thought may also have a strong influence on the process of choice. Specifically, conscious deliberation elicited by environmental or internal cues may cause another action tendency to prevail. Whether this occurs depends on the strength of the motivation behind the tendency. Conscious thought may function as an instigating or resisting force, and any single thought may change a certain course of action.

EMPIRICAL EVIDENCE FOR THE INFLUENCE OF PERSONAL GOALS ON HEALTH BEHAVIOR

Frequently, a certain level of conflict between the current behavior and highly valued long-term goals is necessary to initiate behavioral change (Carver & Scheier, 1982). Nevertheless, a "true" adoption of a health behavior depends on a relative lack of conflict between the behavior and other goals. Specifically, the more a health behavior is congruent with perceptions of the self and is associated with the simultaneous enhancement of salient goals that are not related to health, the more likely it is to be adopted and prioritized as a health goal. In a similar vein, the more a health behavior is incongruent with perceptions of the self and is associated with hindrance of prominent non-health related goals, the less likely it is to be adopted and prioritized as a goal. The scarce research on this topic does provide empirical support for these assumptions, some of which is summarized here.

Bagozzi and Edwards (1998) demonstrated that a health behavior such as losing weight is imbedded in a coherent structure of multiple goals of the individual. They asked 197 undergraduates to list five personal reasons why they wanted to lose weight, and also to report for each of the mentioned reasons why this was important for them. The identified goals were found to function in a hierarchical pattern. The aggregation of all associations between reasons as listed by the participants, yielded twelve superordinate goals, such as "enjoy life," "enhance self-esteem," or "live longer." Compared with the other goals, the intermediate goal of "feeling good" had the most associations with all other goals. The authors suggest that the feeling-good goal may be the central goal through which people process new information and make their inferences and decisions (cf., Tice & Bratslavsky, 2000). Based on these findings they conclude that "the hierarchical structure of superordinate goals constitutes a fundamentally different representation of the consequences of goal pursuit and goal achievement than expectancy-value models. Unlike the point-form summation of products of beliefs and evaluations, the hierarchical goal structure models the pattern and interdependence amongst goals. This potentially gives a richer explanation of goal formation and indicates which antecedents should be targeted in any change efforts" (Bagozzi & Edwards, 1998, p. 617).

Testing the Health Behavior Goal Model (Gebhardt, 1997; Gebhardt & Maes, 2001; Maes & Gebhardt, 2000), Gebhardt and Maes (1998) found that goal conflict at a behavioral level was related to exercise behavior in a group of 312 non-exercisers, 466 individuals who trained once or twice a week, and 202 individuals who exercised at least 3 times a week. The three subgroups differed from each other with respect to the number of highly valued activities they anticipated to conflict with exercising 3 or more times a week. Many of the sedentary participants expected that regular exercise would interfere with day-to-day activities, such as social activities, household chores, and watching television. Furthermore, the impediment of these activities was expected to be rather annoying, thus reflecting the relevance of the underlying goals (Gebhardt, Van der Doef & Maes, 1999). In particular activities that take place at home, either to relax (e.g., reading a book) or to fulfill domestic duties (e.g., doing household chores) emerged as prominent obstacles for the sedentary subgroup. Furthermore, those who exercised 3 or more times a week reported a lower number of competing social goals (e.g., visit a friend) than the participants in the 2 other subgroups. In a follow-up study (Gebhardt, 1997) the number of highly valued competing goals appeared to be adequate predictors of the initiation of regular exercise and for relapse to a sedentary lifestyle within the 12 months thereafter. Participants who were sedentary but who became regular exercisers at the follow-up measurement were less likely to have indicated at the baseline measurement that exercise would interfere with other highly valued goals than those who remained sedentary. In addition, those who exercised regularly 3 or more times a week, but who relapsed to being sedentary at the follow-up measurement reported more conflicting goals during baseline measurement than those who continued to be regular exercisers.

McKeeman and Karoly (1991) investigated the role of structural goal conflict in the process of smoking cessation among university undergraduates. They included in their sample 38 smokers who currently smoked at least 15 cigarettes a day and had not made a serious attempt to quit during the previous 8 months, 40 "relapsers" who currently smoked at least 15 cigarettes a day and who had made a serious but unsuccessful attempt to quit in the previous 4 months, and 36 quitters who had stopped smoking for 1 to 4 months but who had been smoking at least 15 cigarettes a day before. These students were asked to indicate the extent to which each of their 5 most important, self-generated, personal goals might have interfered with their smoking cessation attempts. It was found that quitters reported significantly lower levels of inter-goal conflict when compared to the smokers and "relapsers."

In a study by Everett and colleagues (1996) the extent to which bicycle helmet use was perceived to facilitate other goals was examined. In their study, 241 university students completed a questionnaire on bicycle helmet use. Eight different goals related to helmet use were distinguished based on the Ford and Nichols (1987) taxonomy of human goals that includes the following goals: positive bodily sensations, positive self-evaluations, enhancement of self-determination, increased safety, material gain, the acquisition of resources, increased individuality, and social responsibility. The more students perceived that personal goals could be reached by wearing a helmet, the more likely they were to wear one. The authors concluded that, compared to those who do not wear bicycle helmets, those who do wear them appear to value independence and safety, and feel a social obligation to act safely. Clearly, motivation to wear a helmet and actual helmet use were strongly related to the extent to which it was perceived to facilitate other personal goals.

Martin and Leary (2001) investigated self-presentation in relation to risk behaviors among university students. Self-presentation refers to how people wish that others perceive them to be, and to the behaviors they actively choose in order to establish certain impressions of themselves in the eyes of others. The aim of the study was to examine which risk behaviors are commonly used for self-presentational reasons, and the kind of images they wish to create by doing so. One hundred and ten first year university students in their first semester were involved in the study. They were asked to indicate on a list of ten health risk behaviors how often they had engaged in these behaviors during the first semester of university and for what reason. Three quarters of the sample reported to have engaged in at least one risk behavior for self-presentational reasons. They had been drinking and smoking in order to be perceived by others as "cool" or as "fun and social," or had been using drugs in order to be perceived as "cool" or "brave and a risk-taker." These findings relate to work by Gibbons and colleagues (1995; see Gibbons and colleagues, this volume), who argue that health risk behaviors are typically performed in the presence of others, and therefore have direct social consequences. Particularly young people are likely to be influenced by the social implications of their behavior. Accordingly, the perceived prototype associated with the health risk behavior, that is, the image people have of the type of person who engages in the behavior such as the "typical smoker" or the "typical non-smoker," is assumed to affect people's willingness to engage in that behavior. Especially the extent to which the prototype is positively evaluated (prototype favorability), and the extent to which the prototype is perceived to reflect one's self (prototype similarity), are considered to be important. Thus, the social goals of "being accepted by others," "being appreciated by others," and "having a cool image" may be highly significant motivators for (un)healthy behavior.

Gebhardt, Kuyper and Greunsven (2003) found that goals that are not directly related to a specific health behavior could nevertheless influence its occurrence. They conducted a retrospective study on condom use with steady and casual partners among 470 Dutch adolescents. Adolescents who had had casual sex were less likely to pursue intimacy in relationships, and were more likely to have sex to please others, to enhance mood, or to experience pleasure than adolescents who had never had casual sex. Furthermore, adolescents who always used condoms and those who never did differed from each other with regard to the underlying motives for having sex (e.g., to express love, to reduce negative mood, to please others, and/or to experience pleasure) and the need for intimacy in relationships. It appeared that protected sex with a steady partner was associated with a low score on the motive to express love through having sex and a low need for intimacy in relationships. Consistent condom use with casual partners was related to a high need for intimacy in relationships. Particularly for females the meaning attached to having sex or to the relationship within which sex occurs appeared to be of importance for whether or not safe sex was practiced. Thus, the goals people are pursuing within a certain situation, albeit being completely unrelated to health issues, may to a large extent influence the occurrence of health behaviors. In a study with 133 young females, Gebhardt, Kuyper and Dusseldorp (in press) also observed that condom use with a new sexual partner was negatively related to the motive for having sex to cope with negative emotions, but was unrelated to motives such as expressing love, experiencing pleasure, or pleasing others. Clearly, the functionality of behavior, such as the reason for having sex, determines at least partly the choices made with respect to health behaviors, such as using a condom, which takes place within this specific context.

To the best of my knowledge there is only one study in which the effectiveness of a health promotion intervention is examined in relation to the personal goals of the individual. Sanderson and Cantor (1995) designed two different interventions to enhance condom use in young people. In the communication skills intervention, students practiced their communication skills related to sexuality and safe sex through role-playing. In the educational intervention, students were trained how to put on a condom and were asked to participate in a discussion on how to eroticize its use. A randomized treatment-control study with a 12-months follow-up period was conducted involving 166 university undergraduates. It was found that students who pursued identity goals in relationships, that is, goals related to self-reliance and self-exploration, benefited more from the technical intervention than from the communication skills intervention, as expressed by increased condom use. For those who pursued intimacy goals, that is, goals related to mutual dependence and open communication, on the other hand, the communication intervention led to significantly higher levels of reported condom use. Assigning participants to interventions of which the content closely corresponds to their personal goals, therefore, appears to be an effective approach. This finding underscores the potential gain of focusing on the whole personal goals structure of the individual instead of merely considering the health behavior by itself.

CONCLUSION

Personal goals are continuously competing for attention. Any health behavior is merely one possible behavioral goal within a context of multiple goals that are held simultan-eously. Whether or not a health behavior is adopted and given priority over and above other purposes of the individual depends on the strength of its connections to other valued goals, and the relative lack of goal conflict.

Goals and inter-goal conflict certainly have an impact on other phases of behavioral change, such as preparation for action, the initiation of behavioral change and its maintenance over time; a description of which is beyond the scope of this chapter. Clearly, many issues remain to be uncovered related to the dynamic aspects of goal pursuit in the process of health behavioral change. For example, what happens when an individual encounters a conflict in goals when starting a new health behavior? How do the thoughts, feelings, and actions that accompany this conflict influence subsequent actions, and how will these in turn influence the process of change? Such questions will have to be answered by future prospective studies that should include multiple, preferably daily or weekly measurements of goal-related processes and their outcomes.

Finally, the theoretical and empirical evidence presented in this chapter suggests that intervention efforts should aim at: (a) increasing the personal relevance of health goals, (b) reducing the expected or experienced goal conflict, and (c) matching the content of the intervention to the personal goal structure. Health professionals should consider the conflicts that individuals face when a health behavior is not in line with one or more other valued personal goals. Being aware that humans always pursue more than one goal at the same time, it is highly relevant to investigate whether a health behavior is likely to interfere with other short-term or long-term aims. When trying to encourage healthy lifestyles, the following questions should be addressed: What is the nature of these conflicts between goals? How do these conflicts influence the process of behavioral change? And ultimately: How can these conflicts be resolved in order to enhance and sustain a healthy lifestyle? By expanding our knowledge of the role of personal goals and inter-goal conflicts we will be able to increase the effectiveness of our efforts to promote health.

REFERENCES

Abraham, C. & Sheeran, P. (2003). Implications of goal theories for the theories of reasoned action and planned behavior. *Current Psychology, 22,* 264–280.

Anderson, J.A. (1983). *The Architecture of Cognition.* Cambridge, MA: Cambridge University Press.

Ajzen, I. (1985). From intentions to actions: A theory of planned behavior. In J. Kuhl & J. Beckman (Eds), *Action Control: From cognition to behaviour* (pp. 11–39). Heidelberg: Springer.

Armitage, C.J. & Conner, M. (2000). Social cognition models and health behaviour: A structured review. *Psychology and Health, 15,* 173–189.

Atkinson, J.W. & Birch, D. (1970). *The Dynamics of Action.* New York: Wiley.

Austin, J.T. & Vancouver, J.B. (1996). Goal constructs in psychology: Structure, process and content. *Psychological Bulletin, 120,* 338–375.

Bagozzi, R.P. & Edwards, E.A. (1998). Goal setting and goal pursuit in the regulation of body weight, *Psychology and Health, 13,* 593–621.

Bandura, A. (1977). *Social Learning Theory.* Englewood Cliffs, NJ: Prentice Hall.

Bandura, A. (1986). *Social Foundations of Thought and Action: A cognitive social theory.* Englewood Cliffs, NJ: Prentice Hall.

Bandura, A. (1996). Mechanisms of moral disengagement in the exercise of moral agency. *Journal of Personality and Social Psychology, 71,* 364–374.

Bargh, J.A. & Chartrand, T.L. (1999). The unbearable automaticity of being. *American Psychologist, 54,* 462–479.

Baumeister, R.F. & Heatherton, T.F. (1996). Self-regulation failure: An overview. *Psychological Inquiry, 7,* 1–15.

Baumeister, R.F. Heatherton, T.F. & Tice, D. (1994). *Losing Control: How and why people fail at self-regulation.* San Diego, CA: Academic Press.

Becker, M.H. (1974). The health belief model and sick role behaviour. *Health Education Monographs, 2,* 409–419.

Boldero, J. & Francis, J. (2002). Goals, standards, and the self: Reference values serving different functions. *Personality and Social Psychology Review, 6,* 232–241.

Broemer, P. (2002). Relative effectiveness of differently framed health messages: The influence of ambivalence. *European Journal of Social Psychology, 32,* 685–703.

Cantor, N. & Kihlstrom, J.F. (1987). *Personality and Social Intelligence.* Englewood Cliffs, NJ: Prentice Hall.

Cantor, N. (1994). Life task problem solving: Situational affordances and personal needs. *Personality and Social Psychology Bulletin, 20,* 235–243.

Carver, C.S., Lawrence, J.W. & Scheier, M.F. (1999). Self-discrepancies and affect: Incorporating the role of feared selves. *Personality and Social Psychology Bulletin, 25,* 783–792.

Carver, C.S. & Scheier, M.F. (1982). Control theory: A useful conceptual framework for personality—social, clinical, and health psychology. *Psychological Bulletin, 92*, 111–135.

Carver, C.S. & Scheier, M.F. (1999). Stress, coping, and self-regulatory processes. In L.A. Pervin & J.P. Oliver (Eds), *Handbook of Personality Theory and Research* (pp. 553–557). New York: Guilford.

Edwards, W. (1954). The theory of decision making. *Psychological Bulletin, 51*, 380–417.

Emmons, R.A. (1986). Personal strivings: An approach to personality and subjective well-being. *Journal of Personality and Social Psychology, 51*, 1058–1068.

Everett, S.A., Price, J.H., Bergin, D.A. & Groves, B.W. (1996). Personal goals as motivators: Predicting bicycle helmet use in university students. *Journal of Safety Research, 27*, 43–53.

Fazio, R.H. (1990). Multiple processes by which attitudes guide behavior: The MODE model as an integrative framework. In M.P. Zanna (Ed.), *Advances in Experimental Social Psychology* (Vol. 23, pp. 75–109). San Diego, CA: Academic Press.

Fishbein, M. & Ajzen, I. (1975). *Belief, Attitude, Intention, and Behavior: An introduction to theory and research*. Reading, UK: Addison-Wesley.

Fiske, S.T. & Taylor, S.R. (1991). *Social Cognition* (2nd edn). New York: McGraw-Hill.

Ford, M.E. (1992). *Motivating Humans: Goals, emotions and personal agency beliefs*. Newbury Park: Sage.

Ford, M.E. & Nichols, C.W. (1987). A taxonomy of human goals and some possible applications. In D.H. Ford & M.A. Ford (Eds), *Humans as Self-constructing Living Systems: Putting the framework to work* (pp. 289–311). Hillsdale, NJ: Erlbaum.

Gebhardt, W.A. (1997). *Health Behavior Goal Model: Towards a theoretical framework for health behaviour change*. Leiden: Leiden University Press.

Gebhardt, W.A. Van der Doef, M.P. & Maes, S. (1999). Conflicting activities for exercise. *Perceptual and Motor Skills, 89*, 1159–1160.

Gebhardt, W.A., Kuyper, L. & Dusseldorp, E. (in press). Condom use at first intercourse with a new partner in female adolescents and young adults: The role of cognitive planning and motives for having sex. *Archives of Sexual Behavior.*

Gebhardt, W.A., Kuyper, L. & Greunsven, G. (2003). Need for intimacy in relationships and motives for sex as determinants of adolescent condom use. *Journal of Adolescent Health, 33*, 154–164.

Gebhardt, W.A. & Maes, S. (1998). Competing personal goals and exercise behaviour. *Perceptual and Motor Skills, 86*, 755–759.

Gebhardt, W.A. & Maes, S. (2001). Integrating social-psychological frameworks for health behavior research. *American Journal of Health Behavior, 25*, 528–536.

Gibbons, F.X. & Gerrard, M. (1995). Predicting young adults' health risk behaviour. *Journal of Personality and Social Psychology, 69*, 505–517.

Higgins, E.T. (1987). Self-discrepancy: A theory relating self and affect. *Psychological Review, 94*, 319–340.

Higgins, E.T. (1996). Ideals, oughts, and regulatory focus: Affect and motivation from distinct pains and pleasures. In: P.M. Gollwitzer & J.A. Bargh (Eds), *The Psychology of Action: Linking cognition and motivation to behavior* (pp. 91–114). New York: Guilford.

Karoly, P. (1993). Mechanisms of self-regulation: A systems view. *Annual Review of Psychology, 44*, 23–52.

Karoly, P. (1998). Expanding the conceptual range of health self-regulation research: A commentary. *Psychology and Health, 13*, 741–746.

Kearny, M.H. & O'Sullivan, J. (2003). Identity shifts as turning points in health behavior change. *Western Journal of Nursing Research, 25*, 134–152.

Klinger, E. (1977). *Meaning and Void: Inner experience and the incentives in people's lives*. Minneapolis: University of Minnesota Press.

Klinger, E. (1996). Emotional influences on cognitive processing, with implications for theories on both. In P.M. Gollwitzer & J.A. Bargh (Eds), *The Psychology of Action: Linking cognition and motivation to behavior* (pp. 168–189). New York: Guilford.

Kruglanski, A.W. (1996). Goals as knowledge structures. In P.M. Gollwitzer & J.A. Bargh (Eds). *The Psychology of Action: Linking cognition and motivation to behavior* (pp. 599–618). New York: Guilford.

Kuhl, J. (1981). Motivational and functional helplessness: The moderating effect of state versus action orientation. *Journal of Personality and Social Psychology, 40*, 155–170.

Lipkus, I.M., Pollak, K.I., McBride, C.M., Schwartz-Bloom, R., Lyna, P. & Bloom, P.N. (2005). Assessing attitudinal ambivalence towards smoking and its association with desire to quit among teen smokers. *Psychology and Health, 20*, 373–387.

Little, B.R. (1983). Personal projects: A rationale and method for investigation. *Environment and Behavior, 15*, 273–309.

Maes, S., & Gebhardt, W.A. (2000). Self-regulation and health behaviour: The health behaviour goal model. In M. Boekaerts, P.R. Pintrich, & M. Zeidner (Eds). *Handbook of Self-regulation* (pp. 343–368). San Diego, CA: Academic Press.

Markus, H. & Nurius, P. (1986). Possible selves. *American Psychologist, 41*, 954–969.

Martin, K.A. & Leary, M.R. (2001). Self-presentational determinants of health risk behavior among college freshmen. *Psychology and Health, 16*, 17–27.

McKeeman, D., & Karoly, P. (1991). Interpersonal and intrapsychic goal-related conflict reported by cigarette smokers, unaided quitters, and relapsers. *Addictive Behaviors, 16*, 543–548.

Miller, N.E. (1944). Experimental studies of conflict. In J.M. Hunt (Ed.), *Personality and the Behavior Disorders* (pp. 431–465). Oxford, UK: Ronald Press.

Mischel, W., Cantor, N. & Feldman, S. (1996). Principles of self-regulation: The nature of willpower and self-control. In E.T. Higgins & A.W. Kruglanski (Eds), *Social Psychology: Handbook of basic principles* (pp. 329–360). New York: Guilford.

Ogden, J. (2003). Some problems with social cognition models: A pragmatic and conceptual analysis. *Health Psychology, 22*, 424–428.

Riediger, M. (2001). *On the Dynamic Relations Among Multiple Goals: Intergoal conflict and intergoal facilitation in younger and older adulthood.* Berlin: Free University of Berlin (dissertation).

Riediger, M. & Freund, A.M. (2004). Interference and facilitation among personal goals: Differential associations with subjective well-being and persistent goal pursuit. *Personality and Social Psychology Bulletin, 30*, 1511–1523.

Rogers, R.W. (1975). A protection motivation theory of fear appeals and attitude change. *Journal of Psychology, 91*, 93–114.

Rogers, R.W. (1983). Cognitive and physiological processes in fear appeals and attitude change: A revised theory of protection motivation. In J.T. Cacioppo & R.E. Petty (Eds), *Social Psychophysiology: A sourcebook* (pp. 153–176). New York: Guilford.

Rosenstock, I.M. (1974). The health belief model and preventive health behaviour. *Health Education Monographs, 2*, 354–386.

Rothbaum, F., Weisz, J.R. & Snyder, S.S. (1982). Changing the world and changing the self: A two-process model of perceived control. *Journal of Personality and Social Psychology, 42*, 5–37.

Sanderson, C.A. & Cantor, N. (1995). Social dating goals in late adolescence: Implications for safer sexual activity. *Journal of Personality and Social Psychology, 68*, 1121–1134.

Sedikides, C., Gaertner, L. & Toguchi, Y. (2003). Pancultural self-enhancement. *Journal of Personality and Social Psychology, 84*, 60–79.

Sharar, G., Henrich, C.C., Blatt, S.J., Ryan, R. & Little, T.D. (2003). Interpersonal relatedness, self-definition, and their motivational orientation during adolescence: A theoretical and empirical integration. *Developmental Psychology, 39*, 470–483.

Schwarz, N. & Bohner, G. (1996). Feelings and their motivational implications: Moods and the action sequence. In P.M. Gollwitzer & J.A. Bargh (Eds), *The Psychology of Action: Linking cognition and motivation to behavior* (pp. 119–145). New York: Guilford.

Sheldon, K.M. & Kasser, T. (1995). Coherence and congruence: Two aspects of personality integration. *Journal of Personality and Social Psychology, 68*, 531–543.

Sorrentino, R.M. (1996). The role of conscious thought in a theory of motivation and cognition: The uncertainty orientation paradigm. In P.M. Gollwitzer & J.A. Bargh (Eds), *The psychology of action: Linking cognition and motivation to behavior*, (pp. 619–644). New York: Guilford.

Sparks, P., Harris, P.R., & Lockwood, N. (2004). Predictors and predictive effects of ambivalence. *British Journal of Social Psychology, 43*, 371–383.

Stets, J.E. & Burke, P.J. (2000). Identity theory and social identity theory. *Social Psychology Quarterly, 63*, 224–237.

Thompson, M.M. Zanna, M.P. & Griffin, D.W. (1995). Let's not be indifferent about (attitudinal) ambivalence. In J.A. Krosnick & R.E. Petty (Eds), *Attitude Strength: Antecedents and consequences* (pp. 361–386). Hillsdale, NJ: Erlbaum.

Tice, D. & Bratslavsky, E. (2000). Giving in to feel good: The place of emotion regulation in the context of general self-control. *Psychological Inquiry, 11*, 149–159.

Vallacher, R.R. & Wegner, D.M. (1989). Levels of personal agency: Individual variation in action identification. *Journal of Personality and Social Psychology, 57*, 660–671.

Wegner, D.M., Vallacher, R.R. & Dizadji, D. (1989). Do alcoholics know what they're doing? Identifications of the act of drinking. *Basis and Applied Social Psychology, 10*, 197–210.

Weinstein, N.D. (1988). The precaution adoption process. *Health Psychology, 7*, 355–386.

Weinstein, N.D., & Klein, W. (1996). Unrealistic optimism: Present and future. *Journal of Social and Clinical Psychology, 15*, 1–8.

Winell, M. (1987). Personal goals: The key to self-direction in adulthood. In D.H. Ford & M.E. Ford (Eds), *Humans as Self-constructing Living Systems: Putting the framework to work*, (pp. 261–287). Hillsdale, NJ: Erlbaum.

CHAPTER 3

Unintentional Behavior: A Subrational Approach to Health Risk

Frederick X. Gibbons, Meg Gerrard,
Rachel A. Reimer, and Elizabeth A. Pomery

Most theories of health behavior and most theories of self-regulation were created to describe and predict the regulatory processes and health-relevant behaviors of adults. Very few of these theories include discussions of how these processes work among adolescents, let alone coverage of developmental issues, or hypotheses about how the behaviors might change over time. In the most recent volume on health and self-regulation (Cameron & Leventhal, 2003), for example, there is practically no mention of children and adolescents. This perspective is a reflection of the fact that these theories generally focus on "mature" health behaviors—those that are rational and intentional, usually involving health promotion. In the current chapter, we present a different perspective on health behavior; one that argues that behaviors that affect health are often not reasoned and *not intentional*, especially when they are performed by young people. The chapter begins with a brief discussion of self-regulation processes, relevant to health. It then describes a model of adolescent health behavior, which includes discussion of self-regulation, and presents some supporting data. We conclude with some suggestions for future research agendas.

SELF-REGULATION AND HEALTH: THE ROLE OF GOALS

The two models of self-regulation most often applied to the study of health behavior are Carver and Scheier's (1981, 1998) Control Theory and Leventhal's Common Sense Model (CSM) (Leventhal, Brissette & Leventhal, 2003; Leventhal, Meyer & Nerenz, 1980). The former presents a general view of self-regulation, whereas the CSM is more

Self-regulation in Health Behavior.   Edited by Denise T.D. de Ridder and John B.F. de Wit.
© 2006 John Wiley & Sons Ltd.

focused, mostly because it was intended as a heuristic for understanding how individuals monitor their health status and how they respond to health threats.

Control Theory

The Carver and Scheier theory, which is based on their earlier work on attention and self-consciousness (Carver, 1979; Scheier, 1980), draws from classic self-regulation theories (e.g., Powers, 1973), which means it is goal-based: "Central to our view is the notion that people live life by identifying goals and behaving in ways aimed at attaining these goals." (Scheier & Carver, 2003, p. 17). In the case of health, an obvious general goal is staying healthy. Thus, health self-regulation consists, essentially, of periodic assessments of current health status *vis à vis* that higher-order goal. The model has been applied very effectively to health promotion and health maintenance and to both approach and avoidance goals. Examples are: Staying in shape (through exercise regimens), or just staying healthy (through proper diet, including eating good foods and avoiding bad ones), as well as avoiding cognitive deterioration (e.g., by staying mentally active). It also works very well in outlining reactions to health problems, such as dealing with diabetes or coping with illness.

Goals exist at different levels of abstraction in the Carver and Scheier model. At the highest level would be general goals such as being healthy—what they call "be" goals. Next are what they call "do" goals, which comprise courses of action, such as medical regimens or exercise plans. Finally, at the lowest level are the motor control goals, which involve specific actions like, for instance, signing up at the fitness center or setting out one's daily pill box before going to bed at night. Higher level goals provide guidance and direction for the lower level goals, which are instrumental in reducing the perceived discrepancy between current status and the goal.

The Common Sense Model

Leventhal's model was created in an effort to explain how people detect and react to the presence of a health threat or problem. The initial realization of a problem triggers a dual response, characteristic of other dual-process models (see Chaiken & Trope, 1999, for a review of these models) that have a cognitive and an affective component. Thus, the individual will consider the threat from a more *rational* perspective, in terms of what corrective or coping actions are called for and/or might be implemented, as well as a more *emotional* level, which includes formulating a strategy for dealing with the negative affective response that awareness of the problem has elicited. Individuals' perceptions of the problem (symptom identification, for example) and their plans of action (the preferred coping process) often reflect their common sense models or beliefs about the problem (e.g., "heart attacks include pain running down the left arm") and its appropriate treatment (e.g., "in these situations, people usually ... take nitroglycerin ... lie down"). Progress or development of the problem as well as the coping strategy, if there is one, are monitored periodically in a process not unlike that described in the Carver and Scheier and other self-regulatory models, with more or less the same higher level goal, that is, good health.

The Common Sense Model also includes a significant social influence component (Leventhal et al., 2003). Determining whether a particular symptom is cause for concern, for example, often involves (social) comparison with others who have experienced similar symptoms (Suls, Martin & Leventhal, 1997). The same is true when trying to estimate the impact of the event and/or its corrective action on the self (e.g., the impact of surgery; Kulik & Mahler, 1987, 1997). Even the goal itself—staying healthy—may be partly a reflection of presumed needs and desires of significant others (Leventhal, Hudson & Robataille, 1997). Thus, the perspectives of others are considered, at least potentially, at each step of the health-status assessment process.

The Common Sense Model and Carver and Scheier's attention-based theory are similar in many respects and typical of self-regulation models. In particular, they share three basic assumptions about health behavior: (a) it is goal-based, reflecting a general overarching goal of good health, (b) people periodically assess their health status *vis à vis* their goals, and do so more often under some circumstances (e.g., illness) than others, and (c) self-regulation is a dual process that involves cognition and affect. More generally, both models describe a self-monitoring process that requires basic knowledge and cognitive capacity and takes time.

Health Impairing Behaviors: Goals?

Consistent with their focus on higher-order goals, such as staying healthy, the Common Sense Model and the Carver and Scheier model have been applied mostly to logical (or "common-sense") kinds of health-relevant behavior. Higher-order goals can conflict, however (Gebhardt, this volume), and both models do have something to say about behaviors that are potentially health-impairing, such as drug use or alcohol consumption. In the Carver and Scheier model, a higher level goal could be entertainment or pleasure. A drink or two with dinner or at a cocktail party would be consistent with this type of goal. Because of its focus on health threat, the Common Sense Model does not apply directly to substance use, except as a means of coping with illness. For example, substance (ab)use might be an emotion-focused strategy that effectively mutes the physical and psychological pains that accompany a diagnosis of terminal illness. Related to this last point, both models also address the issue of how individuals respond to a realization that they have not made satisfactory progress toward a meaningful goal. An inability to reduce an important discrepancy can lead to an increase in negative affect, which, again, can result in a desire to self-medicate in order to reduce the disappointment and concern. In short, health-risk behaviors among adults can be self-destructive or counterproductive, and they may not be logical or rational, but they are not necessarily outside the purview of self-regulatory models. Rational or not, they often are instrumental actions that serve a particular purpose. Thus, adults usually drink (sometimes too much), use drugs, or gamble excessively, because they have made a decision at some level that these actions will help achieve a particular goal. For some, those instrumental behaviors may become addictive, but *in most instances*, they remain within the control of the individual—unwise, perhaps, but certainly not unpredictable.

The Expectancy Value Perspective

With regard to health behavior, self-regulation models also share a perspective with expectancy-value theories of decision-making in cognitive and social psychology (Feather, 1990). These theories are based on an assumption that social behavior is the result of a deliberate decision-making process. That process involves an assessment of behavioral options, which includes the expected outcomes or consequences associated with each one (Loewenstein, Weber, Hsee & Welch, 2001, call this approach the "consequentialist" perspective). This assessment results in the formulation of a plan of action. Examples of expectancy value theories that have been applied effectively to health behavior include the Health Belief Model (Rosenstock, 1974), Protection Motivation Theory (Rogers, 1983), and the Theory of Reasoned Action (Fishbein & Ajzen, 1975) and its derivative, the Theory of Planned Behavior (Ajzen, 1991). The Theory of Reasoned Action is the most popular such theory and so can be used as an illustration of the general category.

The plan of action in the Theory of Reasoned Action is the individual's behavioral intention to engage in the behavior. According to the Theory of Reasoned Action and other expectancy value theories, behavioral intention is the only proximal antecedent to social behavior—health or otherwise. Intentions have been defined variously as: Plans to achieve a particular behavioral goal (Ajzen, 1996), proximal goals (Bandura, 1997), or an indication of how much effort one is willing to exert to reach a particular goal (Ajzen, 1991). In other words, they reflect goal states, which, because they involve specific plans of action, resemble the "do" goals outlined in control theory (more so than higher level "be" goals).[1] There are two antecedents to behavioral intention in the theory. The first is attitude, which results from a consideration of possible outcomes associated with a behavior (hence the term expectancy value), as well as an assessment of one's affective reaction to the behavior. The second antecedent, labeled subjective norms, is more social: It comprises individuals' beliefs about whether important others do or do not want them to perform the behavior. Thus, the decision to engage in testicular or breast self-examination is likely to reflect a determination that the behavior is effective, that it is affectively acceptable, and that significant others think it should be done. Other similar models designed more specifically for health behavior, such as the Health Belief Model or Protection Motivation theory, also include a *perception of vulnerability* element—what is my risk for testicular cancer, for example—as an antecedent to intentions. That construct would be subsumed within the attitude component in the Theory of Reasoned Action. The Theory of Planned Behavior adds a self-efficacy factor to the Theory of Reasoned Action in the form of a measure of perceived behavioral control, defined as a perception of one's ability to actually perform the behavior.

Predicting Health Behavior

The Theory of Reasoned Action and Theory of Planned Behavior have proven very successful at predicting a range of health behaviors, from oral hygiene, to seat belt use, to

---

[1] In fact, the principle of "compatibility" (Ajzen & Fishbein, 2005) suggests that measures of higher-level or global goals, such as those described by Carver and Scheier as "be" goals, are not likely to predict subsequent behavior very well because of their non-specific (abstract) nature.

use of birth control. Meta-analyses of the two theories have indicated that the distal antecedents (attitudes and norms) typically account for between 30% and 40% of the variance in intentions (Conner & Sparks, 2005), which, in turn, account for between 20% and 30% of the variance in the relevant behavior (Albarracin, Johnson, Fishbein & Muellereile, 2001; Armitage & Conner, 2001; Conner & Sparks, 2005; Hagger, Chatzisarantis & Biddle, 2002; Sheeran, 2002; Sheeran & Orbell, 1998). Explained variance does vary as a function of a number of factors, however, including age (it is lower for younger people; Albarracin et al., 2001) and type of behavior (Godin & Kok, 1996; Sheeran, 2002).

A recent meta-analysis by Webb and Sheeran (in press) is relevant to this last issue (type of behavior as a moderator). They examined only *experimental* tests of the intention to behavior relation—those in which participants were randomly assigned to a treatment condition to alter their intentions and then behavior was measured subsequently (i.e., interventions). They found 47 such tests. In this more focused analysis, the authors concluded that the relation between behavioral intention and behavior is "a great deal more limited than was previously supposed." They identified three moderators of the behavioral intention—behavior relation that they suggest should be considered in future studies. Specifically, they suggest that intentions have less impact on future behavior when: (a) the participant has little control over the behavior (as the Theory of Planned Behavior would suggest), (b) the behavior is habitual, *and* circumstances promote the habit, and (c) there is potential for "social reaction," that is, the behavior involves health-risk rather than health promotion and has a significant social influence component (see the discussion of social reaction below). In short, expectancy value theories, which are based on an assumption of cognitive deliberation (of options and outcomes), work very well for health behaviors that are instrumental and that have identifiable costs and benefits that can be anticipated—in other words, behaviors that require some planning, such as exercise, contraception, and dieting. Most of these behaviors are health-promoting.

Self-regulation and Age

Self-regulation models acknowledge the possibility of goal conflict. At a fundamental level, the abstract higher level goal, referred to loosely as the "pursuit of happiness" (or pleasure), often conflicts with a slightly more concrete goal of staying healthy (and staying alive). How individuals resolve this conflict can have profound implications for their quality of life—overall happiness, physical fitness, longevity, or marital satisfaction. Moreover, the effectiveness of the resolution, we would argue, depends on the person's ability to *anticipate* the conflict (e.g., "I think I can have four drinks at the office party and still get home safely") and prepare for them ahead of time (e.g., "I'll ask my wife not to drink"). This anticipation comes with experience and maturity. It is likely to vary from one individual to the next, but it is generally characteristic of adult behavior. This is not to suggest that health-relevant behavior among adults is always planned; that is not the case. Adults usually do not plan to drink and drive, over-eat, or engage in (risky) adulterous behavior, and few smokers would claim that smoking is a goal for them (cutting down may be, of course). Thus, higher-order "be" goals (stay healthy) and even mid-level "do" goals (stay sober, stay fit, stay married) can succumb to competing needs and ressures—often in social contexts, such as office parties, dinner engagements, or vacations. Although often not intentional, these behaviors are anticipated and premeditated, and therefore usually predictable. The situation is different for young people, however.

Adolescent Health Behavior

There are a number of ways in which the regulatory processes of adolescents *vis à vis* health differ from those of adults. First, health is much more of a social phenomenon for young people. Their health-relevant behaviors are more likely to involve risk—substance use, risky driving, risky sex—*and* these behaviors are much more likely to take place in groups or social settings (Simpson, 1996; Udry, 1998; Zimring, 1998). More generally, adolescents are more responsive to social influence than are adults (Gardner & Steinberg, 2005; Pasupathi, 1999), especially when it comes to risky behaviors (Rivis & Sheeran, 2003). Second, lack of experience makes it more difficult for young people to anticipate the conflicts mentioned above (Fischhoff, 1992) and to arrange for alternative responses or simply avoidance of the temptation. Third, adolescents' cognitive processing styles differ from those of adults in a variety of ways, including a tendency to be more impulsive and less introspective (Beyth-Marom & Fischhoff, 1997; Steinberg & Cauffman, 1996). Fourth, there is some evidence that the area of the brain responsible for executive functioning (such as considering risks), is not completely mature until age 25 (Giedd, 2004), which suggests there may be a biological substrate to the risky behavior of adolescents.

What goals factor into adolescents' regulating process involving health? Most adolescents do not have clearly-defined health maintenance goals of the nature found in adults. Many are physically active, for example, but they do not have exercise regimens. Few monitor their diets or caloric-intake—in spite of an obvious and increasing need to do so, as indicated by recent statistics on childhood obesity in the USA (Hedley et al., 2004). The problem does not appear to be unique to the USA, however. A recent cross-cultural study of four countries suggested that exercise behavior is more prevalent among American adolescents—ages 14 to 18—than it is among Hungarian, Polish, or Turkish adolescents (Luszczynska, Gibbons, Piko & Tekozel, 2004). Similarly, American adolescents are more likely to state that they think about nutrition than are their Hungarian and Polish counterparts. Nonetheless, nutrition is still not a concern for the vast majority of adolescents: When asked how many of their friends watch their diet, 86% of the Americans said half or fewer; the figure was greater than 90% in Poland. Also, although very few studies have examined the issue, we suspect that very few young people maintain a regular physical check-up routine, choosing instead to rely on parents and others to remind them when it is time. Finally, illness is relatively rare among young people and therefore not likely to be a salient assessment dimension (or "referent value" in the Carver & Scheier model).

This is not to suggest that adolescents do not have health goals. Certainly if asked, many would claim that they do. What we are suggesting, instead, is that, relative to adults, health-maintenance goals are not very salient for adolescents. They may exist in an abstract sense, but if so, they are usually not accompanied by implementation plans (Gollwitzer, 1999), and therefore not very likely to influence their day to day actions.

Thus, traditional self-regulation and attitude-behavior consistency approaches cannot be applied as effectively at understanding and predicting these behaviors.

So what goals do guide adolescents' behavior? Many of them have to do with the self, especially the self *vis à vis* others. In other words, they are *social* goals. At a basic level, developing a sense of self—answering the question "Who am I?"—and finding out how that self fits in to their social environment are dominant concerns (Erickson, 1968; Sebald, 1989). Being popular, having good relationships, and being attractive are all lower level goals subsumed by the overall goal of social acceptance. Other goals do exist—personal accomplishment in academics and athletics, perhaps financial success—but these goals are seldom related to their health behavior. For the most part, they are healthy and they expect to stay that way, so they don't think much about it.

Conclusion

Expectancy value theories and most theories of self-regulation are based on an assumption that individuals' health behavior, like other behaviors, is the result of a deliberative process that includes consideration of options and outcomes and involves a more or less logical, deductive reasoning—this is what I want, this is what I will do, this is what will happen. These assumptions do not hold as well for health-relevant behaviors that are risky, especially if they include a significant social influence component, and many health-risk behaviors do (Webb & Sheeran, in press). Thus, health behavior is not always planned or intentional; but for adults, it is at least anticipated and therefore usually predictable. For adolescents, however, health-risk behavior is often unanticipated—it is a social reaction. As such, it may be part of a general desire for social acceptance, but for the most part, it is usually not goal-based.

A SOCIAL-REACTION MODEL OF ADOLESCENT HEALTH

In an effort to improve the predictive power of existing theories of health behavior, we have developed a model that differs from extant theories in several ways. It is a social-reaction model, named after its two focal constructs (Gibbons & Gerrard, 1997; Gibbons, Gerrard & Lane, 2003). The prototype-willingness model is based on a belief that adolescent health behavior is often a reaction to social stimuli and social situations—situations that are quite common for adolescents, increasingly so as they age. For this reason, we believe that a social-psychological perspective with an emphasis on social cognition is very useful in trying to understand these behaviors.

Unplanned Behavior?

Although the answer may seem obvious to many parents (see Steinberg, 2003), there are very few studies that have directly assessed the question of whether adolescent health-risk behavior is always intentional; much of the evidence is indirect and/or anecdotal. For example, surveys with unwed pregnant teenage girls have suggested that the sexual

Table 3.1 Risk behavior as a function of previously stated behavioral intention and behavioral expectation

	Behavior	
	Casual sex	DUI
Did it at T2[a]	24 %	58 %
No BI at T1[b]	39 % (1)	40 % (1)
No BI or BE at T1[b]	24 % (3)	23 % (3)
No BW at T1[b]	5 % (2)	9 % (3)

$N = 381$ (218 females; Mean age at T2 $= 19$)
Note:
[a]Percentage saying at T2 that they had done the behavior in the past year.
[b]Numbers reflect the percentage of those who said at T2 that they had engaged in the behavior (i.e., the top row) that reported no BI, BI/BE, or BW at the previous wave (T1). See text for further explanation. BI = Behavioral Intention to have casual sex (column 1) and also to drive under the influence of alcohol (column 2); BE = Behavioral Expectation to have casual sex and also to drive under the influence; BW = Behavioral Willingness to have casual sex and also to drive under the influence; DUI = driving under the influence (of alcohol); The number of items used to measure BI, BI/BE, and BW are shown in the parentheses.

behavior that resulted in their condition was not intentional (Erickson, 2003; Ingham, Woodcock, & Stenner, 1991; cf. Gerrard & Warner, 1990). Similar results emerge from studies of adolescent smoking (Kremers, Mudde, De Vries, Brug & De Vries, 2004), drunk driving, and risky sexual behavior (Murry, 1994; Zabin, Stark & Emerson, 1991). Kremers and colleagues (2004) argue that many adolescents do not have intentions one way or the other with regard to smoking and that it is only after they have tried it a few times that they start engaging in a decision making process that eventually results in an intention to smoke or not smoke.

More direct evidence of the issue can be seen in our own research. The data in Table 3.1 come from a panel of white adolescents (mean age 14 at Wave 1, 250 males and 250 females) who were assessed annually for 8 years. The general question is whether these adolescents' risk behaviors were intentional. The specific question was whether the proximal antecedents of behavioral intention and behavioral expectation would predict risk behavior in young people.

Behavioral expectation is a construct very similar to behavioral intention that assesses perceived likelihood of engaging in a behavior ("How likely is it that you will do X?"; Warshaw & Davis, 1985). Thus, it includes assessment of factors that may influence performance of the behavior—either in a facilitating or inhibiting fashion (e.g., "I don't intend to drink too much at the party, but I expect I probably will"). In fact, the two proximal constructs of behavioral intention and behavioral expectation are often used interchangeably in research within the Theory of Reasoned Action and the Theory of Planned Behavior; when both are used they appear to define a single factor (Armitage & Conner, 2001).

At T2, which was Wave 6 for the panel (age 19), and the first wave at which we had all of the relevant measures, we asked them if they had engaged in sex with a casual partner in the previous year, and if they had driven after drinking several drinks. As Table 3.1 indicates, about a quarter of the sample had engaged in casual sex and about half had driven while under the influence of alcohol. We then looked back at their behavioral predictions at the previous wave, at which time we had asked them if they had any intention of doing these behaviors in the next year (1 item: "Do you intend to have sex with a casual partner in the next 12 months?" from 1 = *definitely not* to 7 = *definitely*) and if they had any expectation that they would do them (2 items: e.g., "How likely is it that you will have sex with a casual partner?" from 1 = *not at all likely* to 7 = *very likely*; the behavioral willingness items are described below). The percentages listed are those who said they did the behavior and had responded with a 1 on *each one* of these three questions. One would assume if they had any inkling at all that they were thinking of doing the behaviors or even that the behaviors might happen, let alone if these behaviors were goals for them, then that would show up as something other than a series of "1" responses on the three scales.

In general, when we ask these "active non-intenders" why they did what they did, a typical response has been something like "It just happened" (Mitchell & Wellings, 1998; Steinberg, 2003). So, we asked this question directly in a second panel of approximately 125 male and 125 female African American adolescents (ages 13, 15, and 18 at the 3 waves). We asked them if they had smoked and, if so, whether the behavior was intentional or not: "Think about the last time you smoked cigarettes. Had you planned (ahead of time) to do it or did it just happen?" followed by a 4 point scale (from 1 = *it just happened* to 4 = *I planned to do it*). Over the 3 waves, percentages reporting they had smoked ranged from 35% to 49%. Within these groups, the percentage answering "1" ranged from 67% to 72%, whereas the percentage claiming it was planned ("4") was 6% at the first 2 waves. The latter percentage climbed to 18% at wave 3, when they were 18 and smoking was most likely habitual for the intentional group. In short, the responses of many adolescents who engage in risky behaviors suggest either directly or indirectly that they had not planned on engaging in the behavior before it happened.

Basic Assumptions of the Model

Our model has two basic assumptions. First, health-risk behavior, in general, tends to be more impulsive than health-promotion behavior, and, therefore, does not fit as well within the consequentialist perspective (Stacy, 1997; Stacy, Newcomb & Ames, 2000). Again, that is especially true for novice risk-takers, such as adolescents. In other words, much adolescent health-risk behavior is the result of a decision making process that is done "on-line" in response to environmental circumstances; it is "subrational." By the same token, these behaviors are usually not goal-oriented. They may facilitate a general goal of stimulation and excitement, and they may be consistent with other goals, such as social inclusion (Beyth-Marom & Fischhoff, 1997), but they are not instrumental actions that are planned and implemented under anticipated conditions. In contrast (as discussed in the chapter by Gerrard and colleagues in this volume), the decision to *not engage* in these behaviors, when it occurs, is more deliberative and goal-based and often a reflection of a self-regulatory process. The second assumption of the model is that most adolescent health-risk behavior is socially oriented. The details of the model have been presented elsewhere (Gibbons & Gerrard, 1997; Gibbons et al., 2003). A brief overview here will facilitate understanding of the new material that will be discussed.

Reasoned Processing

Ours is a modified dual process model—actually, it is a dual pathway model. One path comes directly from expectancy value theories and proceeds to behavior through the standard proximal antecedent of behavioral intention. This is the *reasoned* pathway. It reflects the fact that some adolescent risk behavior is planned, even at a very young age. We have found, for example, that some 10-year-olds will indicate that they are planning (and expecting) to smoke or drink and, in fact, 2 years later they tell us they have done that (Gibbons, Gerrard, Cleveland, Wills & Brody, 2004). These children have thought about the behavior and decided they want to do it; and chances are very good that they will. Antecedents to behavioral intention in the prototype model are similar to those in the Theory of Reasoned Action, but operationalized somewhat differently given the more specific focus on adolescents and health. The first antecedent is *attitude*, which is defined as outcome expectancies—or, more specifically, perceived risk ("How dangerous is the behavior?") and perceived result ("What will happen?"). The second antecedent is *norms*, which in this case are descriptive (i.e., perceptions of what peers and others are doing) rather than injunctive (what do other people want me to do), as is the case with the Theory of Reasoned Action or the Theory of Planned Behavior.[2] The processing that is thought to occur in this path is similar to that seen in the more analytic processing modes in dual process models, variously labeled as cognitive, systematic, or central (see Chaiken & Trope, 1999). It is also similar to the type of processing outlined in self-regulatory models; it is deliberative, usually goal-based, and involves a regulatory feedback loop.

Reactive Processing

The second pathway to health risk is the social reaction path. It adds a second proximal antecedent, called "behavioral willingness" which is defined as an openness to risk opportunity—what an individual would be willing to do under certain (risk-conducive) circumstances. When assessing behavioral willingness, risk-conducive circumstances are described (e.g., a party at which marijuana or alcohol is available; a new, interested potential sex partner) and then a series of options are presented that increase in risk level: e.g., try some, get stoned, take/buy some for later. These are combined into a behavioral willingness index. As one would expect, behavioral willingness and behavioral intention are correlated (*r*s range from 0.20 to 0.70), but they are distinct constructs that predict behavior independently as well as jointly. In fact, a number of studies have shown that this construct has good predictive validity—better than behavioral intention for younger people. Evidence of that can be seen in the bottom row of Table 3.1: Very few of those adolescents who engaged in the two risky behaviors reported no willingness to do so at the previous wave. What this means is that even adolescents have an idea of what their *capabilities* are ("Under the right circumstances, I might have casual sex with someone I

---

[2] Because of their questionable predictive validity, many researchers have avoided using injunctive subjective norm measures, often replacing them with some form of descriptive norm measures (Rivis & Sheeran, 2003). Ajzen and Fishbein (2005) suggest that both types should be used.

just met") before they actually encounter any opportunity. This level of self-awareness increases as they mature.

Behavioral willingness shares two antecedents with behavioral intention: descriptive norms and perceived risk. It has two additional antecedents, however, that are unique to the model. The first is *personal vulnerability*, which is also part of the attitude construct: "Will *I* get caught / hurt / in trouble *if I were to do the behavior*?"[3] Relative to perceived danger or risk, which involves more systematic or analytic processing, personal vulnerability involves more heuristic processing. Sometimes, this leads to a sense of personal immunity, which is a form of *optimistic bias* (Weinstein, 1980): "If I did it, I could get away with it." Thus, perceived danger is part of the reasoned path and so is related more to behavioral intention than behavioral willingness, whereas personal vulnerability is part of the social reaction path and therefore is related to behavioral willingness more than behavioral intention (Gibbons, Gerrard, Blanton & Russell, 1998; Gibbons et al., 2005).

Risk Images

The second unique antecedent to behavioral willingness is the *image* (prototype) the person associates with the behavior: The type of person (their age) who uses drugs, for example, or drinks heavily, or "sleeps around." The images are part of a *typology*. What is influential is not so much the visual image that the adolescent associates with the behavior, but more his or her sense of the *type* of person who does it. When asked, adolescents can describe these typologies, oftentimes in vivid detail. The less favorable the description and the less similar to the self it is thought to be ("I'm not that type"), the less willing the person is to do the behavior. The images develop at a very early age, influenced by media, peers, and family, which means they are malleable and therefore good targets for preventive interventions intended to delay onset of the behaviors among adolescents (see Gerrard et al., this volume). The model is presented in Figure 3.1.

Processing in the social reaction path is similar to that associated with heuristic modes in dual processing models, also labeled experiential, emotive, or peripheral. More specifically, it involves more affect, is more heuristic (e.g., images are part of it), and is less deliberative. The social reaction model differs from previous prototype-based models of behavior in that it is assumed that risk images are not seen as goals—boys usually do not start smoking because they are trying to acquire a *Marlboro Man* image for example (cf. Leventhal & Cleary, 1980; Chassin et al., 1981), or start using drugs because they want to look like Kurt Cobain. But they may avoid drugs or tobacco because they believe the image is not consistent with their self-concept or the social image they wish to project (Gerrard et al., 2002). In this sense, the images are *social consequences* of the actions. The decision making involves rapid and often truncated consideration: What will others think of me? Am I that kind of person? Further evidence of processing style is presented in the Gerrard et al. chapter (this volume). Suffice it to say that rather than include consideration of consequences (other than social consequences), behavioral willingness is actually associated with *avoidance* of such consideration (Gerrard et al.,

---

[3] Because they are presented in the subjunctive—"If you *were* to do..."—these items are also referred to as *conditional* perceived vulnerability measures (Gibbons et al., 2002).

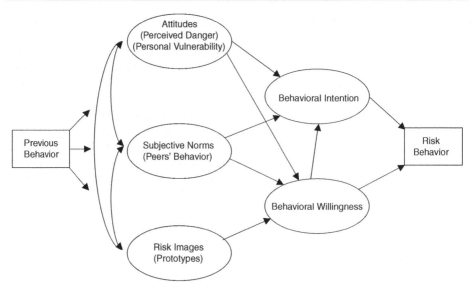

Figure 3.1   The Prototype/Willingness Model

2002). In many instances, adolescents are willing to engage because they have not thought about the behavior much ahead of time. Thus, inducing such thought should reduce behavioral willingness.

To recap, the prototype model maintains that adolescents generally find risky behaviors, such as drug use or casual sex, to be enticing, but they are also aware that these behaviors have costs associated with them—not just health costs, but social costs as well. Engaging in public, which is where these behaviors usually occur, means being associated with a particular image and the group it represents. Concern about this social cost deters many young people from the behavior. For some, however, the images are not inconsistent with self-concept. That belief, combined with a (relative) sense of personal immunity and a belief that others are engaging in the behavior (often exaggerated; Gibbons, Helweg-Larsen & Gerrard, 1995; Marks, Graham & Hansen, 1992), will often lead to participation. Finally, the model says little about *amount* of participation—how much alcohol will be consumed or how many sex partners will be involved, for example. However, if the adolescent is comfortable with the label, once he or she has engaged, there is little additional consequence to increased participation, unless, of course, public *over*indulgence becomes a common and very visible occurrence.

MODERATORS OF PATH DETERMINATION

An important question for the model, with implications for interventions and also for self-regulation, is what factors influence path determination? As the model indicates, the paths are not mutually exclusive. For a given individual, some behavior may be intentional and some willingness-based; the ratio will vary from one individual to the next. Logically, the developmental trend is toward intentional behavior, and the ratio of behavioral intention:behavioral willingness increases with age. We will discuss four factors that moderate path determination: personality, context, experience, and affect or emotional state.

Personality: Self-control

Using theory and research by Tarter and Vanyukov (1994) and Rothbart (Rothbart & Ahadi, 1994), Wills has conducted a series of studies examining self-control in adolescents, focusing specifically on how it predicts health behavior (e.g., Wills, Sandy & Yaeger, 2001; Wills, Windle & Cleary, 1998). Factor analyses indicate that there were two self-control dimensions: "good" self-control and "poor" self-control (Wills et al., 2001). Although correlated (typically around -0.40), they are distinct constructs that appear to be linked to separate neuropsychological systems (Rothbart & Bates, 1998). Both are reasonable indicators of self-regulatory functioning. Good self-control includes traits such as planfulness ("I like to plan things ahead of time," in fact, the trait is also referred to as "planfulness"); soothability, and attentional control ("I think before I act"). As might be expected, good self-control correlates with future orientation: Adolescents who are high in good self-control are more capable of regulating their emotional states and more likely to avoid risky situations. In short, they think ahead, which means, relatively speaking, they are proficient at self-regulation.

Poor self-control comprises 3 factors: impulsiveness ("I like to switch from one thing to another"), impatience, or poor delay of gratification ("If I find that something is really difficult, I get frustrated and quit"), and distractability. Obviously, adolescents who are high on these traits struggle with self-regulation issues. Wills's work has shown that the two traits are good predictors of health-risk behavior, and the relations are intuitive: good self-control is negatively associated with use, poor self-control is positively associated (Wills et al., 1998; Wills & Stoolmiller, 2002). Similarly, the 2 traits correlate with early and risky sexual behavior (Wills, Gibbons, Gerrard, Murry & Brody, 2003). These relations exist controlling for the trait of risk-taking, which correlates moderately with poor self-control ($rs = 0.30$ to 0.40), but only weakly with good self-control ($rs = 0.10$ to 0.20). Thus, adolescents who are high in good self-control are not simply timid; they do seek out stimulation, but they do it in a more controlled fashion. In short, their behavior is more internally driven.

How does this fit in with the prototype model? The behavior of adolescents with poor self-control appears to be more reactive; that is, they are more likely to be influenced by circumstances and events surrounding them. Those with good self-control, on the other hand, are more likely to think ahead about possible behavioral options and to anticipate problems and opportunities. Thus, we would expect adolescents who are high in poor self-control to be more predisposed toward the social reaction path, whereas those high in good self-control should be more inclined toward the reasoned path. Table 3.2 presents data relevant to this question. These data come from another one of our panels (124 female and 110 male African American 15 year-olds), which included measures of good and poor self-control as well as substance use (alcohol, drugs, and tobacco), behavioral willingness, and risk prototypes (smokers, drinkers, drug users). There were also two social influence constructs: norm items ("How many of your friends and peers are using drugs/alcohol/tobacco?") and a direct measure of social influence, which asked to what

Table 3.2 Correlations of good and poor self-control (SC) with risk cognitions and behavior

	Good SC	Poor SC
Substance Use	−0.15*	0.16*
Behavioral Willingness	−0.13*	0.31**
User Prototype	−0.24**	0.26**
Social Influence	−0.07	0.29**
Friends' Use	−0.06	0.17*

$N = 234$ (124 Females); *$p < 0.05$, **$p < 0.001$.
User Prototype = target's image of the type of adolescent who uses substances (smoking, drinking and drugs); Social Influence = target's report of friends' influence on their own substance use (same three substances); Friends' Use = target's report of how many of their friends use substances (averaged across the three substances).

extent they thought their friends influenced their decisions to use or not use each one of the substances.

The relations with use are modest, but significant. The relations with the various cognitions were stronger, however. Poor self-control was related to behavioral willingness, as well as the substance user images (combined across the three substances), and social influence (all $ps < 0.001$). The relations with good self-control were negative and somewhat weaker (see Gerrard et al., this volume, for additional analyses on non-user images and healthy cognitions). Regression analyses also indicated that the relation between these adolescents' behavioral willingness and their substance use was significantly stronger for those who were high in poor self-control ($p < 0.008$). Overall, then, adolescents high in poor self-control did have more willingness than those low in poor self-control or those high in good self-control, but the most pronounced difference was in whether or not they acted on that willingness. Put another way, behavioral willingness is more likely to translate into substance use among adolescents who have poor self-control.

Conclusion

Good self-control and poor self-control are both indicators of self-regulation. Adolescents who are high in good self-control are more planful and deliberative about their actions. They are less likely to engage in risky behavior, in part, because they are more likely to avoid risk-conducive situations. Their processing is more typical of the reasoned path to risk. In general, their behavior is less risky, but when they do engage it is with some forethought. Those who are high in poor self-control are more likely to follow the reactive route to risk. They are less planful about their actions, which tend to be more impulsive and more influenced by social and environmental factors (i.e. externally driven).

Context: Risk "Opportunity"

As suggested earlier, behavioral willingness is an openness to risk opportunity, which means it is responsive to social and contextual factors. Thus, context (risk) should moderate the relation between amount of behavioral willingness and risk behavior. This hypothesis was examined in a recent study using structural equation modeling with another panel consisting of the younger siblings (age 10.5 at Wave 1; N = 897) of the black teenagers mentioned above (Gibbons et al., 2004). Behavioral willingness, behavioral intention, risk prototypes, and substance use (including self-reports and reports of friends' use) were assessed at T1 and at T2 (however, there was virtually no use at T1, so the two T1 use measures were dropped from the model). In addition, there was a measure of environmental risk that included items on crime, gang activity, and substance availability. The model turned out consistent with hypotheses. Social factors (peer use) were much more strongly related to behavioral willingness than to behavioral intention, whereas use in the home by parents was more strongly related to behavioral intention. Our interpretation of this latter effect was that observing use by the parents induced consideration of the behavior and led to the development of a plan to use or not use—even at the age of (Gerrard, Gibbons, Brody, Murry & Wills, 2005). This was one reason why behavioral intention at T1 predicted use two years later, at age 12.

Context Modulation

In general, behavioral willingness was a better predictor of use at this age than was behavioral intention, as has been the case in previous studies with adolescents under the age of 16 or 17 (e.g., Gibbons et al., 1998). However, this relation was moderated by context (see Figure 3.2): It was significantly stronger in high-risk neighborhoods than it was in low-risk neighborhoods. In fact, if we look at the subset of the sample that was high (above the median) in behavioral willingness, but had no behavioral intention at all, more than half of this group was using substances at T2 if *they lived in a high risk environment*. If they lived in a lower risk environment, only 20% were using. Thus, there was more use in the high-risk neighborhoods, but this was attributable almost entirely to the high-willing adolescents. In contrast, behavioral intention was equally effective at predicting use in high and low risk neighborhoods. In other words, those who were high in

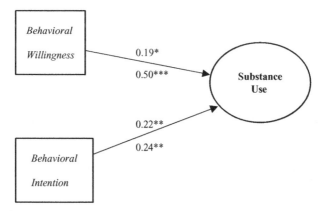

Figure 3.2   Risk opportunity (i.e., neighborhood risk) as a moderator of relations between substance use (alcohol, tobacco, and drugs) with behavioral willingness and behavioral intention

Low risk neighborhoods are above the line, high risk neighborhoods below the line. Figures represent standardized regression coefficients; *$p < 0.05$ **$p < 0.01$ ***$p < 0.001$.

behavioral intention (and there weren't very many of them) ended up using whether the substances were readily available or not.

Behavioral willingness and behavioral intention are related but independent proximal antecedents to behavior. Most adolescents are either high or low in both, but some are inconsistent, which can put them at risk for negative outcomes. In particular, those who are high in risk behavioral willingness (above the median) and low in behavioral intention (usually no behavioral intention at all) have not thought much about the behaviors and their *consequences*, which means they are more likely to let environmental factors regulate their behavior. It also means they are less likely to be prepared for these situations—they are not likely to carry condoms, secure a "designated driver," or arrange for a place to "sleep it off." In contrast, the behavior of the consistent groups—those who were high or low in both behavioral intention and behavioral willingness[4]—is more internally determined. In the vast majority of cases, they avoid use (among adolescents, the low–low group is much larger than the high–high group); but some of them do have use as a goal and they will engage in the various lower-order actions necessary to achieve that goal.

Age and Experience

As can be seen in Figure 3.1, there is a hypothesized path from behavioral willingness to behavioral intention. This path illustrates a developmental trend. Many individuals start out with some (low) level of willingness, which eventually develops into at least behavioral expectation if not behavioral intention to engage. More generally, this reflects a shift in processing style that comes with maturity. Epstein (1993) has argued that the cognitive and experiential processing modes continue to function in parallel throughout the life span, and they both continue to develop—people tend to "get better" at both types. However, the *ratio* of the former to the latter increases with age: More decision-making involves rational thought and contemplation as people get older (cf. Chen & Chaiken, 1999). Similarly, behavioral willingness tends to develop sooner than does behavioral intention. Thus, it is a better predictor of risky behavior among pre-adolescents, in part, because they seldom have any intention of engaging. Of course, that, too, changes with age and experience.

Age

Figure 3.3 presents an illustration of the development of the two paths or, more specifically, the relative predictive power of behavioral willingness and behavioral expectation. These data are from a panel of 500 white adolescents, beginning at Wave 1 (mean age 14, range 13–15), and continuing through age 20 (Pomery, Gibbons, Gerrard & Reis-Bergan, 2006, Study 1). It reflects the predictive power of behavioral willingness and behavioral

---

[4] There is an asymmetry between behavioral willingness and behavioral intention in the sense that one can be high in behavioral willingness and low in behavioral intention, but the opposite is unlikely. An adolescent who is high in behavioral intention, will almost always also be high in behavioral willingness. That is reflective of the fact that behavioral willingness usually precedes behavioral intention developmentally.

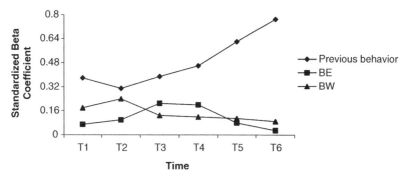

Figure 3.3 Regression coefficients of behavioral willingness, behavioral expectation, and previous behavior predicting smoking across time, controlling for age at T1 (M age at T1 $= 14$; N ranges from 441 at T1 to 265 at T6; waves were annual)

expectation *vis à vis* subsequent smoking (the y-axis shows standardized β coefficients of all three when entered together into the regression equation). As can be seen, behavioral willingness starts out stronger than behavioral expectation, then gives way to behavioral expectation by age 17 or so. Both proximal constructs become non-significant by age 18/19, as previous behavior explains most of the variance. By that time, the behavior is certainly routinized if not habitual. Although not illustrated here, the "superiority" of behavioral willingness as a predictor over behavioral expectation maintains for *initiators*—those adolescents who have not previously tried the behavior. For them, behavioral willingness is a better predictor (of onset) of smoking right up through age 18.

Experience

This latter onset analysis suggests that experience with the behavior, perhaps more than just age, may be a moderating factor in determining which pathway to the risk behavior an adolescent will follow. A second study examined this hypothesis directly, but with a very different type of risk behavior: "skipping" class at university (Pomery et al., 2006, Study 2). The assumption was that all students would maintain a goal of good academic performance (Gibbons et al., 2002), and that attending class would be an instrumental action that could help achieve that goal. In addition, it was assumed that this regulation process would be more internalized for those with a lot of experience in school and more externally-driven for those with less experience. Within the prototype model, that translates into a specific prediction that experience with the behavior (defined in this case as how long they had been in school and therefore how many classes they had attended and skipped) will moderate the respective relations between class skipping and both intention to skip and willingness to skip. In fact, that is what happened: For students with relatively little experience skipping class, behavioral willingness predicted class attendance well, whereas behavioral intention was not related; the opposite pattern occurred among those who had been in school longer and therefore were more experienced at attending (and not attending) class.

Age and experience, which are highly correlated, moderate the self-regulation process and also influence pathway determination in the prototype model. As adolescents age, their ability to process information cognitively improves for several reasons, including increased cognitive capacity and emotional control, more knowledge about events and their antecedents and sequelae, and increased awareness of behavioral alternatives (Fischhoff, 1992). For more or less the same reasons, they also become better at predicting their own behavior. More of it becomes intentional, less of it is an unintended reaction to situations; and they simply spend more time thinking about all relevant elements including the situation, the behavior, and its possible consequences. Similarly, self-regulation becomes more of that—*self* rather than social regulation; more of it is internally driven. Adolescents have the ability to estimate their future (social) reactions at a very young age, but it is only an estimate, not a script. By adulthood, one has had enough experience with risk-conducive situations to effectively predict behavior in these situations when they occur and, presumably, enough maturity to acknowledge that the behavior is internally driven—especially if it has occurred repeatedly in the past. Still, there are some behaviors that remain mostly willingness-based, or opportunistic, through-out life, such as tax evasion, drunk-driving, or adultery. Many who engage in these behaviors do not expect and certainly do not intend to do so; but it does happen.

Emotion

Affect influences processing and regulatory strategies. Positive mood triggers what could be labeled a cautious processing style, oriented toward maintaining the status quo (Eich & Forgas, 2003). Bless (2001; Bless, Clore, Schwarz & Golisano, 1996) suggests that when people are in positive moods, they are more likely to rely on "general knowledge structures," which are essentially heuristics that facilitate rapid, but somewhat superficial scanning of incoming information. The basic idea is that "everything is OK," so there is no pressing need to take the time to carefully examine environmental stimuli. Thus, positive mood is associated with heuristic processing (Epstein, 1985; Tversky & Kahne-man, 1974) that has a general goal of mood maintenance (Isen & Shalker, 1982) and is done more rapidly (Forgas, 1989). It is also mood-congruent. Thus, happy people tend to be more optimistic with regard to outcome expectations and they have lower levels of perceived risk; the opposite is true for unhappy people (Raghunathan & Pham, 1999). This presents a bit of a paradox: Positive moods are associated with more sanguine perceptions and lower levels of perceived risk, and yet they usually lead to *less* risky behavior. In fact, negative affectivity and depression are arguably the most influential antecedents to substance use and abuse (Wills, Sandy, Shinar & Yaeger, 1999). If one's expectations are pessimistic, why engage in behaviors that clearly put the self at risk?

In most self-regulatory models, the existence of a negative mood signals a need for action (Carver & Scheier, 1998; Tesser et al., 1996). Whereas happy people maintain a (relatively) cursory monitoring of the environment, sad people are more vigilant (Forgas, 1989), looking for strategies or actions that might improve their mood states, or at least blunt the dysphoria, and reduce the threat or the identified problem. Thus, the apparent paradox that negative affect leads to more careful processing and also less careful behavior is resolved by the fact that many risky behaviors include at least the *potential* for mood amelioration. Evidence of this can be seen in the literature in the area of "negative state relief" (Cialdini, Darby & Vincent, 1973) and tension reduction (Greeley & Oei, 1999). Feeling better is an immediate goal of unhappy people.

Mood as a Moderator

In a series of studies, Pomery has applied the reasoning from this extensive body of literature examining the impact of mood states on regulation and processing to the prototype model (Pomery, Gibbons & Gerrard 2006). The basic hypothesis here comes directly from the research mentioned above: Mood manipulations will have more impact on the social reaction path than the reasoned path. All dual process models maintain that the heuristic or experiential mode is more sensitive to fluctuations in mood states. The cool, calm processing style that typifies the analytic/cognitive mode (and the formulation of intentions) is more likely to be activated when the individual is, in fact, feeling cool and calm. Thus, behavioral willingness should be more affected by affect manipulations. When asked to consider what they might do in certain risky situations, the negative state relief motive would suggest that students would be invested in feeling better and, therefore, more *willing to consider* taking the risk.

The first step in this investigation involved ascertaining that college students do admit or realize that they may sometimes engage in risky behavior if they are feeling down. This presumption was confirmed in a survey of 1,173 non-virgin students: 68% of them said that having sex with a casual partner could improve their mood, 36% said they had actually done this, and 62% said they had at least thought about doing it. The second step involved correlational analyses assessing the relation between mood states and behavioral willingness. These analyses indicated that behavioral willingness was negatively correlated with mood. The third step required a lab study and experimental manipulations of mood and measures of both proximal antecedents.

In the lab study, college students' mood states were either improved or lowered, and then they were asked whether they would be willing *and* whether they were intending to engage in risky sex. The order of these questions was also varied: half got the behavioral willingness items first, the other half got the behavioral intention items first. Results, illustrated in Figure 3.4, were consistent with predictions. When the behavioral willingness items came first: students in whom a negative mood was induced reported more willingness to have risky sex than did those in whom a positive mood was induced. In contrast, mood had very little effect on intentions, which remained low in both conditions. Moreover, the impact of mood (on behavioral willingness) was eliminated when the behavioral intention items were asked before the behavioral willingness items.[5] This suggests that activating the reasoned pathway (by first asking students to think about their plans, which is what behavioral intention questions do) reduces the

---

[5] The students were asked to indicate their behavioral willingness and behavioral intention on scaled questions and also on open-ended questions ("Please indicate what you would be willing to do ..."), which were content-analyzed. The graph is for the scaled questions, however, the pattern was virtually identical, and the interaction was also significant, on the open-ended questions. All students answered *both* the willingness and the intention questions; the order they answered them in was varied.

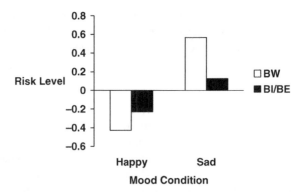

Figure 3.4   Risk willingness and intentions to have unprotected casual sex as a function of (manipulated) mood

N = 83 DV = Standardized responses for behavioral willingness and behavioral intention/behavioral expectation. Higher scores reflect higher willingness or intentions/expectations to engage in unprotected casual sex. From Pomery et al. (2006).

likelihood that the social reaction path will be used. The same is true in dual process theories: Activating the logical or analytic mode reduces use of the heuristic mode (Epstein & Pacini, 1999). The next step will be to determine if these willingness manipulation effects are mediated by, and potentially dampened by, estimates of risk or risk perceptions.

Conclusion

Positive mood induces a more heuristic type of processing aimed at doing whatever is deemed necessary to keep things on track. It is associated with more optimistic expectations, but less risky behavior, because risk can wipe out the bliss. Negative moods lead to more pessimistic risk predictions, but also to more risk behavior, most likely because of a desire to mute the dysphoria. Most important, the impact of mood states on risk behavior appears to be channeled more through the social reaction than the reasoned path, as reflected in greater movement (reaction) on behavioral willingness measures than on behavioral intention measures. This effect has implications for interventions (see Gerrard et al., this volume); but it clearly calls for more empirical attention.

FUTURE RESEARCH

These studies and the model itself suggest a number of empirical questions that can and should be addressed. We are currently looking at data from our panel studies to learn more about what the common and unique antecedents of behavioral willingness and behavioral intention are, as well as what determines when and how behavioral willingness transitions into behavioral intention, as it often does. At a basic level, more experimental work needs to be done to find out exactly how behavioral willingness differs from behavioral intention. Given the often high correlations between the two constructs, issues of discriminant validity remain. This most likely will involve laboratory studies aimed at trying to move or alter one independently of the other. The emotion work is a beginning in this direction.

We are also looking at the impact of priming certain behaviors or stimuli on behavioral intention and behavioral willingness. To the extent that behavioral willingness involves a heuristic type of processing that is activated under conditions of increased affect or arousal—such as when an adolescent is in a risk-conducive situation—then it should be possible to "tap into" these cognitions through implicit cognition types of manipulations (Greenwald & Banaji, 1995). This could include assessing behavioral willingness and prototypes implicitly, through reaction time measures, for example (e.g., how quickly do individuals respond to behavioral willingness items when in different mood states?; and does reaction time to risk prototype measures signal proclivity to risk?), and also manipulating them implicitly (e.g., Does priming risk prototypes, perhaps subliminally, increase behavioral willingness? Similarly, it might be possible to determine whether different types of risk behaviors (sex and drugs, for example) are linked through "risky cognitive networks" that involve heuristic processing, including images and willingness. For example, does priming a favorable sexual prototype lead to more willingness to use drugs? This might explain why risky health behaviors tend to covary.

Finally, this work on altering behavioral willingness also has intervention implications (see the Gerrard et al. chapter). One important question being explored is how can we make adolescents aware of their behavioral willingness—given that it is associated with a tendency to avoid consideration of outcomes and risk? More generally, can adolescents be taught to self-regulate? These questions are being examined in an ongoing preventive-intervention with African-American children that is based, in part, on the social reaction model (Brody et al., 2004; Gerrard et al., in press), as well as the self-control work of Wills. The curriculum involves a number of components, including exercises intended to get them to realize that behavioral willingness can result in behavior even in the absence of behavioral intention, and to encourage them to consider the possible consequences of their actions (see Gerrard et al., in press).

Health self-regulation generally increases with age, in part, because there is more need for it as we get older. For the most part, adolescents do not engage in goal-oriented health regulation. The behaviors that they do engage in that are health-relevant often involve some potential risk. Moreover, these risk behaviors are usually social "events," occurring in public in the presence of peers and friends. Traditional self-regulation models, which view health behavior as goal-based, do not capture this social reaction element of the behavior. Similarly, expectancy value theories, which assume behaviors are premeditated and/or planned, often come up short when applied to actions that are irrational and/or impulsive—actions that are more common among adolescents than adults. Social-cognitive approaches that are based on social-psychological principles are likely to provide a more complete understanding of what motivates these behaviors, and therefore improve our ability to predict and perhaps change them. Future work in this area should acknowledge the limitations of the goal-based approach and focus more attention on external influences on adolescent health behavior and on their cognitive processing (cf. Webb & Sheeran, in press).

REFERENCES

Ajzen, I. (1991). The theory of planned behavior. *Organizational Behavior & Human Decision Processes, 50*, 179–211.

Ajzen, I. (1996). The social psychology of decision making. In E.T. Higgins & A.W. Kruglanski (Eds), *Social Psychology: Handbook of Basic Principles* (pp. 297–328). New York: Guilford.

Ajzen, I. & Fishbein, M. (2005). The influence of attitudes on behavior. In D. Albarracín, B.T. Johnson & M.P. Zanna (Eds), *The Handbook of Attitudes* (pp. 173–221). Mahwah, NJ: Erlbaum.

Albarracín, D., Johnson, B.T., Fishbein, M. & Muellerleile, P.A. (2001). Theories of reasoned action and planned behavior as models of condom use: A meta-analysis. *Psychological Bulletin, 127*, 142–161.

Armitage, C.J., & Conner, M. (2001). Efficacy of the theory of planned behaviour: A meta-analytic review. *British Journal of Social Psychology, 40*, 471–499.

Bandura, A. (1997). *Self-efficacy: The exercise of control.* New York: Freeman.Times Books.

Beyth-Marom, R. & Fischhoff, B. (1997). Adolescents' decisions about risks: A cognitive perspective. In J. Schulenberg, J.L. Maggs & K. Hurrelmann (Eds), *Health Risks and Developmental Transitions During Adolescence* (pp. 110–135). New York: Cambridge University Press.

Bless, H. (2001). Mood and the use of general knowledge structures. In L.L. Martin & G.L. Clore (Eds), *Theories of Mood and Cognition: A user's guidebook*, (pp. 9–26). Mahwah, NJ: Erlbaum.

Bless, H., Clore, G.L., Schwarz, N. & Golisano, V. (1996). Mood and the use of scripts: Does a happy mood really lead to mindlessness? *Journal of Personality & Social Psychology, 71*, 665–679.

Brody, G.H., Murry, V.M., Gerrard, M., Gibbons, F.X., Molgaard, V., McNair, L., Brown, A.C., Wills, T.A., Spoth, R.L., Luo, Z., Chen, Y. & Neubaum-Carlan, E. (2004). The Strong African American Families Program: Translating research into prevention programming. *Child Development, 75*, 900–917.

Cameron, L.D. & Leventhal, H. (2003). *The Self-regulation of Health and Illness Behaviour.* New York: Routledge.

Carver, C.S. (1979). A cybernetic model of self-attention processes. *Journal of Personality and Social Psychology, 37*, 1251–1281.

Carver, C.S. & Scheier, M.F. (1981). Self-consciousness and reactance. *Journal of Research in Personality, 15*, 16–29.

Carver, C.S. & Scheier, M.F. (1998). *On the Self-regulation of Behavior.* New York: Cambridge University Press.

Chaiken, S. & Trope, Y. (1999). *Dual-process Theories in Social Psychology.* New York: Guilford.

Chassin, L., Presson, C.C., Sherman, S.J., Corty, E. & Olshavsky, R.W. (1981). Self-images and cigarette smoking in adolescence. *Personality and Social Psychology Bulletin, 7*, 670–676.

Chen, S. & Chaiken, S. (1999). The heuristic-systematic model in its broader context. In S. Chaiken & Y. Trope (Eds), *Dual-process Theories in Social Psychology*, (pp. 73–96). New York: Guilford.

Cialdini, R.B., Darby, B.L. & Vincent, J.E. (1973). Transgression and altruism: A case for hedonism. *Journal of Experimental Social Psychology, 9*, 502–516.

Conner, M. & Sparks, P. (2005). Theory of planned behavior and health behaviour. In M. Conner & P. Sparks (Eds), *Predicting Health Behaviour: Research and practice with social cognition models* (2nd edn, pp. 170–222). Maidenhead, UK: Open University Press.

Eich, E. & Forgas, J.P. (2003). Mood, cognition, and memory. In A.F. Healy & R.W. Proctor (Eds), *Handbook of Psychology: Experimental psychology* (Vol. 4, pp. 61–83). New York: John Wiley & Sons, Inc.

Epstein, S. (1985). The implications of cognitive-experiential self-theory for research in social psychology and personality. *Journal for the Theory of Social Behaviour, 15*, 283–310.

Epstein, S. (1993). Implications of cognitive-experiential self-theory for personality and develop- mental psychology. In D.C. Funder, & R.D. Parke (Eds), *Studying Lives Through Time: Personality and development* (pp. 399–438). Washington, DC: American Psychological Association.

Epstein, S. & Pacini, R. (1999). Some basic issues regarding dual-process theories from the perspective of cognitive-experiential self-theory. In S. Chaiken & Y. Trope (Eds), Dual *Process Theories in Social Psychology* (pp. 462–482). New York: Guilford.

Erickson, E.H. (1968). *Identity: Youth and crisis.* New York: Norton.

Erickson, P.I. (2003). Cultural factors affecting the negotiation of first sexual intercourse among Latina adolescent mothers. In M.I. Torres & G.P. Cernada (Eds), *Sexual and Reproductive Health Promotion in Latino Populations: Parteras, promotoras y poetas: Case studies across the Americas* (pp. 63–79). Amityville, NY: Baywood.

Feather, N.T. (1990). Bridging the gap between values and actions: Recent applications of the expectancy-value model. In E.T. Higgins (Ed.), *Handbook of Motivation and Cognition: Founda- tions of social behavior* (Vol. 2, pp. 151–192). New York: Guilford.

Fischhoff, B. (1992). Risk taking: A developmental perspective. In J.F. Yates (Ed.), *Risk-taking Behavior* (pp. 133–162). Chichester, UK: John Wiley & Sons, Ltd.

Fishbein, M. & Ajzen I. (1975). *Belief, Attitude, Intention, and Behavior: An introduction to theory and research.* Reading, (MA: Addison-Wesley.

Forgas, J.P. (1989). Mood effects on decision making strategies. *Australian Journal of Psychology, 41,* 197–214.

Gardner, M. & Steinberg, L. (2005). Peer influence on risk-taking, risk preference, and risky decision-making in adolescence and adulthood: An experimental study. *Developmental Psychology, 41,* 625–635.

Gerrard, M., Gibbons, F.X., Brody, G.H., Murry, V.M. & Wills, T.A. (in press) Theory-based dual focus alcohol intervention for pre-adolescents: Social cognitions in The Strong African American Families Program. *Psychology of Addictive Behaviors.*

Gerrard, M., Gibbons, F.X., Reis-Bergan, M., Trudeau, L., Vande Lune, L. & Buunk, B. (2002). Health cognitions and adolescent alcohol consumption: Inhibitor effects of drinker and non- drinker prototypes. *Health Psychology, 21,* 601–609.

Gerrard, M. & Warner, T.D. (1990). Antecedents of pregnancy among women Marines. *Journal of the Washington Academy of Sciences, 80,* 1–15.

Gibbons, F.X. & Gerrard, M. (1997). Health images and their effects on health behavior. In B.P. Buunk & F.X. Gibbons (Eds), *Health, Coping, and Well-being: Perspectives from social compar- ison theory* (pp. 63–94). Mahwah, NJ: Erlbaum.

Gibbons, F.X., Gerrard, M., Blanton, H. & Russell, D.W. (1998). Reasoned action and social reaction: Willingness and intention as independent predictors of health risk. *Journal of Personality and Social Psychology, 74,* 1164–1181.

Gibbons, F.X., Gerrard, M., Cleveland, M.J., Wills, T.A. & Brody, G.H. (2004). Perceived discrimination and substance use in African American parents and their children: A panel study. *Journal of Personality and Social Psychology, 86,* 517–529.

Gibbons, F.X., Gerrard, M. & Lane, D.J. (2003). A social reaction model of adolescent health risk. In J. Suls, & K.A. Wallston (Eds), *Social Psychological Foundations of Health and Illness* (pp. 107– 136). Malden, MA: Blackwell.

Gibbons, F.X., Gerrard, M., Vande Lune, L.S., Wills, T.A., Brody, G. & Conger, R.D. (2004). Context and cognition: Environmental risk, social influence, and adolescent substance use. *Personality and Social Psychology Bulletin, 30,* 1048–1061.

Gibbons, F.X., Helweg-Larsen, M., & Gerrard, M. (1995). Prevalence estimates and adolescent risk behavior: Cross-cultural differences in social influence. *Journal of Applied Psychology, 80,* 107–121.

Gibbons, F.X., Lane, D.J., Gerrard, M., Reis-Bergan, M., Lautrup, C.L., Pexa, N. & Blanton, H. (2002). Comparison level preferences after performance: Is downward comparison theory still useful? *Journal of Personality and Social Psychology, 83*, 865–880.

Gibbons, F.X., Stock, M.L., Gerrard, M., Eggleston, T.J., Dykstra, J.L., Kulik, J.A. & Mahler, H.I.M. (2006). Reactance as heuristic responding: Moderators of reactions to health persuasion (Manuscript submitted for publication).

Giedd, J.N. (2004). Structural magnetic resonance imaging of the adolescent brain. *Annals of the New York academy of science, 1021*, 77–85.

Godin, G. & Kok, G. (1996). The theory of planned behavior: A review of its applications to health-related behaviors. *American Journal of Health Promotion, 11*, 87–98.

Gollwitzer, P.M. (1999). Implementation intentions: Strong effects of simple plans. *American Psychologist, 54*, 493–503.

Greeley, J. & Oei, T. (1999). Alcohol and tension reduction. In K.E. Leonard & H.T. Blane (Eds), *Psychological Theories of Drinking and Alcoholism* (2nd edn, pp. 14–53). New York: Guilford.

Greenwald, A.G. & Banaji, M.R. (1995). Implicit social cognition: Attitudes, self-esteem, and stereotypes. *Psychological Review, 102*, 4–27.

Hagger, M.S., Chatzisarantis, N.L.D. & Biddle, S.J.H. (2002). The influence of autonomous and controlling motives on physical activity intentions within the theory of planned behaviour. *British Journal of Health Psychology, 7*, 283–297.

Hedley, A.A., Ogden, C.L., Johnson, C.L., Carroll, M.D., Curtin, L.R. & Flegal, K.M. (2004). Overweight and obesity among US children, adolescents, and adults, 1999–2002. *Journal of the American Medical Association, 291*, 2847–2850.

Ingham, R., Woodcock, A. & Stenner, K. (1991). Getting to know you. Young people's knowledge of their partners at first intercourse. *Journal of Community and Applied Social Psychology, 1*, 117–132.

Isen, A.M. & Shalker, T.E. (1982). The effect of feeling state on evaluation of positive, neutral, and negative stimuli: When you "accentuate the positive," do you "eliminate the negative"? *Social psychology quarterly, 45*, 58–63.

Kremers, S.P.J., Mudde, A.N., De Vries, N.K., Brug, J. & De Vries, H. (2004). Unplanned smoking initiation: new insights and implications for interventions. *Patient Education and Counseling, 55*, 345–352.

Kulik, J.A. & Mahler, H.I.M. (1987). Effects of preoperative roommate assignment on preoperative anxiety and postoperative recovery from coronary-bypass surgery. *Health Psychology, 6*, 525–543.

Kulik, J.A. & Mahler, H.I.M. (1997). Social comparison, affiliation, and coping with acute medical threats. In B.P. Buunk & F.X. Gibbons (Eds), *Health, Coping, and Well-being: Perspectives from social comparison theory* (pp. 227–261). Mahwah, NJ: Erlbaum.

Leventhal, H., Brissette, I. & Leventhal, E.A. (2003). The common-sense model of self-regulation of health and illness. In L.D. Cameron & H. Leventhal (Eds), *The Self-regulation of Health and Illness Behavior* (pp. 42–65). New York: Routledge.

Leventhal, H. & Cleary, P.D. (1980). The smoking problem: A review of the research and theory in behavioral risk modification. *Psychological Bulletin, 88*, 370–405.

Leventhal, H., Hudson, S. & Robitaille, C. (1997). Social comparison and health: A process model. In B.P. Buunk, & F.X. Gibbons (Eds), *Health, Coping, and Well-being: Perspectives from social comparison theory* (pp. 411–432). Mahwah, NJ: Erlbaum.

Leventhal, H., Meyer, D. & Nerenz, D. (1980). The common-sense representation of illness danger. *Medical psychology, 2*. New York: Pergamon.

Loewenstein, G.F., Weber, E.U., Hsee, C.K. & Welch, N. (2001). Risk as feelings. *Psychological Bulletin, 127*, 267–286.

Luszczynska, A., Gibbons, F.X., Piko, B.F. & Tekozel, M. (2004). Self-regulatory cognitions, social comparisons, and perceived peers' behaviors as predictors of nutrition and physical activity: A comparison among adolescents in Hungary, Poland, Turkey and USA. *Psychology and Health, 19*, 577–593.

Marks, G., Graham, J.W. & Hansen, W.B. (1992). Social projection and social conformity in adolescent alcohol use: A longitudinal analysis. *Personality and Social Psychology Bulletin, 18*, 96–101.

Mitchell, K. & Wellings, K. (1998). First sexual intercourse: Anticipation and communication. Interviews with young people in England. *Journal of Adolescence, 21*, 717–726.

Murry, V.M. (1994). Black adolescent females: A comparison of early versus coital initiators. *Family Relations: Interdisciplinary Journal of Applied Family Studies, 43*, 342–348.

Pasupathi, M. (1999). Age differences in response to conformity pressure for emotional and non-emotional material. *Psychology and Aging, 14*, 170–174.

Pomery, E.A., Gibbons, F.X. & Gerrard, M. (2006). The influence of positive and negative affect on willingness and intentions to engage in risky health behaviors. (Manuscript in preparation).

Pomery, E.A., Gibbons, F.X. Gerrard, M. & Reis-Bergan, M. (2006). Experience as a moderator of the developmental shift from willingness to intentions. (Manuscript in preparation).

Powers, W.T. (1973). *Behavior: The control of perception.* Chicago: Aldine.

Raghunathan, R., & Pham, M.T. (1999). All negative moods are not equal: Motivational influences of anxiety and sadness on decision making. *Organizational Behavior and Human Decision Processes, 79*, 56–77.

Rivis, A. & Sheeran, P. (2003). Social influences and the theory of planned behaviour: Evidence for a direct relationship between prototypes and young people's exercise behaviour. *Psychology and Health, 18*, 567–584.

Rogers, R.W. (1983). Cognitive and physiological processes in fear appeals and attitude change: A revised theory of protection motivation. In T.T. Cacioppo & R.E. Petty (Eds), *Social psychophysiology* (pp. 153–176). New York: Guilford.

Rosenstock, I.M. (1974). Historical origins of the Health Belief Model. *Health Education Monographs, 2*, 1–8.

Rothbart, M.K. & Ahadi, S.A. (1994). Temperament and the development of personality. *Journal of Abnormal Psychology, 103*, 55–66.

Rothbart, M.K. & Bates, J.E. (1998). Temperament. In. W. Damon & N. Eisenberg (Eds), *Handbook of Child Psychology*, (5th edn, Vol. 3, pp. 105–176). New York: John Wiley & Sons, Inc.

Scheier, M.F. (1980). Effects of public and private self-consciousness on the public expression of personal beliefs. *Journal of Personality and Social Psychology, 39*, 514–521.

Scheier, M.F. & Carver, C.S. (2003). Goals and confidence as self-regulatory elements underlying health and illness behavior. In L.D. Cameron & H. Leventhal (Eds), *The Self-regulation of Health and Illness Behavior* (pp. 17–41). London: Routledge.

Sebald, H. (1989). Adolescents' peer orientation: Changes in the support system during the past three decades. *Adolescence, 24*, 937–946.

Sheeran, P. (2002). Intention-behavior relations: A conceptual and empirical review. In W. Stroebe & M. Hewstone (Eds), *European Review of Social Psychology* (Vol. 12, pp. 1–36). Chichester, UK: John Wiley & Sons, Ltd.

Sheeran, P. & Orbell, S. (1998). Do intentions predict condom use? Meta-analysis and examination of six moderator variables. *British Journal of Social Psychology, 37*, 231–250.

Stacy, A.W. (1997). Memory activation and expectancy as prospective predictors of alcohol and marijuana use. *Journal of Abnormal Psychology, 106*, 61–73.

Stacy, A.W., Newcomb, M.D. & Ames, S.L. (2000). Implicit cognition and HIV risk behavior. *Journal of Behavioral Medicine, 23*, 475–499.

Simpson, R. (1996). Neither clear nor present: The social construction of safety and danger. *Sociological Forum, 11,* 549–562.

Steinberg, L. (2003). Is decision making the right framework for research on adolescent risk taking? In D. Romer (Ed.), *Reducing Adolescent Risk: Toward an integrated approach* (pp. 18–34). Thousand Oaks, CA: Sage.

Steinberg, L. & Cauffman, E. (1996). Maturity of judgment in adolescence: Psychosocial factors in adolescent decision making. *Law and Human Behavior, 20,* 249–272.

Suls, J., Martin, R. & Leventhal, H. (1997). Social comparison, lay referral, and the decision to seek medical care. In B.P. Buunk, & F.X. Gibbons (Eds), *Health, Coping, and Well-being: Perspectives from social comparison theory* (pp. 195–226). Mahwah, NJ: Erlbaum.

Tarter, R.E. & Vanyukov, M.M. (1994). Alcoholism as a developmental disorder. *Journal of Consulting and Clinical Psychology, 62,* 1096–1107.

Tesser, A., Martin, L.L. & Cornell, D.P. (1996). On the substitutability of self-protective mechanisms. In P.M. Gollwitzer & J.A. Bargh (Eds), *The psychology of action: Linking cognition and motivation to behavior* (pp. 48–68). New York: Guilford.

Tversky, A. & Kahneman, D. (1974). Judgment under uncertainty: Heuristics and biases. *Science, 185,* 1124–1131.

Udry, J.R. (1998). *The National Longitudinal Study of Adolescent Health (Add Health), Waves I & II,* 1994–1996 (Data Sets 48–50, 98, A1-A3, Kelley, M.S. & Peterson, J.L.) [machine-readable data file and documentation]. Chapel Hill, NC: University of North Carolina at Chapel Hill, Carolina Population Center.

Warshaw, P.R. & Davis, F.D. (1985). Disentangling behavioral intention and behavioral expectation. *Journal of Experimental Social Psychology, 21,* 213–228.

Webb, T.L. & Sheeran, P. (in press). Does changing behavioral intentions engender behavior change? A meta-analysis of the experimental evidence. *Psychological Bulletin.*

Weinstein, N.D. (1980). Unrealistic optimism about future life events. *Journal of Personality and Social Psychology, 39,* 806–820.

Wills, T.A., Gibbons, F.X., Gerrard, M., Murry, V.M. & Brody, G.H. (2003). Family communication and religiosity related to substance use and sexual behavior in early adolescence: A test for pathways through self-control and prototype perceptions. *Psychology of Addictive Behaviors, 17,* 312–323.

Wills, T.A., Sandy, J.M., Shinar, O. & Yaeger, A. (1999). Contributions of positive and negative affect to adolescent substance use: Test of a bidimensional model in a longitudinal study. *Psychology of Addictive Behaviors, 13,* 327–338.

Wills, T.A., Sandy, J.M. & Yaeger, A.M. (2001). Time perspective and early-onset substance use: A model based on stress-coping theory. *Psychology of Addictive Behaviors, 15,* 118–125.

Wills, T.A. & Stoolmiller, M. (2002). The role of self-control in early escalation of substance use: A time-varying analysis. *Journal of Consulting & Clinical Psychology, 70,* 986–997.

Wills, T.A., Windle, M. & Cleary, S.D. (1998). Temperament and novelty seeking in adolescent substance use: Convergence of dimensions of temperament with constructs from Cloninger's theory. *Journal of Personality & Social Psychology, 74,* 387–406.

Zabin, L.S., Stark, H.A. & Emerson, M.R. (1991). Reasons for delay in contraceptive clinic utilization: Adolescent clinic and nonclinic populations compared. *Journal of Adolescent Health, 12,* 225–232.

Zimring, F.E. (1998). Toward a jurisprudence of youth violence. *Crime and Justice, 24,* 477–501.

CHAPTER 4

Social Influences on Adolescent Substance Use: Insights into How Parents and Peers Affect Adolescent's Smoking and Drinking Behavior

Rutger C.M.E. Engels and Sander M. Bot

National surveys in Europe showed that experimentation with risk behaviors, such as cigarette smoking, marijuana use, and alcohol consumption is rather normal, and almost normative, among adolescents (Hibell et al., 2004). The majority of adolescents at least try smoking and the overwhelming majority of adolescents experiment with alcohol, which results in more or less regular drinking habits (Hibell et al., 2004; Poelen, Scholte, Engels, Boomsma & Willemsen, 2005). However, there are strong individual differences, for example, regarding the age at which people start experimenting with smoking, the pace with which they get dependent on nicotine, or the frequency of binge drinking and drunkenness. In this chapter we address recent studies on the impact of people in the immediate social environments of young people on individual differences in smoking and drinking in adolescents. We assume that in particular parents and peers, as significant social referent persons in the environments of adolescents, affect the way adolescents are able to refrain from cigarette and alcohol use.

SELF-CONTROL AND ADOLESCENT SUBSTANCE USE

If we define self-control as the ability to control impulses and to delay gratification (Finkenauer, Engels & Baumeister, 2005), initiating smoking and drinking may be perceived as lack of control, but only when individual adolescents did not intend to

Self-regulation in Health Behavior. Edited by Denise T.D. de Ridder and John B.F. de Wit.

use substances in the first place. One may take a moral perspective, arguing that smoking and alcohol misuse are generally considered to be deviant behaviors, and therefore could be seen as a form of low self-control. From an "individual perspective" it is problematic to see substance use merely as the outcome of low self-control as adolescents might engage in these behaviors because they plan to do so. For instance, when an individual goes out on a Saturday evening with friends and "plans" to engage in binge drinking, one might question whether actually drinking 10–15 glasses is an indication of low self-control. However, when someone intends to drink only a few glasses, but is persuaded by peers to drink more than planned, this might be seen as a form of low self-control. The same holds for smoking of course. If, for instance, a non-smoking youth's attitudes towards smoking become positive in the adolescent years and, at a certain moment, in the company of peers with pro-smoking norms, he or she tries a few puffs, one might wonder whether this can be seen as an effect of low self-control. In this chapter, we do not explicitly discuss whether substance use should be seen as a form of low self-control. In addition, it should be noted that in our studies on adolescent substance use we also do not measure self-control directly. However, if one perceives initiation of substance use in adolescence as a strong indication of low self-control and poor regulation of emotions and behaviors, one might read this chapter from the perspective that we examine the role of peers and parents in the regulation of substance use in youths.

Furthermore, in our opinion, it remains an open question whether regulation of substance use by *not* becoming involved should be valued as positive or negative. To give an example, moderate alcohol use may put some persons at risk for alcohol dependency or make them (more) aggressive, whereas for others, moderate alcohol consumption may be stress relieving and promote social behavior. Concerning the latter, there is some evidence that adolescents who are involved in substance use are more sociable, have a larger and more supportive peer network, and have more experiences with intimate relationships (see review by Engels & Van den Eijnden, in press). Not only the adolescents themselves perceive this as socially beneficial but their peers do as well (Engels, Scholte, Van Lieshout, Overbeek & De Kemp, in press).

It is a fact that adolescents are more involved in risk taking behaviors than other age groups. This can be explained by taking into account that adolescents are on the border of becoming adults. They realize that they are capable of unfolding the same activities that other people in society are involved in (like having a profession, having sex, starting a family life) without being intensively controlled by parents and teachers anymore (Pape & Hammer, 1996). On the other hand, they are still insecure of their own identity and their relationships with others. Risk-taking is an excellent activity to explore one's own boundaries, and provides boys as well as girls with a sense of belonging to the group of peers that is involved in the activity. In a sense, exploring boundaries can be considered healthy behavior for adolescents. In other words, engagement in substance use might be seen as a form of loosening control and exploring certain boundaries (for example, in the relationship with parents), but it might also be perceived as a form of control, namely keeping control over social relationships, as drinking and smoking are so strongly intertwined with social contexts.

Concerning the pros and cons of engagement in substance use, it is clear that there is some evidence that drinking may provide youngsters with opportunities to become socially active and experienced. On the other hand, consuming large amounts of alcohol (e.g. through binge drinking), may lead to many unfavorable outcomes such as drunk driving, aggression, or problem drinking later in life.

With respect to smoking, it is quite evident that there is hardly any evidence for the positive effects of cigarette use on people's health. Furthermore, it has been revealed that early smoking initiation increases the risk of developing nicotine dependence at a later age. There is, not surprisingly, only very limited research on the social consequences of smoking uptake in adolescence. In one study we found that smokers in early adolescence were more strongly perceived as being social and extrovert by their peers than non-smokers, but these effects were smaller than for alcohol use (see Engels, Scholte et al., in press). In other words, although youth involvement in substance use might be seen as socially adaptive in a sense (especially alcohol) and fulfils some developmental tasks, such as catching up with adult-like behaviors, it is important to realize that it has short and long term negative consequences as well.

Summarizing, in our opinion, it is difficult and possibly unnecessary to draw conclusions about whether adolescent engagements in substance use should be seen as lack of control, and therefore an outcome of dysfunctional behavioral regulation. As substance use becomes almost normative in a sense in late adolescence, it might even be that lack of involvement in substance use can be seen as lack of control and social adaptation. On the other hand, evidence clearly shows that the uptake of regular smoking and heavy and problematic drinking is associated with mortality and morbidity in adulthood.

Theoretical Models

This chapter may differ from the other ones in this book, as we did not formulate one or two explicit theoretical models that we empirically tested. Although we refer in the following to theoretical models, such as the Prototype/Willingness Model, Theory of Planned Behavior, Social Learning Theory, or Attachment Theory, we did not start from an a priori extensive and overarching theoretical framework to examine the impact of parents and peers on adolescent substance use. We decided not to do so because of two reasons. The first is that a substantial part of the literature on the role of parents is so preliminary that it might be wise to first examine various, separate parts of assumptions underpinning social influences on adolescent substance use, before testing a general model. Secondly, when it comes to how young people's complex and ongoing interactions with persons in their immediate social environments affect their initiation and development of substance use patterns, it is almost impossible to develop a general model at all. Thus, in this chapter we will delineate findings of recent studies on parental and peer influences on adolescent substance use, address the shortcomings in research, and discuss some of the directions for further research.

PARENTS AND ADOLESCENT SUBSTANCE USE

Empirical evidence shows that parents directly and indirectly affect their adolescent children's substance use through parenting and through their own patterns of substance use (e.g., Chassin, Presson, Todd, Rose & Sherman, 1998; Henriksen & Jackson, 1998).

Although adolescents strive for independency and autonomy they also want to maintain a good relationship with their parents. As a result, parents remain influential during the period of adolescence and continue to affect adolescents' behavior, including substance use.

Parenting is one way by which parents affect their children's substance use and can be divided into two kinds of parenting: general and substance-specific parenting. Research usually examines the direct effects of general parenting on adolescents' substance use. *General parenting* can be divided into two dimensions: support and control. The support dimension refers to the affective and supportive behavior of the parent, while the control dimension varies from supervision and monitoring (i.e., strict control) to more manipulative, suppressing control (i.e., psychological control) of the parent (Darling & Steinberg, 1993). Empirical studies, in general, indicate that adolescents with parents who support and control them without using manipulative strategies are less likely to smoke (e.g., Chassin et al., 1998; Cohen, Richardson & La Bree, 1994). With regard to general parenting practices, support appears to prevent early onset as well as frequent and heavy alcohol use among adolescents. For example, Barnes, Reifman, Farell and Dintcheff (2000) reported that adequate parental support and positive parent-child communication were related to lower levels of heavy drinking. Moreover, many authors have advocated the relationships between parental behavioral control, notably setting limits on children's activities and whereabouts (e.g., Barnes et al., 2000; Raskin White, Johnson & Buyske, 2000), and substance use. The problem with many of these studies is that they: (a) employed cross-sectional designs not permitting causal interpretations, (b) have only interviewed adolescents or parents on parenting behaviors, or (c) did not explicitly examine predictors of specific stage transitions in adolescent substance use.

General Parenting

Over the past years we conducted several longitudinal studies into the effects of general parenting on adolescent substance use. Concerning smoking, it is quite clear that the control dimension of parenting is hardly related to smoking onset in offspring. In other words, whether parents enact firm (or psychological, manipulative) control or not, it has hardly any effects on smoking. In short-term longitudinal studies among 12 to 14-year-old adolescents and their parents (with a 6-month interval between the waves), we found no significant associations between strict or psychological control on the one hand and adolescent smoking onset on the other (Den Exter Blokland, Hale, Meeus & Engels, in press; Harakeh, Scholte, De Vries, Vermulst, & Engels, 2004; Engels, Finkenauer, Kerr & Stattin, in press). With respect to alcohol use the picture is slightly different. Using cross-lagged Structural Equation Modeling (SEM) analyses on three waves of data of early adolescents, we find consistent preventive effects of parental enforcement of strict control on the development of adolescent alcohol use (Van der Vorst, Engels, Meeus, Deković & Vermulst, in press). These effects are rather small, however; parental control only predicted a small percentage of the variance in drinking over time. Further, it should be stressed that some lay people assume that enforcing firm control may lead to a counter-reaction by offspring; they might start becoming engaged in drug use partly to get out from under the wings of parents. We never found support for this assumption in any of our analyses. In analyses of other dimensions of parenting, such as providing warmth, support and being responsive, the findings are somewhat in contrast with those described above for parental control. We found in the same sample of early adolescents that parental support and warmth has a preventive effect on smoking (Den Exter Blokland, Hale, Meeus & Engels, 2005; Harakeh et al., 2004; Otten, Engels & Van den Eijnden, 2005). No effects of parental support on the development of alcohol use are found in early adolescents (Van der Vorst, Engels, Deković & Meeus, 2005) or in mid-adolescents (Van Zundert, Van der Vorst, Vermulst & Engels, in press).

Substance-specific Parenting

Substance-specific parenting refers to the explicit activities that parents undertake to discourage or prevent their offspring from smoking or drinking (Engels & Willemsen, 2004). Although few studies have investigated smoking-specific parenting, empirical evidence shows that smoking-specific parenting practices are important in preventing adolescents from smoking. For example, Clark, Scarisbrick-Hauser, Gautam and Wirk (1999) carried out a cross-sectional study in the US among 311 parents of children aged 6 to 17, concerned with house rules on smoking and the presence of tobacco advertisements in the home. Their findings showed that 87% of the parents reported they had some kind of house rules concerning smoking at home and 11% indicated that they had explicitly forbidden their offspring to smoke at home. In a study among 1,213 adolescents, Jackson and Henriksen (1998) demonstrated that when parents have certain anti-smoking strategies, such as establishing non-smoking rules, warnings about smoking risks, and punishments when they found out that their child smoked, these children are less likely to smoke.

Only a few studies have explored alcohol-specific socialization (see Van der Vorst, Engels, Deković, Meeus & Van Leeuwe, 2005). With respect to alcohol use, up to now most attention has been focused on enforcement of rules regarding underage drinking. Wood, Read, Mitchell and Brand (2004) showed that late adolescents drank less alcohol if their parents disapproved of their drinking behavior. In line with this finding, Yu (2003) observed that being strict about children's alcohol use at home prevented heavy drinking of youngsters. Jackson, Henriksen and Dickinson (1999) found that children who were permitted to consume alcohol at home were more likely to drink two years later. In another study, Jackson (2002) pointed out that it is important that adolescents consider parental authority to be legitimate. Adolescents who did not acknowledge their parents' authority were nearly four times as likely to consume alcohol compared to adolescents who did. Thus, if adolescents think that their parents are not effective in their efforts this will rarely lead to lower levels of drinking in youths. Another strategy that parents might use to deal with adolescents' alcohol consumption is communication about alcohol. According to Ennett, Bauman, Foshee, Pemberton and Hicks (2001), parents talk more often with their offspring about alcohol use if both parents are non-users than if one or both of the parents drink. However, in both using and non-using parents, frequency of communication on alcohol matters was not related to adolescents' alcohol use (see also Jackson et al., 1999).

What Do Parents Know?

Before we come into the details of studies on alcohol and smoking-specific socialization we address the findings of two studies on parental knowledge regarding adolescent engagement in substance use. If many parents do not even know that their child is experimenting with substance use, or is even using heavily, they might be less likely to undertake actions to prevent their child from continuing to use. Our analyses in which we compared adolescent and parental reports on adolescent smoking and drinking behavior showed that: (a) parents strongly underestimate their child's engagement in drinking and smoking, (b) this underestimation is generally stronger for the younger child, (c) fathers generally make stronger errors than mothers, and (d) the magnitude of underestimations are related to parental involvement in alcohol-specific socialization efforts; the stronger the errors, the less parents are engaged (see Engels, Van der Vorst, Deković & Meeus, 2005; Harakeh, Engels, Scholte & De Vries, 2005). Thus, the study clearly shows that many parents hardly know whether their child is engaged in substance use or not.

Rules on Smoking

Our own studies on the effects of substance-specific socialization of adolescent use do not always provide a clear, straightforward picture. In initial explorative cross-sectional analyses on smoking-specific socialization we found that some parental controlling efforts, like warning children for the negative consequences of smoking, or acting constructively and in a problem-solving manner when being confronted with a child that experiments with smoking, seem to be effective in preventing adolescents from starting to smoke (Engels & Willemsen, 2004). However, in prospective analyses among large samples of early adolescents and their parents, Den Exter Blokland et al. (in press) found that parental rules on smoking, parental warnings on smoking frequency, and parental monitoring were not related to the adolescent's smoking onset (see also Engels, Finkenauer et al., in press). For instance, parents with clear house rules on no-smoking do not necessarily end up with children who smoked more than parents who did not have these rules at all.

Communication on Smoking-related Issues

There are ambiguous findings concerning the effects of the frequency of parent-adolescent communication on adolescents' smoking. Some of the studies showed that it is a protective factor against adolescent smoking (e.g., Engels & Willemsen, 2004; Ennett et al., 2001), whereas others indicated it is a risk factor (e.g., Chassin et al., 1998; Clark et al., 1999; Jackson & Henriksen, 1998). In most of our cross-sectional analyses we found that higher frequency of communication is related to higher risks of adolescent smoking (Den Exter Blokland et al., in press; Otten, Harakeh, Vermulst, Engels & Van Den Eijnden, 2005; Harakeh, Scholte, De Vries & Engels, 2005; Harakeh, Scholte, De Vries, Vermulst & Engels, 2005). A reasonable explanation for this 'unexpected' finding has to do with the causal direction of the relationship. Perhaps when adolescents already start experimenting with smoking, parents start to communicate more with their children about smoking in an effort to prevent them from continuing the habit (Ennett et al., 2001). The results might also indicate that many parents communicate with their adolescents in a rather unconstructive way. Perhaps some parents talk so often and ineffectively with their adolescents about smoking topics, that it results in increased likelihood of smoking. In our longitudinal analyses we found no or few *positive* effects of frequency of communication about smoking on adolescent smoking. In sum, this suggests that the message underlying many prevention efforts that focus on parental involvement, namely "talk with your children," should be approached cautiously.

Nonetheless, besides frequency of parent-adolescent communication about smoking it is also important whether the discussions or communications on smoking take place in a constructive and respectful manner. Perhaps manner is more important than frequency. There is no previous research on quality of smoking-related communication and adolescent smoking. In our own studies amongst a sample of 826 early and mid-adolescents, we found that when parents talk in a positive and constructive way about smoking, children are less likely to smoke (Harakeh, Scholten, De Vries & Engels, 2005), or initiate smoking (Otten, Harakeh et al., 2005). The strength of these findings is underlined by the fact that we found consistency in both children and parents' reports on quality of communication. In addition, in longitudinal analyses over a two-year period in our full family study, Den Exter Blokland, Harakeh, Engels, Meeus and Hale (2005) showed that non-smoking children at the first wave, who had parents who talked about no-smoking in a positive and constructive way, were three times less likely to start smoking at a subsequent wave, two years later, than children who had parents who could not talk constructively. Summarizing, our findings clearly show that it is not important to talk frequently about smoking, but that it has to happen in a positive, constructive way. Simply put, it is not frequency but quality of communication that matters.

Non-smoking Agreement

Many parents think it is wise at a certain moment in adolescence to establish a no-smoking agreement with their child; some parents promise their offspring money or gifts when they would not smoke before the age of 18. If this would appear to be effective, it would be a relatively easy and constructive tool for parents to stimulate children to refrain from smoking. In longitudinal analyses on two data sets we tested whether parents who have this non-smoking agreement are effective in preventing their children from smoking (Den Exter Blokland, Harakeh, Engels et al., 2005). We did not find evidence for this. In contrast, it appears that sometimes children who have this agreement with their parents are *more* likely to smoke. This might be explained by the fact that: (a) some parents make this no-smoking agreement with their child when they find out that their child experiments with smoking, (b) some parents do not have to have this agreement as they know from the start that their child will not start smoking at all, or (c) parents who have made this agreement might think it is set and done and do not spend time and efforts in discussing the topic of smoking any more; they think the agreement will do the trick. In none of the longitudinal analyses, that span periods of six months to two years and cover the entire period of early to late adolescence, we found that this no-smoking agreement indeed prevented children from starting to smoke.

Alcohol Rules

As said before, the literature on alcohol-specific socialization is even more limited than that concerning smoking. To some extent, it is strange to realize that there is so much work done on the role of the social environment in adolescent substance use, but only few scholars have actually looked at what parents do to prevent children from smoking or drinking, and whether these efforts are effective. One of the most important alcohol-specific socialization practices seems to be imposing strict rules on adolescents' alcohol use. In cross-sectional analyses Van der Vorst et al., (2005) revealed a strong negative association between providing strict rules on alcohol use and adolescent drinking. This association was found on the basis of separate reports of different family members (father, mother, and siblings), and for older (on average 14.3 years old) as well as younger (on average 12.5 years old) siblings in one family, demonstrating the robustness of the findings. Furthermore, the results clearly show that parents treated their adolescents differently concerning rule setting. Parents imposed stricter rules on younger adolescents than on older ones. However, the magnitude of the associations between setting rules on alcohol and adolescent drinking was similar for both siblings. We found the preventive effects of rule enforcement on youth alcohol use again in a sample of adolescents following special education, underscoring the robustness of these findings (Van Zundert et al., in press). In additional longitudinal SEM analyses on this data set, we found that enforcement of rules especially prevents adolescents from starting to drink; so alcohol specific rules seem to postpone the age of onset (Van der Vorst, Engels, Meeus & Deković, 2005).

Communication about Alcohol

With respect to other parental socialization efforts to prevent children from drinking (heavily), we found that, as with smoking, frequency of communication on drinking issues is positively related to alcohol use, and the reactions of parents, in the case an adolescent comes home drunk, are not significantly related to the adolescent's alcohol consumption; this applied to parental negative reactions and to neglecting reactions (Van der Vorst et al., 2005).

Parental Own Substance Use

Parents' own smoking behavior is another way through which parents have an effect on their children's smoking either directly or indirectly. According to Social Learning Theory (Bandura, 1977) a direct influence may be explained in a sense that parents set an example or function as (role) model for their children, that is children observe and imitate their parents' behavior. Therefore, children with parents who smoke are more likely to start smoking or to remain smokers (e.g., Avenevoli & Merikangas, 2003). Parents' smoking can also indirectly affect their offspring's smoking through the smoking-specific parenting practices. An assumption is that smoking parents, contrary to non-smoking parents, engage less in smoking-specific parenting practices. A possible explanation may be that smoking parents worry that their children perceive them as barely credible sources of anti-smoking messages because of the inconsistency between their attitudes and behaviors (e.g. Henriksen & Jackson, 1998). Thus, it is possible that children of smoking parents are more likely to smoke compared to children of non-smoking parents, because smoking parents engage less in smoking-specific parenting practices than non-smoking parents.

Parental Drinking and Parenting

Alcohol use of parents has proven to be positively associated with adolescent alcohol involvement. One can also imagine that not merely the actual observation of drinking by parents encourages children to drink, but the drinking may also affect their parenting. Engels, Vermulst, Dubas, Bot and Gerris (2005) argued that heavy drinking parents are less supportive and more aggressive towards their children, and provide less structure than not-heavy drinking parents. Further, if parents are heavy drinkers themselves they may be less inclined, or able, to enforce strict rules regarding adolescent drinking. Therefore, parental drinking may indirectly affect adolescent drinking through inadequacy of parenting practices.

Like Father Like Son?

There is substantial evidence for the direct effects of parental own substance use on adolescent use (Engels, Knibbe, De Vries, Drop & Van Breukelen, 1999; Engels, Knibbe & Drop, 1999). To give an example, in prospective analyses predicting adolescent and young adult alcohol use over a period of two and seven years, we found small consistent effects of parental use on adolescent use over time, even after controlling for sibling and peer group drinking (Poelen, Scholte, Willemsen, Boomsma & Engels, 2005). Similar long-term effects are found for smoking (De Vries et al., 2003; Engels, Knibbe, De Vries et al., 1999; Engels, Knibbe & Drop, 1999; Engels, Vitaro, Den Exter Blokland, De Kemp & Scholte 2004; Vink et al., 2003). In a different type of analytic approach, we showed that when parents quit smoking it decreases the chance that children start to smoke (Den Exter Blokland, Engels, Hale, Meeus & Willemsen, 2004). Even more interestingly, the duration of exposure to a smoking parent was linearly related to adolescent smoking; when parents quit smoking it appears to be most effective if they do that before the child reaches the age of seven.

Parental Substance Use and Parenting Practices

Concerning the indirect effects, we very consistently found in all our analyses that parents who drink or smoke are less involved in efforts to withdraw their children from substance use (see Den Exter Blokland, Hale et al., 2005; Harakeh, Scholte, De Vries & Engels, 2005; Harakeh, Scholte, De Vries, Vermulst et al., 2005; Van der Vorst et al., 2005; Van Zundert et al., in press). However, multi-group analyses in SEM, in which we systematically tested whether the magnitude of paths between socialization on the one hand and adolescent substance use on the other differs between using and non-using parents, do not show that using parents are *less* effective in preventing children from smoking or drinking (Harakeh, Engels et al., 2005; Van der Vorst, Engels, Deković & Meeus, 2005). In other words, even parents who smoke or drink themselves can still undertake successful efforts to prevent their children from substance use.

The Link between General and Substance-specific Parenting

On a theoretical level, it is reasonable to assume that substance-specific and general parenting practices are related (Darling & Steinberg, 1993). For example, parents who control their offspring's activities in general, will be more likely also to control their children's smoking. However, there is not much known about how substance specific practices are exactly related to general parenting practices.

Two of our studies explicitly focused on the link between general and specific parenting. In analyses of the full-family sample, we found that high levels of parental control are related to higher enforcement of alcohol-specific rules (Van Zundert et al., in press). This indeed suggests that alcohol-specific rule enforcement intervenes in the relationship between behavioral control and adolescent alcohol use. Concerning smoking, we found that high levels of parental support are related to higher quality of communication on smoking issues (Otten, Harakeh et al., 2005). Parent and adolescent reports indicated that high levels of parental support were related to a high quality of parent-child communication on smoking-related issues; resulting in turn in lower likelihood of smoking in both siblings. The perception of parental support was also related to an increased frequency of parent-child communication. In other words, if parents maintain a positive, supportive, and stimulating relationship with their children, this will generally result in good quality and more frequent parent-child communications about smoking-specific related issues.

Adolescent Cognitions

Parents may not only directly affect children's addictive behaviors but also indirectly by shaping their cognitions on substance use. The Theory of Planned Behavior is designed to predict and explain human behavior in specific contexts (Ajzen, 1991). In terms of smoking, the Theory of Planned Behavior postulates that smoking-related cognitions (i.e., attitude, self-efficacy, and social norm) predict intentions to start smoking, and intention in turn predicts actual smoking onset. In addition, self-efficacy directly predicts actual smoking onset as well. Various studies have found support for the predictive validity of the Theory of Planned Behavior with respect to smoking.

We tested whether, and which, parental practices are related to smoking-related cognitions. In a longitudinal study among Dutch high school students, anti-smoking parenting practices, measured by parental reactions to use, house rules about smoking, and communication about smoking, were associated with smoking-related cognitions, which were in turn related to smoking (Huver, Engels & De Vries, in press). Furthermore, in another study, Huver, Engels, Van Breukelen and De Vries (2005) showed that maternal and paternal strictness had positive effects on smoking and these effects were mediated by smoking attitudes and intentions to smoke. In a one-year follow up study Otten, Harakeh et al. (2005) showed that frequency of communication on smoking appeared to be indirectly related to adolescent smoking through smoking cognitions; more frequent communication was related to higher pro-smoking attitudes, lower self-efficacy, and lower perceived parental approval. Furthermore, they found that higher quality of communication on smoking issues was associated with lower pro-smoking attitudes, perceived approval of friends, and higher self-efficacy. In longitudinal analyses on the links between general parenting practices and smoking cognitions, we found that effects of quality of the parent-child relationship on smoking initiation were mediated by attitudes towards smoking, self-efficacy, social norm, and intentions to smoke (Harakeh et al., 2004). Moreover, parental knowledge about offspring's whereabouts predicted smoking initiation through self-efficacy and social norm, in turn mediated by intentions to smoke.

We only conducted one study on the role of parental norms and adolescent cognitions on alcohol use (Spijkerman, Van den Eijnden, Overbeek & Engels, in press). In this longitudinal study among early adolescents, we used prototypes as mediating cognitive concept (for further elaboration see Gibbons and colleagues, this volume). These analyses clearly showed that parental norms on appropriateness of drinking for adolescents are related to the development of less favorable prototypes of adolescents of peers who drink which in turn affect adolescent drinking over time.

Summarizing, although our findings are preliminary in nature and future research should reveal how systematic these mediating effects of smoking and drinking-related cognitions are, they seem to suggest that parenting practices partly affect adolescent substance use by shaping their related cognitions, such as norms, attitudes, prototypes, and feelings of self-efficacy.

Parents' Influence on Adolescents' Functioning in Peer Relationships

The influence of parents may be underestimated for most studies concentrated exclusively on the impacts of parental alcohol use and parenting on adolescent alcohol consumption. Parents may also play a role in affecting the peer environment of adolescents. In that sense, part of the peer influences may be attributed to indirect parental influences. Firstly, parents may affect the selection of potential peers by making explicit or implicit "choices" concerning neighborhood and school, and providing rules about leisure time activities. Secondly, parents may try to direct children to affiliate with specific peers or try to obstruct affiliation with, in the perspective of the parent, non-attractive peers ("do not hang around with that guy, because he is bad influence"). In other areas of problem behaviors it has been shown that: (a) high parental monitoring prevents adolescents from affiliating with deviant peers, and (b) parents' negative reactions to friendships may affect the continuation of those friendships. Related to this issue, parents may affect adolescent's feelings of self-efficacy. For example, when parents provide children with confidence and knowledge on how to resist peer pressure, this may strengthen their children's self-efficacy. Thirdly, intergenerational transference of parental norms on offspring may direct young people's affiliations with peers (Engels, Knibbe, De Vries et al., 1999).

Only a few empirical studies have concentrated on the link between parent and adolescent's peer contexts in relation to substance use. We examined the influence of parental smoking behavior on selective peer associations. The findings showed that the selection of new friends in late adolescence could be predicted by the smoking status of the parents after controlling for the effects of the adolescent's own smoking (Engels et al., 2004). When parents smoked, children were more likely to affiliate with a smoker when establishing a new friendship. In other analyses we found that parental communication and setting rules were related to higher levels of self-efficacy to resist (peer) pressure to smoke (see Engels & Willemsen, 2004; Huver et al., in press; Otten, Harakeh et al., 2005).

Unfortunately we have not examined whether specific parenting practices or general parenting styles affect selective peer affiliation yet. It is rather essential in our opinion to carry out these types of longitudinal analyses as they may provide not only further insight into the complex mechanisms underlying parental behaviors and adolescent substance use, but they may also provide a better understanding of the relative roles of peers in adolescent substance use.

Bi-directional Relationships

From the way we address the role of parents in the development of adolescent substance use, one might guess that our theoretical models underpinning parental actions on adolescent behaviors primarily involve parent-to-child effects and no child-to-parent effects. We definitely do not want to give this impression and it is also not what some of our longitudinal data show. From a statistical point of view, it is essential to realize that cross-sectional correlations between parent and child behaviors are often interpreted in terms of *effects* of parental actions on adolescents' development, but it could easily be the other way round; parents *responding* to adolescent behaviors. In various analyses we found strong indications for the existence of these so-called child effects. For example, the reason for finding a positive association between frequency of communication on substance use and adolescent use is probably parents responding to adolescent behaviors.

In cross-lagged longitudinal models on adolescent alcohol use, Van der Vorst et al., (2005) found that parental support did not predict adolescent engagement in drinking over time, but the other way round, when adolescents start to drink heavily in an early age, parents respond by providing less support (see also Stice & Barrera, 1995). This may sound peculiar as one might expect that when parents find out their child is involved in problematic behaviors, which parents mostly will dislike, they would increase their actions to try to withdraw their child from further engagement. However, this is not what we found. Parents seem to be just ordinary people who respond to child disengagement (parents often interpret adolescent engagement in problem behaviors as disengagement from the family) by disengaging themselves.

In a way it is ludicrous to try to discriminate between parent-to-child effects and child-to-parent effects for various reasons. First, it is essential to realize that the specific measurements we normally take as researchers when we interview parents and adolescents on their relationships with each other are the results of millions and millions of micro-social interactions that took place from child's birth on up to adolescence. It is in some way impossible to disentangle parent and child effects; it is all about social interactions. Children's regulation of behavior and emotions affect their social environment responses, and these responses subsequently affect their regulation. And so on. And so forth. Second, it might be possible that it is not the mean level of parental actions, such as enforcement of rules on alcohol, which are important, but the flexibility (or rigidity) of parental actions. Perhaps when parents strongly fluctuate in daily life when dealing with adolescent drinking, sometimes permitting their adolescent child to drink and at other occasions not, this does not provide a clear signal for children, leading to higher likelihood of adolescent drinking. On the other hand, rigidity of parents might be perceived as an indication of inflexibility to deal with their child's needs, and subsequently lead to higher involvement of adolescents in problem behaviors. These types of mechanisms can only be studied with designs in which there are multiple assessments of parental actions as well as child responses available. We currently lack studies with these kinds of designs in the field of addiction.

Finally, in all our studies we aim to study family communication patterns and their subsequent effects on adolescent substance use *without* actually studying these interactions in real time. When it comes to, for example, how parents set and enforce rules on alcohol use, how their children respond to the way parents set rules, how children and parents talk about substance use at home, or what positive and constructive communication exactly consist, and how it works, then we totally lack knowledge. In our opinion, the best way to proceed is to combine survey designs with observational studies in which micro-social interactions in real time as well as over time can be observed when it comes to communication on substance use in families.

Complexity of Family Interactions

Most research has concentrated on between-family differences in substance use, and not on within-family differences. This is not a problem if: (a) siblings would not differ much in substance use and if (b) parents would not treat their children differently, or if they do, the children would not perceive these differences. Both conclusions are probably incorrect. To fully understand the complexity of family factors when investigating smoking and alcohol use, it is important to gain insight into the shared and non-shared effects of parental actions and reactions towards adolescents in between and within family designs (see also Darling & Cumsille, 2003).

When it comes to shared and non-shared parental influences we did some preliminary work. Most fascinating are the differences between smoking and drinking. As for smoking, parents did not vary between siblings in their smoking-specific socialization efforts; when they were strict towards one child they were equally strict to the other. So, it made no difference for parents whether their child was in early or mid-adolescence (Harakeh, Scholte, De Vries & Engels, 2005). The effects of parental actions on adolescent smoking did not differ between the two siblings in one family: parents are generally strict or not. As for alcohol use, the picture was completely the opposite.

Concerning alcohol-specific rules, parents were much more permissive towards their oldest child than towards their youngest (Van der Vorst et al., 2005). Longitudinal data over three waves indeed showed that when children become older, parents were loosening their ties when it comes to drinking (Van der Vorst et al., 2005). Nevertheless, despite these differences in parental treatment between children, the effects of parental rules on adolescent drinking were no different for the two adolescent siblings in our study.

THE ROLE OF PEERS

Friends are assumed to be of major importance for the development of cigarette smoking in young people. Throughout adolescence, youngsters experience feelings of uncertainty about their self-image, and consider themselves more or less dependent on the opinions and judgments of friends (Engels, Knibbe, Drop & De Haan, 1997). Meeting the expectations of one's group is crucial to prevent losing friends, become a loner, and eventually lose one's identity. Therefore, associating with friends will be less complicated when one's own behaviors are congruent with others'. People are, in general, more susceptible to conform to prevailing norms in their teenage years than in any other period (Finkenauer et al., 2003), making them vulnerable to initiate or maintain risky habits such as heavy drinking. Studies, carried out in the 1970s and focused on determinants of substance use among young people, show that adolescents have a tendency to be like their friends in behaviors and attitudes (Cohen, 1977). Two processes, influence and selection, could have caused this homogeneity of health related behavior in peer groups. Influence refers to an individual group member's behavior or opinion that is affected by other members. Selection can be divided into two conceptually different mechanisms. First, adolescents might search for new friends with similar characteristics, attitudes, and behaviors. Also, they might avoid contacts with new friends, or even break off friendships, because of differences in opinions and behaviors (i.e., deselection of friends). Not until research will be done that employs longitudinal designs in which changes in smoking and in friendships are traced, can we accurately draw conclusions about: (a) the relative contribution of selection processes and (b) the relative effects of friends' behaviors on individuals' substance use.

In the past decades, several longitudinal studies have examined influence and selection processes in adolescent health behavior (see review by Bauman & Ennett, 1996). For example, a prospective study by De Vries et al. (2003) among 15,705 adolescents in six European countries showed only small effects of best friend and peer group's smoking on smoking onset. These findings are comparable with longitudinal studies of youngsters in the US, and several studies showed that selection processes are largely responsible for homogeneity of smoking in friendships (Bauman & Ennett, 1996).

Fine-grained longitudinal analyses showed that alcohol consumption by best friends, peer group members, or other peers is not strongly predicting initiation and maintenance of juvenile drinking (see review in Poelen, Engels, Van der Vorst, Scholte & Vermulst, 2005). The small to non-significant effects of best friend's alcohol use on the development of drinking in adolescence made Jaccard, Blanton and Dodge (2005, p. 144) conclude that "overall, our data do not support the notion of pervasive peer influence on the part of one's friend with respect to adolescent health behaviors."

Longitudinal Studies on Peer Influences

We found support for Jaccard et al.'s statement in some of our longitudinal studies. Firstly, in a 5-year 3-wave study among 1,063 adolescents, Engels, Knibbe, De Vries et al. (1999) demonstrated very small modeling effects of best friend's alcohol and cigarette use on the development of substance use over time: Best friend's use explained only a few per cent of the variance in smoking and alcohol use at a subsequent wave. Secondly, in a prospective study with a full family design, Poelen, Engels et al. (2005) showed that sibling and best friend's drinking did not affect changes in alcohol use over a 12-month period. In this study, we further examined whether the impact of best friends varied for different drinking stages, as it is possible that peers are for instance more important in the initiation phase of drinking than in the phase of continuation of drinking (Spijkerman et al., in press). We did not find support for this assumption. Thirdly, we conducted a school-based study in which we included early adolescents as well as their reciprocal best friend (Bot, Engels, Knibbe & Meeus, 2005a). In this study we again found only very marginal effects of reciprocal best friend's drinking on adolescent use over a period of six months. In analyses on smoking in early adolescence, we found that reciprocal best friend's smoking hardly predicted individual smoking onset over a period of six and 12 months (Engels et al., 2004). In analyses of the full-family study, Harakeh, Engels, Scholte, De Vries and Vermulst (2005) found, after controlling for the effects of sibling smoking, marginal effects of best friend's smoking on onset and continuation of smoking over a period of 12 months. Also in other prospective studies on the prediction of regular smoking (Engels, Knibbe & Drop, 1999; Vink et al., 2003), heavy drinking and drunkenness (Poelen, Engels et al., 2005), continuation of smoking (Van Zundert et al., in press) and smoking cessation (Engels, Knibbe, De Vries & Drop, 1998) we found non-significant to fairly marginal effects of peer influences.

Summarizing, our survey studies do not provide compelling evidence that modeling of peer substance use plays a substantial role in the development of individual smoking and drinking.

Prototypes and Adolescent Substance Use

In the above-mentioned line of research, the focus is primarily on imitation or modeling effects by peers. However, young people's ideas about the pros and cons of smoking and drinking exhibited by peers might also affect their own substance use. These images or prototypes are of course partly based on perceptions and interpretations of substance use by others (see chapter by Gibbons et al.). In short, the basic assumption is that if somebody positively values the features of a typical smoker or drinker, this person is more likely to start smoking or drinking. Unfortunately the role of prototypes on adolescent substance use has hardly been examined in samples of countries outside North America. In two longitudinal data sets among early and mid-adolescents we looked at the effects of prototypes on different phase transitions in substance use. In general, it can be concluded that Dutch adolescents hold rather negative perceptions of smoking and drinking peers (Spijkerman, Van den Eijnden, Vitale, & Engels, 2004). The assessment of adolescents' smoker and drinker prototypes, when asked which characteristics adolescents associate with smoking and drinking peers, generated rather low scores on characteristics that are in general regarded as favorable features. Our longitudinal findings show that prototypes affect changes in smoking and drinking over time (Van den Eijnden, Spijkerman, & Engels, 2005; Spijkerman et al., in press; Spijkerman, Van den Eijnden & Engels, 2005). Further, our results show significant associations between smoker and drinker prototypes and subsequent substance use, even when tested in relation to other social-cognitive variables, such as the concepts in the Theory of Planned Behavior.

In further analyses, we examined whether adolescents' self-comparison processes affect adolescents' engagement in smoking. As hypothesized in previous research, two types of self-comparison motives may underlie the relationship between smoker prototypes and adolescents' smoking onset: self-consistency motivations and self-enhancement motivations (Aloise-Young et al., 1996). Self-consistency motivations refer to the fact that adolescents would start smoking because the characteristics associated with smoking peers are perceived as similar to their own (real) self-images. Self-enhancement motivations suggest that adolescents would start smoking because the characteristics associated with smoking peers are features adolescents would like to hold or, in other words, are similar to their ideal self-images. According to our longitudinal findings, both self-consistency and self-enhancement motivation explain why adolescents start smoking (Spijkerman et al., 2005). The more adolescents perceive smoking peers, as being similar to themselves and the more adolescents would like to possess characteristics associated with smoking peers, the higher their likelihood of becoming a smoker later on.

However, when taking into account the proportions of variance explained by the concept of prototypes, one could seriously question the importance of prototypes as explanatory concepts for Dutch adolescents' smoking and drinking initiation. In all our analyses the proportions of variance explained by smoker and drinker prototypes were rather low. It should be stressed that cross-sectional findings are ignored as they hold evidential problems with interpretation of the causal direction: A correlation between prototypes and substance use might be interpreted as effects of prototypes on substance use, but it can also be interpreted as people adjusting prototypes when they become engaged in smoking or drinking. Thus, here we are evidently taking exclusively those findings of longitudinal studies into account, in which appropriate corrections are in place for the effects of previous levels of substance use in adolescents as well as the possible bi-directional relationships between prototypes and substance use. When putting the low predictive values and moderate associations in perspective, one can still support the assumption that prototypes provide a meaningful explanation of adolescents' smoking and drinking initiation. After all, a concept can show low levels of explained variance but still have theoretical relevance. Further, other social-cognitive variables assumed to explain adolescents' smoking and drinking onset show quite low predictive values as well (Engels, Knibbe, De Vries et al., 1999; Engels, Knibbe, Drop, 1999; Van den Eijnden, Spijkerman & Engels, in press). Nevertheless, one may still argue that the low levels of explained variance of prototypes imply that they are of minor importance for the explanation of adolescents' substance use.

Methodological Considerations

Does this imply that we should reject the hypothesis that peers affect individual substance use? We have some arguments not to do so. It might be that we have been using insufficient designs to study peer influence. The vast majority of prospective studies are using surveys in which adolescents, and sometimes their peers, are regularly interviewed about their own behaviors and that of their peers. Subsequently, we aim to predict changes in individual drinking and smoking over time by corresponding behaviors of peers. However, theories on imitation of peer behaviors are tested without examining direct interactions between peers. This is presumably the problem in this line of research.

Few studies have employed other designs to test hypotheses regarding peer influences on substance use. First, in the 70s and 80s, a relatively small research tradition existed of experimental studies on alcohol use and modeling (Quigley & Collins, 1999). The findings of these studies generally show that when people are in the company of a drinker, the drinking pace of the other (a confederate) affects individual drinking rates and consumption levels. However, these types of studies examined processes of imitation in pairs of strangers, while adolescents and young adults mainly drink with friends or other peers. Next, they mostly carried out the experiments in a taste-test paradigm limiting the ecological validity of the findings. In our opinion, both aspects strongly limit the generalizability of these experimental studies.

Second, some scholars have been systematically observing communication in chumships. In a series of studies Dishion and colleagues demonstrated that contents and structure of communication between close friends are related to the development of deviant behaviors including drinking (Dishion, Bullock & Nelson, 2002). In a project among 206 boys who were followed from late childhood into young adulthood, videotaped interaction tasks between these boys with their closest friends were coded on contents and structure of communication. Granic and Dishion (2003) showed that friends can be drawn into deviant talks, and that this type of abnormal communication is related to problematic developments later on. In another prospective study Dishion and Owen (2002) revealed that deviant talk in friendships, explicitly dealing with issues related to substance use, in the teenage years was associated with alcohol abuse in young adulthood.

Nonetheless, an important limitation of these studies is that although they focused on observing communications on deviancy in friendships, they did not observe peer influences on alcohol misuse or other problem behaviors in their natural context. In other words, they were not assessing actual social interaction processes in relation to substance use, for example, in a bar, pub, disco, or party. Surprisingly, the role of peer influences on smoking and drinking in its natural context has rarely been studied. We will discuss the findings of a few of our observational studies on substance use in peer groups. In all these studies, we made use of observational data of real time interactions between peers in a bar lab.

Observational Studies on Peers and Alcohol Use

In the first report on our observational study among 238 late adolescents, we aimed to examine the functionality of alcohol expectancies by predicting drinking behaviors in existing peer groups of young adults in a "naturalistic" setting (Bot, Engels & Knibbe, 2005). In other words, we examined whether people's expectations of the outcomes of drinking still affect their drinking levels in a social drinking situation, in which we then controlled for possible peer influences that take place. If these peer influences are operating, they might overshadow people's more rationally based cognitions on alcohol. Young adults were invited to join an experiment with their peer group in a bar annex laboratory. During a "break" of 50 minutes in this experiment, their activities, social behavior and drinking behavior were observed with digital video and audio equipment. A total of 28 peer groups were involved in this study. A peer group consisted of 7–9 persons and the type of relations within these groups range from intimate relations and close friendships to acquaintances. The information of the drinking behavior from the observations, together with questionnaire data on alcohol expectancies, provides the opportunity to look at how and which expectancies are related to actual drinking patterns. Multiple regression and multilevel analyses were applied. We showed that drinking levels in a one-hour ad lib drinking session in a bar lab together with those they normally go out with are strongly related to the average drinking levels of the group. Further, the findings convincingly showed that expectancies of the positive and arousing effects of alcohol consumption predicted alcohol consumptions in a naturalistic, social drinking situation, over and above group effects of drinking. Expectancies of the negative and sedative effects of drinking, however, did not predict drinking. In sum, these findings show that people's actual drinking behavior, as observed in a bar lab context, is related to peer group influences as well as their expectations of the outcomes of drinking.

In a follow-up of these analyses, we tested whether men and women differ in the extent to which they are affected by drinking of peers (Engels, Bot, Van der Vorst & Granic, 2005). There is evidence that in particular among boys, alcohol use is related to social functioning and relational competence. This suggests that not conforming to the group norms has more social consequences for boys than for girls (e.g., Pape & Hammer, 1996). This is in contrast with longitudinal findings of surveys showing no gender differences in the extent to which peer drinking affects alcohol consumption. We again used the data of the observational study in the bar lab ($N = 238$; in 28 groups). The constellation of the groups differed from all men (7%) and all women (7%) to mixed gender (86%). In our observational data, multilevel analyses showed robust gender differences in susceptibility to peer drinking; men are strongly affected by the average drinking levels in the group, but women are not. To find out why women are not strongly affected by peer drinking, we tested a series of hypotheses. The first is that women's drinking is less context-dependent. We found evidence for that. Analyses showed that women's drinking in the bar is more strongly affected by what they normally drink (questionnaire data) than men. The second is that women are more strongly affected by their own expectancies of how alcohol affects them than by the specific social context. Nonetheless, we found no gender differences in the associations between participant's expectations that alcohol makes them more sociable, energetic, sexually aroused, or powerful, and actual alcohol consumption. The third is that when male group members score high on sexual and power expectancies, women are more careful and stop drinking after a few consumptions. Women might do this to keep control over the situation. Multilevel analyses indeed showed that in groups where peer group members are high on sexual expectancies, only women limit their drinking and men do not. Social enhancement, as well as power expectancies by group members did not affect individual drinking.

Third, alcohol consumption typically takes place in a time-out situation; a time-out can be spent by engaging in several leisure time activities (Bot, Engels, Knibbe & Meeus, 2005b). Contextual circumstances like arrangement of a drinking setting might equally strongly affect people's tendencies to consume alcohol as individual characteristics (like alcohol expectancies, intentions to drink, or implementation of intentions) or group characteristics (norms and behaviors of company). In a bar, conversation is the dominant pastime but other activities may take place as well like watching TV or playing games. These activities might inhibit drinking because of the physical difficulties of combining drinking with other activities. In this study, we followed the ad-lib drinking as well as activities of peer groups (consisting of 7–9 persons) during a one hour period. Findings suggest that: (1) selection of activities is not related to initial drinking levels or personality characteristics, (2) active pastime is related to a lower drinking rate than passive pastime (in males), (3) male problem drinkers appear to compensate for the "lost" drinking after an active phase, and (4) involvement in active pastime is unrelated to total alcohol consumption. In other words, it appears that people's drinking levels are indeed affected by the activities they undertake in a bar, but that for a specific group, namely heavy drinking males, this is not the case, as they catch up in terms of drinking more during a less active pastime.

Further Studies

So far, we have not focused on how the various types of relationships existing in groups affect social influence processes. It is very likely that whether people adopt the prevailing drinking norms within their peer group depends on the type of relationships within the group. Some groups consist, like in real life, of weak ties and people hardly know each other, while other groups consist of friends who have known each other for a long time. One might assume that within long-lasting peer groups, in which selection processes already have taken place, it is more likely that deviation from the norm by individual members will be more easily accepted than in groups that were just formed. In the latter groups young people have more risks to be confronted with their deviancy and might be more likely to be socially excluded, and therefore might be expected to conform to group norms. In addition, within each group different types of relationship exist. Some members are more popular than others, and some are seen as more dominant than others. It would be interesting to examine whether social positions within the peer group are related to people's tendencies to adopt drinking behaviors. One might assume that popular and dominant members are more likely to take the lead when it comes to drinking as this is also partly expected by the others (see Engels, Scholte et al., in press). The less popular and more passive and permissive members might be more likely to follow the popular and dominant ones, and might feel more forced to drink when the others are drinking. This aspect, which is in our opinion one of the most interesting features of group processes to study in relation to substance use, will be the topic of further analyses.

Besides the role of different types of relationships within peer groups, it is fascinating to analyze what kind of social influence processes are unfolding in groups. This of course depends to a large extent on the history of the group, the specific set of relationships within the group, the specific context people are in at the moment, the individual expectations people have about what alcohol does to them, and on their regular drinking patterns. These all form requisites for the starting point of the interaction processes. But also the process itself within that one hour in our bar lab is interesting to study. For instance, our findings on women drinking less when they are in a group with members who think that drinking leads to sexual arousal presuppose that women stop drinking at a certain moment. When they realize that a situation might be too dangerous, they seem to stop drinking. This poses the question what some women do in this particular context; do they try to avoid the heavy drinking males and seek company of other men, or do they seek company of other females to get some support? Perhaps what they undertake depends on the group constellation; when girls are with only girls, less control is needed, whereas when a group is dominated by males, they feel obliged to control their drinking rates. This urges for the need to visualize and quantify the order of social interactions over time.

Observational Studies on Peers and Smoking

To our knowledge, there are no systematic observational studies conducted on peer influences and youth smoking behaviors. Recently, we conducted an experimental observational study on imitation by peers and smoking (Harakeh, Engels, Van Baaren & Scholte, 2005). To observe participants in a naturalistic setting, we invited them to our bar lab at the university. A total of 125 participants conducted two tasks in which they had to rate advertisements shown on a television screen together with a confederate. These two tasks were 30 minutes apart and in the break we observed and recorded smoking and social behaviors of the participants with digital video and audio equipment. Trained coders rated the smoking behaviors, in terms of total number of cigarettes, moment of lighting a cigarette, and moment of stopping. Male and female daily smokers were exposed to same-gender confederates who differed on smoking and social behavior during the break. An experimental design with a 3 (smoking behavior of confederate) by 2 (types of social interactions) factorial design was used. The smoking conditions were "non smoking," "light smoking, i.e. 1 cigarette," and "heavy smoking, i.e. 4 cigarettes." Concerning types of interactions during the break, in the "warm model condition" the confederate was open and sociable, and in the "cold model condition" distant, pretty silent, and unsociable. Participants were asked before each session to fill in a questionnaire and at the end of the session to fill in an evaluation form. Just before each session started, confederates were told which condition they should be in.

Findings revealed that the participants modeled the smoking behavior of the confederate. Even after controlling for young people's urge to smoke, the confederate's smoking explains a large proportion of the variance in number of cigarettes smoked. Further, in a warm, sociable interaction, participants are more likely to smoke, and to continue smoking. Both the confederate's smoking and the urge to smoke, affected participants to light up their first cigarette. Concerning the second cigarette, we found that participants in the heavy smoking condition and in the warm model condition were more likely to light up a second. With regard to the third cigarette, only in the heavy smoking condition did participants light up a third one. Thus, findings of this observational experimental study show that young adults imitate the smoking behavior of complete strangers, and the imitation effects also substantially explain why individuals start and continue smoking. Further, young people are more likely to continue smoking if this takes place in a warm and sociable interaction with somebody else.

CONCLUSION

The initiation and further development of substance use are evidently affected by people's actions and reactions in the direct social environment of young people. We have addressed findings of empirical studies on the various ways in which parents affect adolescent substance use, and we have elaborated on a series of our own studies that focus on the interplay between general parenting practices, substance-specific parenting practices, and parental own substance use. In addition, we also discussed some of the limitations in this line of research, such as the lack of longitudinal multi-informant studies, the ignorance of bi-directionality in theoretical models, and the need for observational studies to examine social family interactions in real time.

Regarding peer influences, we have discussed the role of peer substance use as well as the impact of the images people hold regarding substance using peers on adolescent substance use. In our opinion, it becomes quite evident that longitudinal survey studies do not provide convincing evidence for a strong modeling effect of peer substance use. In addition, social images or prototypes held by adolescents did not robustly predict smoking and drinking onset. Before we conclude that peers do not matter, we claim that probably inaccurate research designs have been used to study peer interactions in relation to adolescent and young adult substance use. We further argue that survey designs are less suitable to gain insight into the conditions under which people actually imitate other's drinking behaviors or are susceptible to explicit peer pressure to drink. We assume that longitudinal studies that combine survey and observational data may more successfully shed light on the intriguing matter of how friends affect the individual differently in substance use. We argue that especially observational studies of real-time microsocial interactions between peers in the natural context will provide insight into: (a) whether peers actually have an impact on individual use and (b) the mechanisms underpinning imitation of peer behaviors. We addressed the preliminary findings of a few observational studies on smoking and drinking in youth.

AUTHOR NOTE

During the preparation of this manuscript Rutger Engels was supported by a fellowship of the Dutch Organization for Scientific Research. We would like to thank the PhD students who worked on the studies described in this review; Endy Den Exter Blokland, Zeena Harakeh, Roos Huver, Roy Otten, Evelien Poelen, Renske Spijkerman, Haske Van der Vorst, and Rinka Van Zundert.

REFERENCES

Ajzen, I. (1991). The theory of planned behavior. *Organizational Behavior and Human Decision Processes, 50*, 179–211.

Aloise-Young, P.A., Hennigan, K.M. & Graham, J.W. (1996). Role of the self-image and smoker stereotype in smoking onset during early adolescence: A longitudinal study. *Health Psychology, 15*, 494–497.

Avenevoli, S. & Merikangas, K.R. (2003). Familial influences on adolescent smoking. *Addiction, 98*, 1–20.

Bandura, A. (1977). *Social Learning Theory*. Englewood Cliffs, NJ: Prentice-Hall.

Bauman, K.E. & Ennett, S.E. (1996). On the importance of peer influence for adolescent drug use: Commonly neglected considerations. *Addiction, 91*, 185–198.

Barnes, G.M., Reifman, A.S., Farell, M.P. & Dintcheff, B.A. (2000). The effects of parenting on the development of adolescent alcohol misuse: A six wave latent growth model. *Journal of Marriage and the Family, 62*, 175–186.

Bot, S.M., Engels, R.C.M.E. & Knibbe, R.A. (2005). The effects of alcohol expectancies on drinking behavior in peer groups: Observations in a naturalistic setting. *Addiction, 100*, 1270–1279.

Bot, S.M., Engels, R.C.M.E., Knibbe, R.A. & Meeus, W. (2005a). Friend's drinking and adolescent alcohol consumption: The moderating role of friendship characteristics. *Addictive Behaviors, 30*, 929–947.

Bot, S.M., Engels, R.C.M.E., Knibbe, R.A. & Meeus, W. (2005b). *Pastime in a Pub: Observations of young adults' activities and alcohol consumption*. Manuscript submitted for publication.

Chassin, L., Presson, C.C., Todd, M., Rose, J.S. & Sherman, S.J. (1998). Maternal socialization of adolescent smoking: The intergenerational transmission of parenting and smoking. *Developmental Psychology, 34*, 1189–1201.

Clark, P.I., Scarisbrick-Hauser, A., Gautam, S.P. & Wirk, S.J. (1999). Anti-tobacco socialization in homes of African-American and White parents, and smoking and nonsmoking parents. *Journal of Adolescent Health, 24*, 329–339.

Cohen, J.M. (1977). Sources of peer group homogeneity. *Sociology of Education, 50*, 227–241.

Cohen, D.A., Richardson, J. & La Bree, L. (1994). Parenting behaviors and the onset of smoking and alcohol use: A longitudinal study. *Pediatrics, 94*, 368–375.

Darling, N. & Cumsille, P. (2003). Theory, measurement, and methods in the study of family influences on adolescent smoking. *Addiction, 98*, 21–36.

Darling, N. & Steinberg, L. (1993). Parenting style as context: An integrative model. *Psychological Bulletin, 113*, 487–496.

Den Exter Blokland, A.W., Hale III, W.W., Meeus, W. & Engels, R.C.M.E. (in press). Parental anti smoking socialization and adolescent smoking onset. *European Addiction Research*.

Den Exter Blokland, A.W., Harakeh, Z., Engels, R.C.M.E., Meeus, W. & Hale III, W.W. (2005). *The effectiveness of having a non-smoking agreement*. Manuscript submitted for publication.

Den Exter Blokland, A.W., Hale III, W.W., Meeus, W. & Engels, R.C.M.E. (2005). *Parenting styles and smoking onset*. Manuscript submitted for publication.

Den Exter Blokland, A.W., Engels, R.C.M.E., Hale III, W.W., Meeus, W., & Willemsen, M. (2004). Parental smoking cessation and adolescent smoking onset. *Preventive Medicine, 38*, 359–368.

De Vries, H., Engels, R.C.M.E., Kremers, S., Wetzels, J., & Mudde, A. (2003). Influences of parents and peers on adolescent smoking behavior in six European countries. *Health Education Research, 18*, 617–632.

Dishion, T., Bullock, B.M. & Nelson, S. (2002, July). *A Dynamic System Analysis of Developmental Trajectories: Prosocial and deviant adaptation as an attractor process*. 17th Biennial ISSBD meeting, Ottawa, Canada.

Dishion, T.J. & Owen, L.D. (2002). A longitudinal analysis of friendships and substance use: Bidirectional influence from adolescence to adulthood. *Developmental Psychology, 38*, 480–491.

Engels, R.C.M.E., Bot, S.M., Van Der Vorst, H. & Granic, I. (2005). *Smells like Teen Spirit: Sex differences in susceptibility to peer influences on alcohol use.* Manuscript submitted for publication.

Engels, R.C.M.E., Finkenauer, C., Kerr, M., & Stattin, H. (2005). Illusions of parental control: Parenting and smoking onset in Swedish and Dutch adolescents. *Journal of Applied Social Psychology, 35*, 1912–1935.

Engels, R.C.M.E., Knibbe, R.A., De Vries, H. & Drop, M.J. (1998). Antecedents of smoking cessation among adolescents: Who is motivated to change? *Preventive Medicine, 27*, 348–357.

Engels, R.C.M.E., Knibbe, R.A., De Vries, H., Drop, M.J. & Van Breukelen, G.J.P. (1999). Influences of parental and best friends' smoking and drinking on adolescent use: A longitudinal study. *Journal of Applied Social Psychology, 29*, 338–362.

Engels, R.C.M.E., Knibbe, R.A. & Drop, M.J. (1999). Predictability of smoking in adolescence: Between optimism and pessimism. *Addiction, 94*, 115–124.

Engels, R.C.M.E., Knibbe, R.A., Drop, M.J. & De Haan, J.T. (1997). Homogeneity of smoking behavior in peer groups: Influence or selection? *Health Education and Behavior, 24*, 801–811.

Engels, R.C.M.E., Scholte, R., Van Lieshout, C., Overbeek, G., & De Kemp, R. (in press). Peer group reputation and alcohol and cigarette use. *Addictive Behaviors.*

Engels, R.C.M.E. & Van den Eijnden, R.J.J.M. (in press). The devil in disguise: Functions of substance use in adolescence. In J. Coleman, L. Hendry, & M. Kloep (Eds), *Adolescence and Health.* Chichester, UK: John Wiley & Sons, Ltd.

Engels, R.C.M.E., Van der Vorst, H., Dekovic, M. & Meeus, W. (2005). *Correspondence in Collateral and Self Reports on Alcohol Consumption: A within family analysis.* Manuscript submitted for publication.

Engels, R.C.M.E., Vermulst, A.A., Dubas, J., Bot, S.M. & Gerris, J. (2005). Long term effects of family functioning and child characteristics on problem drinking in young adulthood. *European Addiction Research, 11*, 32–37.

Engels, R.C.M.E., Vitaro, F., Den Exter Blokland, A., De Kemp, R. & Scholte, R. (2004). Parents, friendship selection processes and adolescent smoking behavior. *Journal of Adolescence, 27*, 531–544.

Engels, R.C.M.E. & Willemsen, M. (2004). Communication about smoking in Dutch families: Associations between anti-smoking socialization and adolescent smoking-related cognitions. *Health Education Research, 19*, 227–238.

Ennett, S.T., Bauman, K.E., Foshee, V.A., Pemberton, M. & Hicks, K. (2001). Parent-child communication about adolescent tobacco and alcohol use: What do parents say and does it affect youth behavior? *Journal of Marriage and Family, 63*, 48–62.

Finkenauer, C., Engels, R.C.M.E. & Baumeister, R.W. (2005). Parenting and adolescent externalizing and internalizing problems: The role of self-control. *International Journal of Behavioral Development, 29*, 58–69.

Finkenauer, C., Engels, R.C.M.E., Meeus, W. & Oosterwegel, A. (2002). Self and identity in early adolescence. In T.M. Brinthaupt & R.P. Lipka (Eds), *Understanding the Self of the Early Adolescent.* Albany, NY: State University of New York Press.

Granic, I. & Dishion, T.J. (2003). Deviant talk in adolescent friendships: A step toward measuring a pathogenic attractor process. *Social Development, 12*, 314–334.

Harakeh, Z., Engels, R.C.M.E., Van Baaren, R. & Scholte, R. (2005). *Imitation of Smoking Behavior in Dyads: An experimental observational study.* Manuscript submitted for publication.

Harakeh, Z., Engels, R.C.M.E., Scholte, R., & De Vries, H. (2005). *Concordance in Opinions on Smoking Between Parents and Adolescents.* Manuscript submitted for publication.

Harakeh, Z., Engels, R.C.M.E., Scholte, R., De Vries H., & Vermulst, A.A. (2005). *Best Friend's Smoking Influences on Adolescent Smoking.* Manuscript submitted for publication.

Harakeh, Z., Scholte, R., De Vries, H. & Engels, R.C.M.E. (2005). Anti smoking socialization and smoking behavior: A full family study. *Addiction, 100,* 862–870.

Harakeh, Z., Scholte, R., De Vries, H., Vermulst, A.A. & Engels, R.C.M.E. (2005). *Parenting, Anti-smoking Socialization and Smoking Behavior in Siblings.* Manuscript submitted for publication.

Harakeh, Z., Scholte, R., De Vries, H., Vermulst, A.A. & Engels, R.C.M.E. (2004). Parental factors, smoking specific cognitions and early onset of smoking. *Preventive Medicine, 39,* 951–961.

Henriksen, L. & Jackson, C. (1998). Anti-smoking socialization: Relationship to parent and child smoking status. *Health Communication, 10,* 87–101.

Hibell, B., Andersson, B., Bjarnasson, T., Ahlström, S., Balakireva, O., Kokkevi, A. & Morgan, M. (2004). *The ESPAD Report 2003. Alcohol and Other Drug Use Among Students in 35 European Countries.* The Swedish Council for Information on Alcohol and Other Drugs (CAN), Council of Europe, Co-operation Group to Combat Drug Abuse and Illicit Trafficking in Drugs (Pompidou Group).

Huver, R., Engels, R.C.M.E. & De Vries, H. (in press). Parenting practices, adolescent smoking cognitions and behavior. *Health Education Research.*

Huver, R., Engels, R.C.M.E., De Vries, H. & Van Breukelen, G. (2005). *Associations Between Parenting Style and Smoking Onset.* Manuscript submitted for publication.

Jaccard, J., Blanton, H., Dodge, T. (2005). Peer influences on risk behavior: An analysis on the effects of a close friend. *Developmental Psychology, 41,* 133–147.

Jackson, C. (2002). Perceived legitimacy of parental authority and tobacco and alcohol use during early adolescence. *Journal of Adolescent Health, 31,* 425–432.

Jackson, C., Henriksen, L. & Dickinson, D. (1999), Alcohol-specific socialization, parenting behaviors and alcohol use by children. *Journal of Studies on Alcohol, 60,* 362–367.

Jackson, C. & Henriksen, L. (1998). Do as I say: Parent smoking, antismoking socialization, and smoking onset among children. *Addictive Behaviors, 22,* 107–114.

Otten, R., Engels, R.C.M.E. & Van den Eijnden, R.J.J.M. (2005). *Parenting Styles and Smoking Behavior in Asthmatics.* Manuscript submitted for publication.

Otten, R., Harakeh, Z., Vermulst, A.A., Engels, R.C.M.E. & Van den Eijnden, R.J.J.M. (2005). *Anti-smoking Socialization, Smoking Cognitions and Smoking in Adolescents: A within-family analysis.* Manuscript submitted for publication.

Pape, H. & Hammer, T. (1996). Sober adolescence: Predictor of psychosocial maladjustment in young adulthood? *Scandinavian Journal of Psychology, 37,* 362–377.

Poelen, E.A.P., Scholte, R.H.J., Engels, R.C.M.E., Boomsma, D.I. & Willemsen, G. (2005). Trends in alcohol consumption in Dutch adolescents and young adults. *Drugs and Alcohol Dependence, 79,* 413–421.

Poelen, E.A.P., Engels, R.C.M.E., Van der Vorst, H., Scholte, R., & Vermulst, A.A. (2005). *Best Friends and Alcohol Consumption in Adolescence: A within family analysis.* Manuscript submitted for publication.

Poelen, E.A.P., Scholte, R.H.J., Willemsen, G., Boomsma, D.I. & Engels, R.C.M.E. (2005). *The Effects of Familial and Peer Drinking on Development of Drinking in Dutch Adolescent and Young Adult Twins.* Manuscript submitted for publication.

Quigley, B.M. & Collins, R.L. (1999). The modeling of alcohol consumption: A meta-analytic review. *Journal of Studies on Alcohol, 60,* 90–98.

Raskin White, H., Johnson, V. & Buyske, S. (2000). Parental modeling and parenting behavior effects on offspring alcohol and cigarette use: A growth curve analysis. *Journal of Substance Abuse, 12,* 287–310.

Spijkerman, R, Van den Eijnden, R.J.J.M. & Engels, R.C.M.E. (2005). Self-comparison processes, prototypes and adolescent smoking onset. *Preventive Medicine, 40,* 785–794.

Spijkerman, R., Van den Eijnden, R.J.J.M., Overbeek, G.J. & Engels, R.C.M.E. (in press). The impact of peer and parental norms and behavior on adolescent drinking: The mediating role of drinker prototypes. *Psychology and Health*.

Spijkerman, R., Van den Eijnden, R.J.J.M., Vitale, S. & Engels, R.C.M.E. (2004). Explaining adolescents' smoking and drinking behavior: The concept of smoker and drinker prototypes in relation to variables of the theory of planned behavior. *Addictive Behaviors*, 1615–1622.

Stice, E. & Barrera, M. (1995). A longitudinal examination of the reciprocal relations between perceived parenting and adolescents' substance use and externalising behaviors. *Developmental Psychology*, *31*, 322–334.

Van den Eijnden, R.J.J.M., Spijkerman, R. & Engels, R.C.M.E. (in press). Prototypes and smoking onset in early adolescents. *European Addiction Research*.

Van der Vorst, H., Engels, R.C.M.E., Deković, M. & Meeus, W. (2005). *The Impact of Rules, Parental Norms, and Parental Alcohol Use on Adolescents' Drinking Behavior*. Manuscript submitted for publication.

Van der Vorst, H., Engels, R.C.M.E., Deković, M., Meeus, W. & Van Leeuwe, J. (2005). The role of alcohol specific socialization on adolescents' drinking behavior. *Addiction*, *100*, 1464–1474.

Van Der Vorst, H., Engels, R.C.M.E., Meeus, W. & Deković, M. (2005). *Parents' Rules. An Ecological Analysis on the Link Between Rules and Adolescent Drinking*. Manuscript submitted for publication.

Van der Vorst, H., Engels, R.C.M.E., Meeus, W., Deković, M. & Vermulst, A.A. (in press). Attachment, parental control and alcohol initiation in adolescence. *Psychology of Addictive Behaviors*.

Van Zundert, R., Van der Vorst, H., Vermulst, A.A. & Engels, R.C.M.E. (in press). Parenting and parental alcohol use as related to drinking in children in regular and special education. *Journal of Family Psychology*.

Vink, J.M., Willemsen, G., Engels, R.C.M.E. & Boomsma, D. (2003). Does the smoking behavior of parents, siblings and friends influence smoking behavior in adolescent twins? *Twin Research, 6*, 209–217.

Wood, M.D., Read, J.P., Mitchell, R.E. & Brand, N.H. (2004). Do parents still matter? Parent and peer influences on alcohol involvement among recent high school graduates. *Psychology of Addictive Behaviors*, *18*, 19–30.

Yu, J. (2003). The association between parental alcohol-related behaviors and children's drinking. *Drug and Alcohol Dependence*, *69*, 253–262.

CHAPTER 5

Temperament, Self-regulation, and the Prototype/Willingness Model of Adolescent Health Risk Behavior

Meg Gerrard, Frederick X. Gibbons, Michelle L. Stock, Amy E. Houlihan, and Jennifer L. Dykstra

There is a growing body of research on the development of self-regulation that explores the role of temperament and the social environment in the emergence of self-control and health behaviors. This chapter will briefly review this literature with emphasis on the development of temperament-based self-regulatory processes and their impact on the health and health-risk behavior of adolescents. Next, we will discuss evidence that self-regulatory processes shape the development of organized cognitive systems involving views of the world and people in it. Specifically, we will address the role of a major component of the Prototype/Willingness Model of adolescent health risk behavior, behavioral willingness, as a mediator of the relation between self-control and adolescent risk behavior. Finally, we will discuss the implications of these developmental processes for children's and adolescents' health promoting and health risk behaviors.

EPIGENETIC THEORY: TEMPERAMENT AND THE DEVELOPMENT OF SELF-REGULATION

Temperaments are generally defined as dimensions of personality that appear early in life, are reasonably stable over time, and have a constitutional basis (Buss & Plomin, 1984; Hagekull, 1989; Pedlow, Sanson, Prior & Oberklaid, 1993; Windle & Lerner, 1986). There is ample empirical support for Allport's assertion that temperaments are "largely

Self-regulation in Health Behavior. Edited by Denise T.D. de Ridder and John B.F. de Wit.
© 2006 John Wiley & Sons Ltd.

hereditary in origin" (1961, p. 34; see Braungart, Plomin, DeFries & Fulker, 1992; Emde, Plomin, Robinson & Corley, 1992; Rothbart & Bates 1998). In addition, a number of studies have demonstrated that temperaments are related to adolescent risk behaviors such as substance use (Chassin, Pillow, Curran, Molina & Barrera, 1993; Wills, DuHamel & Vaccaro 1995; Windle, 1991).

In their early research, Buss and Plomin (1975) identified four basic temperaments: activity, emotionality, sociability, and impulsivity. More recent research has led to the re-conceptualization of sociability as positive emotionality because it captures positive reactions to exciting and novel objects as well as people (Rothbart, 1987). Furthermore, negative emotionality (characterized by being easily frustrated, irritated, and intensely upset) has been shown to be a distinct dimension which is orthogonal to positive emotionality rather than the opposite end of the same continuum (Watson & Clark, 1984; Watson & Tellegen, 1985). Likewise, recent research has explored the mechanisms underlying impulsivity, which has led to a change in focus from impulsive behavior to attention to tasks (Rothbart & Ahadi, 1994). Thus, recent research on the relation between temperament and adolescents' health risk and health promoting behaviors has focused on four dimensions of temperament: *activity level*, a tendency to be physically active and have difficulty sitting still; *positive emotionality*, a tendency to easily experience positive mood; *negative emotionality*, a tendency to become easily and intensely upset; and *task attentional orientation*, the ability to focus attention on a task and ignore distracting stimuli. These four temperaments have consistently been associated with adolescent risk behaviors such as substance use and unprotected sex (Lerner & Vicary, 1984; Rothbart & Bates, 1998; Tarter, 1988; Wills et al., 2001; Wills, Gibbons, Gerrard, Murry & Brody, 2003).[1]

It is relatively easy to understand how these basic temperaments would be associated with risk enhancing and risk avoidant behaviors in later childhood and adolescence. For example, the high activity level that contributes to a child's restlessness when required to sit still in class is often associated with exploratory behaviors that can put the child at risk. When high activity level is combined with low task attention orientation, the child's inability to focus on performing and completing tasks could exacerbate his or her tendency to be restless and engage in risky exploratory behavior (Wills & Dishion, 2004).

Epigenetic Theory, however, suggests that basic temperament does not directly affect risk and protective behaviors later in childhood (Goldsmith, Gottesman & Lemery, 1997; Scarr, 1992; Tarter, Moss & Vanyukov, 1995). Although it influences the organization of a child's behavior, behavioral manifestations of these constitutionally-based characteristics change as a function of the development of children's cognitive and social skills and their environment (Barkley, 1997; Kochanska, Murray & Harlan, 2000; Moffitt, 1993; Rothbart & Ahadi, 1994; Tarter et al., 1995). Thus, the theory suggests that the impact of temperament on behavior is moderated by environmental influences such as parenting,

---

[1] In this chapter we use the term "temperament" to refer to a person's (relatively unique) constellation of characteristics that appear early in life, are stable over time, and have a constitutional basis. We will use the terms "temperaments" and "dimensions of temperament" interchangeably to refer to the various components of a person's temperament.

and mediated by a second level of attributes and abilities. These characteristics are based in temperament, but are more complex, and cannot be assessed in early childhood. They are temperament-based cognitions and competencies that represent developmental elaborations of temperament and are an indication of the child's ability to self-regulate cognitions, emotions, and behavior (Wills & Dishion, 2004; Wills et al., 2001; Wills & Stoolmiller, 2002). Once in place, these attributes mediate the expression of temperament in behavior.[2] Other authors have also suggested that self-regulation, at least in part, reflects temperament (Cervone, Mor, Orom, Shadel & Scott, 2004; McCabe, Cunnington & Brooks-Gunn, 2004).

It is not surprising that these self-regulatory attributes have been characterized by different authors in different ways. Rothbart and her colleagues suggest that temperaments facilitate or retard the development of self-regulatory processes (Rothbart & Ahadi, 1994; Rothbart, Derryberry & Posner, 1994). Mischel and Ayduk (2004) refer to self-regulation as both an individual difference variable and a set of processes. Fitzsimmons and Bargh (2004) focus on the non-conscious and automatic aspects of self-regulation (Fitzsimmons & Bargh, 2004), while Eisenberg and her colleagues focus on effortful control (Eisenberg, Smith, Sadovsky & Spinrad, 2004). Like Eisenberg, Epigenetic Theory (and this chapter) primarily addresses self-regulation as conscious impulse and emotional control, or more generally, self-control. Our focus here will be on the three dimensions of self-regulation that have most frequently been linked to substance use in adolescents and young adults: good self-control, poor self-control, and risk-taking (Wills & Dishion, 2004; also see Moffitt, 1993).

Self-control and Risk-taking

Good self-control is characterized by dependability, problem solving, soothability, and focus (Wills et al., 2001; Wills & Stoolmiller, 2002), and includes deliberative responding, and the ability to regulate emotional states and avoid risky situations. Thus, children and adolescents who are high in good self-control are likely to think about potential negative consequences of their behavior, and these cognitions are likely to guide their decision-making. *Poor self-control* comprises three factors: impulsiveness ("I like to switch from one thing to another"), impatience ("If I find that something is really difficult, I get frustrated and quit"), and distractibility. Adolescents who are high in poor self-control tend to respond to situations without reflection or consideration of long-term consequences. Good self-control and poor self-control are clearly related constructs, but they are certainly not redundant (rs range from -0.03 to -0.50; Wills et al., 2001; Wills, Gibbons, Gerrard & Brody, 2000; Wills et al., 2006; Wills, Vaccaro & McNamara, 1994). The idea that good and poor self-control were independent systems was first suggested by Block and Block (1980), and has since been supported by psychometric analyses of self-control instruments and research linking the constructs to separate neuropsychological systems (Rothbart et al., 1994; Wills, Sandy & Yaeger, 2000). *Risk-taking* is characterized by a tendency to enjoy and seek out intense

---

[2] Like Vohs and Baumeister (2004), we will use the terms "self-regulation" and "self-control" interchangeably in this chapter.

stimulation and impulsivity. It is more strongly related to negative emotionality, and more weakly related to activity level than is poor self-control (Wills, Gibbons et al., 2000).

Self-regulation and Adolescent Risk Behavior

The Epigenetic Model suggests that it is these complex self-regulatory characteristics rather than simple temperament dimensions that are the proximal antecedents to adolescent health protection versus risk behaviors. Thus, instead of direct paths from temperament to behavior, the effects of temperament on behavior are mediated by good self-control, poor self-control, and risk-taking. Research by Wills and his colleagues on children aged 10 to 16 has supported these hypothesized relations between the dimensions of temperament and the dimension of self-control, and has demonstrated that self-control is a good predictor of risk behavior, specifically, substance use (Wills et al., 2001). This research has also demonstrated that the relations between temperaments (e.g., activity level) and adolescent risk behavior are mediated through the 3 dimensions of self-control (Wills et al., 1995; Wills et al., 1994; see Figure 5.1).

Both theory and research, however, have suggested that the relation between these dimensions of self-control and adolescent substance use is also not direct, but instead is mediated by more proximal factors (Jessor & Jessor, 1977; Wills, Sandy et al., 2000). More specifically, temperament shapes the development of self-control, which is associated with the more proximal variables of academic competence and peer affiliations. In addition, there is growing evidence that self-control is associated with cognitive structures—what Wills and Dishion (2004) call "organized cognitive systems". These

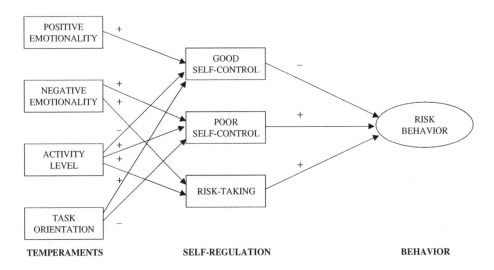

Figure 5.1 Epigenetic Theory
Adapted from Wills, Sandy et al., 2000.

cognitive systems involve views of the world and other people, and include perceptions of vulnerability to potential danger and perceptions of others who engage in risk behaviors. A series of recent studies has demonstrated parallels between these cognitive frameworks and the two key constructs in the Prototype/Willingness Model of Adolescent Health Risk Behavior, specifically, prototypes and behavioral willingness are part of this system (Wills, Gibbons, Gerrard, Murry & Brody 2003; Wills et al., 2006. Before discussing this research, however, we will briefly describe the Prototype Model. (For a more complete description of the model, see the chapter by Gibbons, Gerrard, Reimer & Pomery in this volume.)

THE PROTOTYPE/WILLINGNESS MODEL

Two Paths to Risk Behavior

The Prototype Model is a modified dual process model based on the assumption that there are two "paths" and thus two proximal antecedents, to adolescent risk behavior. The first path, called the *reasoned path*, reflects the fact that some risk behavior is intentional even among young adolescents. This path is described in the Theory of Reasoned Action and the Theory of Planned Behavior as originating in positive attitudes toward performing the behavior and supportive subjective norms, and proceeding to behavior through behavioral intentions (cf. Ajzen, 1991; Fishbein & Ajzen, 1975). The association between intention and behavior, however, is relatively weak in adolescence, a time when many risk behaviors are initiated, but it increases with age (Albarracín, Johnson, Fishbein & Muellerleile, 2001).

The model proposes an additional path to health risk behavior, which involves neither planning nor intentions. This *social reaction path* reflects the fact that adolescents often find themselves in social situations that facilitate (but do not demand) risky behaviors such as drinking, smoking, or unprotected sex. Once in these situations, it is often not their intentions to engage in the behaviors, but their willingness to take a risk that determines their actions. Thus, *behavioral willingness* is defined as a person's openness to risk opportunity, an inclination to engage in certain unintended behaviors when circumstances permit or promote it (e.g., "Suppose you were at a party and there were some drugs available, how willing would you be to try some?"). Hence, it is a reaction rather than a planned (or "reasoned") action. Expressing willingness, therefore, is an acknowledgement that under certain circumstances, one might engage in a risk behavior that was previously not intended or (perhaps) not even considered. Willingness has been shown to predict a variety of risk behaviors, and it does so independent of intention (Gibbons, Gerrard, Blanton & Russell, 1998; Gibbons, Gerrard, Ouellette & Burzette, 1998).

The major antecedent to adolescents' willingness is their risk *prototypes*. These are cognitive representations (or images) of the type of person their age who engages in the specific risk behavior, for example, the "typical" drinker (see Figure 5.2 for an abbreviated version of the model). Assessment of prototypes involves providing research participants with a general definition of prototypes, for instance: "Images are pictures we have in our mind about people and groups. For example, we all have ideas about what

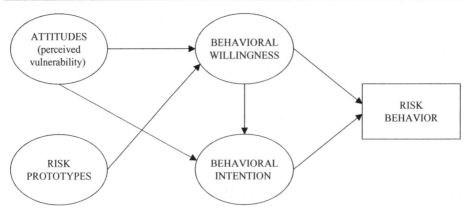

Figure 5.2   The Prototype/Willingness Model

grandmothers are like. We are not saying that all grandmothers are alike, only that some of them are similar in some ways ..." They are then asked to "... think for a minute about the type of person your age who ... [drinks frequently]," and indicate how much each of a list of adjectives describes their image of that person, including smart, confused, popular, immature, "cool" [sophisticated], self-confident, independent, careless, unattractive, dull [boring], considerate, and self-centered.

Young people maintain clear images of the type of person their age who engages in various risk behaviors, and there is general agreement among them as to the characteristics associated with these prototypes (e.g., independence, rebelliousness). Because of this social consensus, adolescents realize that if they were to engage in the behaviors in public, they would acquire aspects of the image themselves; they would be seen by others as being a drinker, smoker, etc. In this sense, the images are social consequences of the behavior. The more favorable the adolescent's risk image, the more willing he or she is to accept these consequences by engaging in the behavior and/or affiliating with others who do. Prospective research on adolescents' prototypes (of drinkers, smokers, reckless drivers, etc.), their willingness to engage in the risk behaviors, and their subsequent behavior has demonstrated these links (see Gibbons, Gerrard & Lane, 2003, for a review).

Two Types of Processing

Like Leventhal's Common Sense Model (Leventhal, 1970; Leventhal, Brissette & Leventhal, 2003), a core assumption in the prototype model is that the reasoned and social reaction paths are associated with different types of cognitive processing. The reasoned path is characterized by relatively deliberative, analytic reasoning similar to that outlined in expectancy value models (e.g., Protection Motivation Theory, Theory of Reasoned Action). The social reaction path, however, has elements of heuristic processing outlined by dual-process models of self-regulation (see Gibbons et al.,

2003, for a more complete discussion of this issue). More specifically, the social reaction path is image-based in that it is linked to adolescents' perceptions of what peers who engage in risk behavior are like. These images prompt, and, therefore are influential through a social comparison process, the self vis-à-vis the image or prototype (i.e., "Am I the type of person who ...?").

In addition, there is evidence of truncated processing with regard to consideration of potential risks associated with specific behaviors (Gibbons, Gerrard, Ouellette et al., 1998). Evidence of the different types of processing involved in the reasoned versus reactive paths can be seen in a study by Gerrard, Gibbons, Reis-Bergan, Trudeau, Vande Lune & Buunk (2002), which assessed both the drinker and *non-drinker* (abstainer) images of adolescents across 3 annual waves (age 16 at T1). The adolescents were also asked direct questions about the amount they had thought about each type of image: for instance, "How often have you thought about this type of person?" The assumption was that the drinker image would involve more heuristic or experiential processing, whereas the non-drinker image would involve more systematic or reasoned processing. More generally, we assumed that, relatively speaking, health promotion involves more reasoned processing, whereas health risk involves more reactive or heuristic processing.

The data fit the pattern outlined by the prototype model, and thus, expanded it by providing a more complete picture of the processes by which images influence behavior. Specifically, results replicated previous research suggesting that favorable risk images are associated with avoidance of thoughts about potential physical dangers (Gibbons, Gerrard, Ouellette, et al., 1998), and demonstrated that risk and non-risk images influence behavior via very different processes. Unlike risk images (e.g., the typical smoker), non-risk images operate through a relatively reasoned or contemplative path, similar to that outlined by earlier prototype matching studies (Mosbach & Leventhal, 1988). That is, (some) adolescents think about positive social consequences associated with these non-risk images, and this consideration is associated with lower levels of willingness to engage in risk behavior when opportunities arise, and subsequently with less risk behavior. In short, risk images appear to influence risk behavior via a social reaction process whereas non-risk images inhibit risk behavior via a more contemplative process.

Risk Prototypes as Goals?

The prototype model suggests that risk images (e.g., the image of the typical smoker) represent the social consequences of the behavior: "If I smoke, I will be seen by others as being like other smokers my age." Thus, the favorability of the image determines whether an adolescent smokes when an opportunity arises. The original model, however, did not directly address the extent to which adolescents are motivated to acquire the characteristics associated with these images. In other words, are these images positive enough to represent goals for adolescents? Gerrard, Gibbons, Reis-Bergan et al., (2002) also addressed this question in that drinkers and abstainers had less favorable images of drinkers than of non-drinkers. Furthermore, drinkers' and abstainers' images of drinkers

Table 5.1   Adolescent abstainers' and drinkers' prototypes and self images

	Abstainers	Drinkers	Between-group t
Drinker Prototype	3.67	4.04	3.66*
Non-drinker Prototype	5.29^a	4.84^a	5.08*
Self Image	5.10^{ab}	5.09^{ab}	0.23
Ideal Self	6.25^{ab}	6.25^{ab}	0.04

Data from Gerrard, Gibbons, Reis-Bergan et al., 2002; all scales = 1–7 with high numbers reflecting positive ratings;
^{a}Significantly different from drinker prototypes, $p < 0.01$;
^{b}Significantly different from non-drinker prototypes, $p < 0.01$.

were significantly less favorable than their images of themselves and their ideal-selves (see Table 5.1).

Thus, it appears that the non-drinker image has some of the characteristics of a goal for those who abstain, and also (to a lesser extent) for those who drink. In contrast, the drinker image was not correlated with the drinkers' self images, or ideal selves. In addition, the data revealed an unexpected direct, negative path from favorable non-drinker image to subsequent consumption that was not mediated by willingness or contemplation of the image. This path suggests that for some adolescents, these (negative) non-drinker images may be so well established that they inhibit subsequent risk behavior without further contemplation of the social consequences of the behavior.

Differential Influence of Intentions and Willingness over Time

Like most dual-processing models, the Prototype/Willingness Model maintains that both processing modes continue throughout the life span, but that the ratio of heuristic to analytic processing tends to decrease with age (Chen & Chaiken, 1999; Epstein & Pacini, 1999; however, see Reyna, 2004). In other words, adolescents are more likely than adults to respond in an experiential or heuristic manner. Our model also argues that this is particularly true when it comes to enticing but dangerous activities such as substance use and risky sex. The data appear to support this. A recently completed analysis of 7 annual waves of panel data from adolescents who were 13 or 14 at Wave 1 revealed that willingness was a better predictor of smoking and change in smoking than was intention up to age 16 (Pomery, Gibbons, Gerrard & Reis-Bergan, 2006). From age 16 up to about 18, expectation became a better predictor than willingness as the behavior became more intentional. By age 18 or 19, previous behavior, which was controlled in all analyses, became the dominant predictor as the behaviors became habitual. Content analyses (ongoing) of open-ended responses by these adolescents also suggest that willingness is associated with more heuristic processing that slowly gives way to more analytic reasoning, and that is true for reasoning about engaging as well as not engaging in the behavior.

All of the relations outlined in Figure 5.2 have been documented in a series of studies over the last decade (see Gibbons et al., 2003, for a review). Briefly, research on substance use has demonstrated that adolescents' images of the type of person who uses substances predict their willingness to use substances, and that these images and willingness have been linked with changes in substance use (Blanton, Gibbons, Gerrard, Conger & Smith, 1997; Gerrard, Gibbons, Stock, Vande Lune & Cleveland, 2005; Ouellette, Gerrard, Gibbons & Reis-Bergan, 1999). Early prospective research on caucasian American adolescents' prototypes of drinkers, willingness to drink, and subsequent alcohol consumption also supported these assumptions (Blanton et al., 1997). More recent research has demonstrated that the model is also useful in explaining the behavior of African American adolescents and pre-adolescents (Cleveland, Gibbons, Gerrard, & Pomery, 2005; Gerrard et al. in press).

POOR SELF-CONTROL AND WILLINGNESS

As indicated above, adolescent behavior can follow either the social reaction pathway, characterized by a lack of premeditation about consequences, or the reasoned pathway, characterized by more deliberative or analytic processing that includes some consideration of consequences. It appears that the behavior of adolescents high in poor self-control is more reactive: their behavior is more likely to be influenced by circumstances and events surrounding them. Adolescents who are high in good self-control, however, are more likely to think ahead about risk-conducive situations, anticipate problems and opportunities, and consider possible behavioral options (see Gibbons et al., this volume). Thus, we would expect that adolescents with high poor self-control would be more predisposed toward the social reaction path, whereas those with high good self-control should be more inclined toward the reasoned path. Data from one of our ongoing studies of African American families, the Family and Community Health Study (FACHS), are relevant to this question. (For a description of the sample, measures, and procedures of FACHS, see Gerrard et al., 2005; Gibbons, Gerrard, Cleveland, Wills & Brody, 2004.)

Willingness as a Proximal Mediator of the Poor Self-Control to Risk Behavior Link

Analysis of data from the older siblings in FACHS (African American 15-year-olds) examined relations between good and poor self-control, prototype favorability, resistance efficacy, and willingness related to substance use (alcohol, drugs, and tobacco). In this analysis, resistance efficacy was defined as a lack of willingness to take advantage of a risk-conducive situation. Poor self-control was positively correlated with favorable risk prototypes and willingness, and negatively correlated with the non-risk prototype (image of the typical young person who does not use substances). In contrast, good self-control was positively correlated with the favorability of the non-risk prototype and resistance efficacy. It was negatively correlated with favorable risk prototypes and willingness to use substances. The relation between these adolescents' willingness and their substance use was significantly stronger for those who were high in poor self-control. In addition, adolescents with high poor self-control appear to have more willingness than those with low poor self-control or those with high good self-control, suggesting that willingness is more likely to translate into use among adolescents who are high in poor self-control. Additional analyses examined whether poor self-control was a moderator of the relation between willingness and escalation in substance use. The pattern was as predicted: the relation between willingness and use was significantly stronger for those adolescents who were high in poor self-control. These analyses, then, suggested that self-regulation theory and the prototype model are not only compatible, but that behavioral willingness is a likely candidate as a proximal mediator of the relation between self-control and behavior.

A structural equation model (SEM) of these data provided further evidence that the effects of self-control on risk behavior are indirect rather than direct, and that willingness is an important proximal mediator of this relation (Wills et al., 2003). More specifically, this analysis revealed a direct and positive path between good self-control and resistance in situations conducive to using substances. It also demonstrated that resistance mediated the relation between good self-control and substance use. It is worth noting that these findings existed controlling for religion, temperament, risk-taking, parents' education, parent-child relationship, and parent-child communication.

A more recent study with a different sample of African American youth has provided additional and stronger evidence that the relation between self-control and risk behavior is mediated by willingness (Wills et al., 2006). This study examined the relation between self-control, willingness, and two risk behaviors, unprotected sex and substance use, among 11-year-old African American youth in the Strong African American Families Project (SAAF; a family-based, universal preventive intervention for ten-year-old African American children based in part on the prototype model.) The data for this paper were collected as part of a pre-intervention battery before the children were assigned to either an early alcohol intervention or a control group. The analyses included separate SEMs predicting substance use and sexual behavior. The model of the substance use data revealed a direct and negative relation between good self-control and willingness to use substances (cigarettes, marijuana, and alcohol). In addition, willingness mediated the relation between good self-control and substance use. The model on the sexual behavior data revealed a direct positive relation between poor self-control and willingness to have unprotected sex, and a weaker indirect negative relation between good self-control and willingness. Consistent with the substance use analyses, willingness mediated the influence of good and poor self-control on unprotected sex.

Contemplation of Consequences

A number of theorists have suggested that one of the characteristics that differentiates good and poor self-regulation in general, and good and poor self-control in particular, is the ability to engage in deliberative responding and consideration of potential negative consequences of behavior. Thus, it is not surprising that the reasoned and reactive paths of the prototype model involve different types of cognitive processing; the reasoned path from non-risk prototypes to willingness is associated with contemplation of the social consequences of engaging in the behavior (the nature of the risk prototype), and the social reaction path from risk prototypes to willingness is not (Gerrard, Gibbons, Reis-Bergan et al., 2002). Recent analyses of FACHS data have revealed similar differences in thinking about another kind of consequence, the potential riskiness of the behavior, as reflected in the item: "How much do concerns about your health and safety influence your behavior." These analyses indicated that adolescents who were high in good self-control were more likely to report that they typically consider health and safety issues when deciding whether to engage in a risky behavior, and this consideration, in turn, led to lower risk willingness. Those who were high in poor self-control were much less influenced by consideration of health and safety, and their willingness was not related to such concerns. In short, these differences demonstrate a key distinction between adolescents who have developed self-regulatory skills and those who have not: an ability to think about the potential consequences of their behavior.

Summary

The distinctions between adolescents high in poor self-control and those high in good self-control appear to be consistent with distinctions between the reasoned and social reaction paths in the prototype model. In particular, those high in poor self-control have more favorable images of peers who engage in risk behavior, are more responsive to social influences, and are less likely to think about the social and physical consequences of their behavior than are those high in good self-control. These similarities between good self-control and the reasoned path, and poor self-control and the social reaction path, suggest an individual difference perspective on the Prototype Model that has not been explored before. Thus, they raise a number of important questions about the relations between the Epigenetic Model (based on individual differences), models of self-regulation, and the prototype model that have only been hinted at in prior research. For example, is temperament a distal antecedent to behavioral willingness? Given that willingness is not redundant with good or poor self-control, is it a proximal mediator of the relation between self-regulation and subsequent risk behavior? How does willingness relate to the third self-regulatory trait, risk-taking? In other words, how does behavioral willingness fit into Epigenetic Theory?

BEHAVIORAL WILLINGNESS AND THE EPIGENETIC MODEL

A Cross-sectional Analysis

As noted above, several analyses (cf. Wills et al., 2003) have explored the relation between self-control and elements of the prototype model. Only one published paper, however, has directly addressed the relations between temperament, self-regulation, and behavioral willingness (Wills, Gibbons, et al., 2000). In this study SEM was employed to examine the relation between temperament, all three components of self-regulation and hypothesized mediators on the one hand, and willingness to use and resist substance use on the other. The paths of interest to us here are those that link temperament (protective and difficult) to self-regulation (good and poor self-control, risk taking), and those that link self-regulation to willingness and resistance. The sample was the FACHS younger siblings at wave 1 (mean age 10.5).

In this model, the paths from temperament to self-regulation were as predicted by Epigenetic Theory: good self-control was predicted by task orientation and positive emotionality, (low) activity level and negative emotionality; poor self-control was predicted by activity level and negative emotionality; risk taking was predicted by activity level. Consistent with other analyses of our data, willingness was predicted by risk-taking, (high) poor self-control, and (low) good self-control, and resistance was predicted by risk taking and poor self-control. Thus, this model provided evidence that temperament is related to willingness, and that this relation is mediated by good and poor self-control, and risk-taking. In other words, this cross-sectional model suggests that temperament is associated with the development of self-regulation, which in turn is linked to behavioral willingness, and to subsequent risk behavior.

A Prospective Analysis

Since the Wills, Gibbons, et al. (2000) article was published, we have collected two additional waves of FACHS data that have allowed us to expand our exploration of this individual difference perspective on the development of willingness employing a prospective analysis. Thus, we have extended the model reported in the Wills et al. paper to test the hypothesis that temperament in middle childhood predicts pre-teen self-regulation, which in turn, predicts risk behavior at age 15, and that willingness mediates the relation between self-regulation and subsequent risk behavior. This analysis was conducted on the younger FACHS participants who had not used substances at wave 1 (N = 621). It used the same measures of temperament employed in the Wills et al. paper, plus the adolescents' self-reports of smoking, drinking, and drug use. The temperament variables were assessed at age 10–11, self-regulation and willingness were measured approximately two years later, and substance use was assessed at age 15. This analysis was a more direct test of the hypothesis that willingness mediates the self-regulation to behavior path than the Wills et al. model because they covered 4–5 years of the participants' development.

This analysis replicated all but one of the previous paths between temperament and self-regulation: the path between negative emotionality and poor self-control (see Figure 5.3). It also provided more evidence that the dimensions of self-regulation and willingness are not redundant, and replicated the previous paths from good self-control and risk-taking to willingness. More important, this model supported the hypothesis that the paths from good self-control and risk-taking to subsequent substance use were mediated by willingness to use substances; the path from good self-control was totally mediated and that from risk-taking was partially mediated. In addition, a second model that included participants who had and had not used substances, and controlled for wave 1 use, was not significantly different in spite of a direct (stability) path from wave 1 substance use to wave 3 substance use.

These studies provide evidence that there are conceptual parallels between the role of self-regulation in Epigenetic Theory and the reasoned and social reaction paths in the prototype model. In addition, it appears that a combination of the two models can be

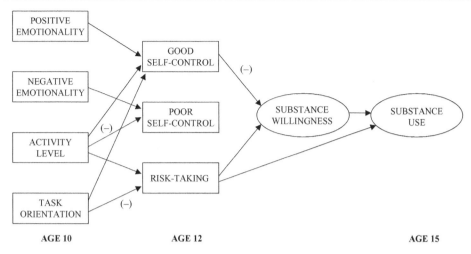

Figure 5.3 The Epigenetic Model predicting substance use with mediation by willingness

used to explain the developmental paths to adolescent health and risk behaviors more completely. More specifically, temperament is antecedent to the development of self-control, which is associated with favorability of risk images and willingness to take advantage of risk-conducive situations. Good and poor self-control are associated with differences in behavior patterns and cognitive processing that are central elements of the social reaction versus the reasoned pathways of the prototype model. Finally, behavioral willingness is a more proximal mediator of the relation between self-regulation and risk behavior. The question, then, is what are the implications of such a combination of theoretical approaches? Do the parallels between the models change our thinking about Epigenetic Theory? Or the prototype model? Are there practical implications of combining these two theoretical approaches?

THEORETICAL IMPLICATIONS

There are two ways in which the current research suggests that it could be productive to apply an individual difference perspective to the Prototype/Willingness Model. First, a number of analyses have provided support for the parallels between the type of responses evinced by adolescents who are high in good and poor self-control, and the responses associated with the social reaction and reasoned paths in the model. Adolescents who are high in good self-control tend to be planful and deliberative, and, therefore, are more likely to focus on future consequences. Thus, their processing is more typical of the reasoned path to risk than the social reaction path. In contrast, high poor self-control is associated with less deliberation and consideration of consequences, and being more responsive to social and environmental factors. These differences suggest that prototype perceptions and behavioral willingness may be influenced by individual differences, a perspective that is not incompatible with the prototype model, and has been implicit in previous research, but one which has not previously been an explicit part of the model.

Data linking early temperament to prototypes and willingness also suggest the utility of applying an individual difference perspective to these risk cognitions, and raise a question about genetic and environmental factors that might influence adolescents' cognitive processing related to risk behavior. More specifically, the prototype model maintains that adolescents generally find risky behaviors such as alcohol use and unprotected sex to be enticing, but it recognizes that they are aware that these behaviors are associated with potential social and health costs (Gerrard, Gibbons, Benthin & Hessling, 1996; Gerrard & Luus, 1995). The model also suggests that there are two primary differences between the social reaction and reasoned pathways. The first has to do with the amount of precontemplation of the behavior and its outcomes; the social reaction path is character-ized by a lack of attention to these negative cognitions whereas the reasoned path includes them. The second is that experiential (image-based) or reactive processing (as outlined by dual-process models of self-regulation) is linked to adolescents' perceptions of peers who engage in specific risk behaviors, and is more likely than reasoned processing to predict risk behavior. In part, this is the result of truncated processing with regard to the potential risks associated with behaviors. Several studies have supported this contention by demonstrating that willingness is associated with avoidance of consideration of risk, which, in turn, leads to unrealistic and a superficially-considered sense of personal immunity (e.g., Gerrard, Gibbons, Vande Lune, Pexa & Gano, 2002; Gibbons, Gerrard, Ouellette et al., 1998). Poor self-control is associated with the same pattern of cognitive processing: reactive rather than proactive responding to environmental stimuli, greater emotionality in responding and susceptibility to social influence, and reduced ability/ willingness to consider future consequences of current actions. Thus, given the clear association between temperament and self-control, it would be wise to explore the possibility that the tendency to avoid consideration of potential risks and have an optimistic bias regarding vulnerability is also linked to individual differences that are constitutional, or represent gene X environment interactions. More specifically, are differences associated with adolescents' willingness to engage in risk behaviors and their ability to regulate their own behavior, associated with genetic predispositions and moderated by environmental influence?

PRACTICAL IMPLICATIONS

Even though temperament is relatively stable over time, there are several reasons to expect that both self-control and the cognitions associated with adolescents' risk behaviors can be changed, and that these changes can influence risk behavior. Primary among these is existing research indicating that adolescents' and young adults' prototypes and willingness are malleable, and that altering them is related to subsequent behavior change. The second reason is that research suggests that parents can play an active role in the development of their children's self-control (Wills et al., 2001; Wills, Windle & Cleary, 1998; Wills, Sandy et al., 2000), and their risk and non-risk cognitions (Blanton et al., 1997; Gerrard, Gibbons, Zhao, Russell & Reis-Bergan, 1999; Ouellette et al., 1999).

Manipulating Image Favorability and Behavioral Willingness

Several lab and field studies have demonstrated the applied utility of the prototype model. These studies have provided evidence of the malleability of risk and non-risk prototypes, and the beneficial effects of prototype alteration. For example, Blanton et al. (2001; Study 4) presented college students with bogus survey results indicating that people who use condoms were perceived as less selfish and more responsible than those who do not. As expected, the students who read this information reported significantly less willingness to engage in casual sex than did those who had not read the material. Similarly, a second study demonstrated that willingness to engage in casual sex increases when sexually permissive individuals (prototypes) are described in positive terms (Gibbons, Stock, Gerrard, Dykstra, Mahler, Eggleston & Kulik 2006). Another series of studies has demonstrated the efficacy of interventions designed to change behavior by manipulating prototypes. In one of these studies, college students, many of whom were using tanning booths, were shown ultraviolet (UV) photographs of their faces, which revealed the underlying skin damage they had already sustained from UV exposure, damage that is not visible to the naked eye (Gibbons, Gerrard, Lane, Mahler & Kulik, 2005). Viewing this damage was associated with a significant decline in attitudes toward tanning, including favorability of the prototype of the typical tanned person, and willingness to tan. This change, in turn, predicted decreases in tanning in the next three to four weeks.

The most persuasive evidence of the impact of altering prototypes, however, comes from research on SAAF, our family-based intervention program intended to change children's prototypes and willingness, and thereby prevent or delay onset of alcohol use and abuse among African American adolescents (Gerrard et al., in press). The theoretical basis for the intervention included the prototype model, previous research by Brody and Murry on the protective aspects of regulated and supportive home environments (Brody, Flor & Gibson, 1999; Brody et al., 2004; Brody, Stoneman & Flor, 1996), and Wills and colleagues' research on the role of temperament and self-control in early substance use (Wills et al., 2001; Wills, Sandy et al., 2000; Wills & Stoolmiller, 2002). Findings from these three lines of research were translated into a seven-session curriculum intended (among other things) to: (a) demonstrate that youths generally associate more negative than positive characteristics with early drinkers, and to identify and reinforce the participants' negative images of young drinkers, (b) convey the distinction between intentional and willingness-based behavior, and degrees of willingness, (c) promote recognition of risk-conducive situations and the formation of plans to avoid such situations, and (d) correct participants' misperceptions that their peers hold favorable images of young drinkers. In addition, SAAF was designed to facilitate contemplation of the consequences of drinking and consideration of potential responses to risk-conducive situations. The program has been successful. Controlling for pre-test assessments, post-test drinker prototypes are more negative, non-drinker images are more positive, and willingness is significantly lower in the intervention than the control condition at a 24-month follow-up. More important, as the prototype model would predict, there was significantly less alcohol use by the intervention group, and changes in drinker images mediated changes in willingness and behavior. (For more detail about the curriculum see Brody et al., 2004; Murry et al., 2005; Wills et al., 2006).

Parenting and Epigenetic Theory

The SAAF data also provided evidence of the prototype model's dual-process hypothesis by demonstrating mediation of intervention effects through both the social reaction and the reasoned/intention paths. More specifically, in addition to altering the favorability of drinker prototypes and thereby changing willingness to drink, the intervention was designed to increase parental involvement, monitoring, and communication about alcohol. The hypothesis was that increasing these parenting behaviors would effect a change in the children's intentions to drink, rather than their willingness to drink. Thus, the study was designed to alter the social reaction path to alcohol use by altering prototypes and willingness, and to alter the reasoned path by altering parental behaviors, and childrens' intentions. The data supported the hypothesis: The intervention was successful in changing parenting, and changes in parenting mediated the effect of the intervention on changes in the children's intentions to drink. In addition, these changes were linked to changes in consumption 29 months later (when the children were 13 or 14), independent of the changes in prototypes and willingness. Thus, the study provided further evidence that these two processes are independent, but complementary, and demonstrated the efficacy of a dual-process approach; one that strives to reduce reactive behavior and to facilitate reasoned behavior. In addition, however, this study provides evidence of the applicability of the dual-process approach to Epigenetic Theory.

CONCLUSION

It is not surprising that a number of epigenetic studies have demonstrated that parents can play an active role in the development of their children's self-control and subsequent behavior (Wills, Blechman & McNamara, 1996; Wills, Sandy et al., 2000). The relation between children's temperament, their development of self-regulatory skills, the parenting they receive, and their risk behavior, however, is complex. Wills and Dishion (2004) suggest that children with easy and affectionate dispositions elicit very different kinds of parenting than do those with difficult temperaments. In addition, parenting can moderate the effects of children's temperaments on self-control, making some children more or less resilient than would be predicted by their temperament, that is, parenting can facilitate the process of learning self-control (Barkley, 1997; Dishion & Patterson, in press; Rothbart & Bates, 1998). Thus, a child's temperament can elicit a specific kind of parenting (cf. Rothbart & Ahadi, 1994), and parenting can affect how temperament is translated into self-regulation (Wills, Cleary, et al., 2001).

Parenting can also moderate the relation between temperament and children's images of peers who engage in risk behaviors. For example, parents' behavior (e.g., drinking) and the nature of the parent-child relationship (e.g., communication of values and expectations regarding drinking) can facilitate or inhibit the formation of strong, favorable non-risk images and unfavorable risk images. This influence can have effects that the children carry with them and maintain long after other (more direct) methods of parental influence (e.g., monitoring) are no longer viable (Gibbons et al., 2003). The goals of family-based interventions, however, are often limited to facilitating parents' involvement in strengthening youths' intentions to avoid risk behavior through teaching monitoring and clear communication of expectations and rules (Tobler et al., 2000). The SAAF intervention suggests that family-based interventions can be more effective when they are informed by the complex nature of the relations between temperament, self-control, parenting, and the more reactive, less contemplative proximal antecedents of risk behavior. Furthermore, it suggests that because of the complex nature of the relation between temperament, parenting, self-control, and both the social reaction and the reasoned path to adolescent risk behaviors, interventions should be informed by further research on the interaction between temperament and parenting factors, and both the social reaction and reasoned paths to risk behavior. In sum, although there is clearly a need for more research on how risk cognitions develop in adolescence (Beyth-Marom & Fischhoff, 1997), and the processes by which they influence behavior, these interventions provide encouraging evidence of the utility of altering health cognitions that can directly or indirectly translate into more healthy behavior among adolescents.

REFERENCES

Ajzen, I. (1991). The theory of planned behavior. *Organizational behavior and human decision processes*, *50*, 179–211.

Albarracín, D., Johnson, B.T., Fishbein, M. & Muellerleile, P.A. (2001). Theories of reasoned action and planned behavior as models of condom use: A meta-analysis. *Psychological Bulletin*, *127*, 142–161.

Allport, G.W. (1961). *Pattern and Growth in Personality*. New York: Holt, Rinehart and Winston.

Barkley, R.A. (1997). Behavioral inhibition, sustained attention, and self-control functions: Constructing a unifying theory of ADHD. *Psychological Bulletin*, *121*, 65–94.

Beyth-Marom, R., & Fischhoff, B. (1997). Adolescents' decisions about risks: A cognitive perspective. In J. Schulenberg, J.L. Maggs & K. Hurrelmann (Eds), *Health Risks and Developmental Transitions during Adolescence* (pp. 110–135). New York: Cambridge University Press.

Blanton, H., Van den Eijnden, R.J.J.M., Buunk, B.P., Gibbons, F.X., Gerrard, M. & Bakker, A. (2001). Accentuate the Negative: Social Images in the Prediction and Promotion of Condom Use. *Journal of Applied Social Psychology*, *31*, 274–295.

Blanton, H., Gibbons, F.X., Gerrard, M., Conger, K.J. & Smith, G.E. (1997). Development of health risk prototypes during adolescence: Family and peer influence. *Journal of Family Psychology*, *11*, 271–288.

Block, J.H. & Block, J. (1980). The role of ego-control and ego-resiliency in the organization of behavior. In W.A. Collins (Ed.), *Minnesota Symposium on Child Psychology*, (Vol. 13, pp. 39–101). Hillsdale, NJ: Erlbaum.

Braungart, J.M., Plomin, R., DeFries, J.C. & Fulker, D.W. (1992). Genetic influence on tester-rated infant temperament as assessed by Bayley's Infant Behavior Record: Nonadoptive and adoptive siblings and twins. *Developmental Psychology*, *28*, 40–47.

Brody, G.H., Flor, D.L. & Gibson, N.M. (1999). Linking maternal efficacy beliefs, developmental goals, parenting practices, and child competence in rural single-parent African-American families. *Child Development*, *70*, 1197–1208.

Brody, G.H., Murry, V.M., Gerrard, M., Gibbons, F.X., Molgaard, V., NcNair, L., Brown, A.C., Wills, T.A., Spoth, R.L. Luo, Z., Chen, Y. & Neubaum-Carlan, E. (2004). The Strong African American Families Program: Translating research into prevention programming. *Child Development*, *75*, 900–917.

Brody, G.H., Stoneman, Z. & Flor, D. (1996). Parental religiosity, family processes, and youth competence in rural, two-parent African-American families. *Developmental Psychology, 32,* 696–706.

Buss, A.H. & Plomin, R. (1975). *A Temperament Theory of Personality Development.* New York: John Wiley & Sons, Inc.

Buss, A.H. & Plomin, R. (1984). *Temperament: Early Developing Personality Traits.* Hillsdale, NJ: Erlbaum.

Cervone, D., Mor, N., Orom, H., Shadel, W.G. & Scott, W.D. (2004). Self-efficacy beliefs on the architecture of personality: On knowledge, appraisal, and self-regulation. In R.F. Baumeister & K.D. Vohs (Eds), *Handbook of Self-regulation: Research, theory, and applications* (pp. 188–210). New York: Guilford.

Chassin, L.A., Pillow, D.R., Curran, P.J., Molina, B. & Barrera, M. (1993). Relation of parental alcoholism to early adolescent substance use: A test of three mediating mechanisms. *Journal of Abnormal Psychology, 102,* 3–19.

Chen, S. & Chaiken, S. (1999). The heuristic-systematic model in its broader context. In S. Chaiken & Y. Trope (Eds), *Dual-Process Theories in Social Psychology* (pp. 73–96). New York: Guilford.

Cleveland, M.J., Gibbons, F.X., Gerrard, M. & Pomery, E.A. (2005). The impact of parenting on risk cognitions and risk behavior: A study of mediation in a panel of African American adolescents. *Child Development, 76,* 1–17.

Dishion, T.J. & Patterson, G.R. (in press). The development and ecology of antisocial behavior. In D. Cicchetti & D.J. Cohen (Eds), *Developmental Psychopathology, Vol. 3: Risk, disorder, and adaptation.* New York: John Wiley & Sons, Inc.

Eisenberg, N., Smith, C.L., Sadovsky, A. & Spinrad, T.L. (2004). Effortful control: Relations with emotional regulation, adjustment, and socialization in childhood. In R.F. Baumeister & K.D. Vohs (Eds), *Handbook of Self-regulation: Research, theory, and applications* (pp. 259–282). New York: Guilford.

Emde, R.N., Plomin, R., Robinson, J. & Corley, R. (1992). Temperament, emotion, and cognition at fourteen months: The MacArthur Longitudinal Twin Study. *Child Development, 63,* 1437–1455.

Epstein, S. & Pacini, R. (1999). Some basic issues regarding dual-process theories from the perspective of cognitive-experiential self-theory. In S. Chaiken & Y. Trope (Eds), *Dual-Process Theories in Social Psychology* (pp. 73–96). New York: Guilford.

Fishbein, M. & Ajzen, I. (1975). *Belief, Attitude, Intention, and Behavior: An introduction to theory and research.* Reading, MA: Addison-Wesley.

Fitzsimmons, G.M. & Bargh, J.A. (2004). Automatic self-regulation. In R.F. Baumeister & K.D. Vohs (Eds), *Handbook of Self-regulation: Research, theory, and applications* (pp. 151–170). New York: Guilford.

Gerrard, M., Gibbons, F.X., Brody, G.H., Murry, V.M., Cleveland, M.J. & Wills, T.A. (in press). A Theory-based Dual Focus Alcohol Intervention for Pre-adolescents: The Strong African American Families Program. *Psychology of Addictive Behavior.*

Gerrard, M., Gibbons, F.X., Benthin, A. & Hessling, R.M. (1996). A longitudinal study of the reciprocal nature of risk behaviors and cognitions in adolescents: What you do shapes what you think and vice versa. *Health Psychology, 15,* 344–354.

Gerrard, M., Gibbons, F.X., Reis-Bergan, M., Trudeau, L., Vande Lune, L.S. & Buunk, B. (2002). Inhibitory effects of drinker and nondrinker prototypes on adolescent alcohol consumption. *Health Psychology, 21,* 601–609.

Gerrard, M., Gibbons, F.X., Stock, M.L., Vande Lune, L.S. & Cleveland, M.J. (2005). Images of Smokers and Willingness to Smoke among African American Pre-adolescents: An Application of the Prototype/Willingness Model of Adolescent Health Risk Behavior to Smoking Initiation. *Pediatric Psychology, 30,* 305–313.

Gerrard, M., Gibbons, F.X., Vande Lune, L.S., Pexa, N.A. & Gano, M.L. (2002). Adolescents' substance-related risk perceptions: Antecedents, mediators, and consequences. *Risk Decision and Policy, 7,* 175–191.

Gerrard, M., Gibbons, F.X., Zhao, L., Russell, D.W. & Reis-Bergan, M. (1999). The effects of peers' alcohol consumption on parental influence: A cognitive mediational model. *Journal of Studies on Alcohol, 13,* 32–44.

Gerrard, M. & Luus, C.A.E. (1995). Judgments of vulnerability to pregnancy: The role of risk factors and individual differences. *Personality and Social Psychology Bulletin, 21,* 160–171.

Gibbons, F.X., Gerrard, M., Blanton, H. & Russell, D.W. (1998). Reasoned action and social reaction: Willingness and intention as independent predictors of health risk. *Journal of Personality and Social Psychology, 74,* 1164–1181.

Gibbons, F.X., Gerrard, M., Cleveland, M.J., Wills, T.A. & Brody, G. (2004). Perceived discrimination and substance use in African American parents and their children: A panel study. *Journal of Personality & Social Psychology, 86,* 517–529.

Gibbons, F.X., Gerrard, M. & Lane, D.J. (2003). A social reaction model of adolescent health risk. In J.M. Suls & K. Wallston (Eds), *Social Psychological Foundations of Health and Illness* (pp. 107–136). Oxford, UK: Blackwell.

Gibbons, F.X., Gerrard, M., Lane, D.J., Mahler, H.I.M. & Kulik, J.A. (2005). Using UV photography to reduce use of tanning booths: A test of cognitive mediation. *Health Psychology, 24,* 358–363.

Gibbons, F.X., Gerrard, M., Ouellette, J.A. & Burzette, T. (1998). Cognitive antecedents to adolescent health risk: Discriminating between behavioral intention and behavior willingness. *Psychology and Health, 13,* 319–339.

Gibbons, F.X., Stock, M.L., Gerrard, M., Dykstra, J.L., Mahler, H.I.M., Eggleston, T.J. & Kulik, J.A. (2006). *Reactance as heuristic responding.* Manuscript preparation.

Goldsmith, H.H., Gottesman, I.I. & Lemery, K.S. (1997). Epigenetic approaches to developmental psychopathology. *Development and Psychopathology, 9,* 365–387.

Hagekull, B. (1989). Longitudinal stability of temperament within a behavioral style framework. In G.A. Kohnstamm, J.E. Bates & M.K. Rothbart (Eds), *Temperament in Childhood* (pp. 283–297). New York: John Wiley & Sons, Inc.

Jessor, R. & Jessor, S. (1977). *Problem Behavior and Psychosocial Development.* New York: Academic Press.

Kochanska, G., Murray, K.T. & Harlan, E.T. (2000). Effortful control in early childhood: Continuity and change, antecedents, and implications for social development. *Developmental Psychology, 36,* 220–232.

Lerner, J.V. & Vicary, J.R. (1984). Difficult temperament and drug use. *Journal of Drug Education, 14,* 1–8.

Leventhal, H. (1970). Findings and theory in the study of fear communications. *Advances in Experimental Social Psychology, 5,* 119–186.

Leventhal, H., Brissette, I. & Leventhal, E.A. (2003). The common-sense model of self-regulation of health and illness. In L.D. Cameron & H. Leventhal (Eds), *The Self-Regulation of Health and Illness Behavior* (pp. 42–65). New York: Routledge.

McCabe, L.A., Cunnington, M. & Brooks-Gunn, J. (2004). The development of self-regulation in young children: Individual characteristics and environmental contests. In R.F. Baumeister & K.D. Vohs (Eds), *Handbook of self-regulation: Research, theory, and applications* (pp. 357–372). New York: Guilford.

Mischel, W. & Ayduk, O. (2004). Willpower in a cognitive-affective processing system: The dynamics of delay of gratification. In R.F. Baumeister & K.D. Vohs (Eds), *Handbook of Self-regulation: Research, theory, and applications* (pp. 99–129). New York: Guilford.

Moffitt, T.E. (1993). The neuropsychology of conduct disorder. *Development and Psychopathology, 5,* 135–151.

Mosbach, P. & Leventhal, H. (1988). Peer group identification and smoking. *Journal of Abnormal Psychology*, 97, 238–245.

Murry, V.M., Brody, G.H., McNair, L.D., Lu, Z., Gibbons, F.X., Gerrard, M. & Wills, T.A. (2005). Promoting self-pride and sexual self-concept among rural African American pre-adolescents through the Strong African American Families Program. *Journal of Marriage and the Family*, 67, 627–642.

Ouellette, J.A., Gerrard, M., Gibbons, F.X. & Reis-Bergan, M. (1999). Parents, peers, and prototypes: Antecedents of adolescent alcohol expectancies, alcohol consumption, and alcohol-related life problems in rural youth. *Psychology of Addictive Behaviors*, 13, 183–197.

Pedlow, R., Sanson, A., Prior, M. & Oberklaid, F. (1993). Stability of maternally reported temperament from infancy to 8 years. *Developmental Psychology*, 29, 998–1007.

Pomery, E.A., Gibbons, F.X., Gerrard, M. & Reis-Bergan, M. (2006). *Experience as a moderator of the developmental shift from willingness to intentions*. Unpublished manuscript.

Reyna, V. (2004). How people make decisions that involve risk: A dual-process approach. *Current Directions in Psychological Science*, **13**, 60–66.

Rothbart, M.K. (1987). A psychobiological approach to the study of temperament. In G. Kohnstamm (Ed.), *Temperament Discussed* (pp. 63–72). Amsterdam: Swetz & Zeitlinger.

Rothbart, M.K. & Bates, J.E. (1998). Temperament. In W. Damon (Series Ed.) & N. Eisenberg (Vol. Ed), *Handbook of Child Psychology, Vol. 3: Social, Emotional, and Personality Development*, (5th edn, pp. 105–176). New York: John Wiley & Sons, Inc.

Rothbart, M.K. & Ahadi, S.A. (1994). Temperament and the development of personality. *Journal of Abnormal Psychology*, 103, 55–66.

Rothbart, M.K., Derryberry, D. & Posner, M.J. (1994). A psychobiological approach to the development of temperament. In J.E. Bates & T.D. Wachs (Eds), *Temperament: Individual differences at the interface of biology and behavior* (pp. 83–116). Washington, DC: American Psychological Association.

Scarr, S. (1992). Developmental theories for the 1990s: Development and individual differences. *Child Development*, 63, 1–19.

Tarter, R.E. (1988). Are there inherited behavioral traits that predispose to substance abuse? *Journal of Consulting and Clinical Psychology*, 56, 189–196.

Tarter, R.E., Moss, H.B. & Vanyukov, M.M. (1995). Behavior genetic perspective of alcoholism etiology. In H. Begleiter & B. Kissin (Eds), *Alcohol and Alcoholism* (Vol. 1, pp. 294–326). New York: Oxford University Press.

Tobler, N.S., Roona, M.R., Ochshorn, P., Marshall, D.G., Streke, A.V. & Stackpole, K.M. (2000). School-based adolescent drug prevention programs: 1998 meta-analysis. *Journal of Primary Prevention*, 20, 275–336.

Watson, D. & Clark, L.A. (1984). Negative affectivity: The disposition to experience aversive emotional states. *Psychological Bulletin*, 96, 465–490.

Watson, D. & Tellegen, A. (1985). Toward a consensual structure of mood. *Psychological Bulletin*, 98, 219–235.

Wills, T.A., Blechman, E.A. & McNamara, G. (1996). Family support, coping, and competence. In E.M. Hetherington & E.A. McNamara (Eds), *Stress, Coping, and Resiliency in Children and Families. Family Research Consortium: Advances in family research* (pp. 107–133). Hillsdale, NJ: Erlbaum.

Wills, T.A, Cleary, S., Filer, M. Shinar, O., Mariani, J. & Spera, K. (2001). Temperament related to early-onset substance use: Test of a developmental model. *Prevention Science*, 2, 145–163.

Wills, T.A. & Dishion, T.J. (2004). Temperament and Adolescent Substance Use: A Transactional Analysis of Emerging Self-Control. *Journal of Clinical Child and Adolescent Psychology*, 33, 69–81.

Wills, T.A., DuHamel, K. & Vaccaro, D. (1995). Activity and mood temperament as predictors of adolescent substance use: Test of a self-regulation mediational model. *Journal of Personality and Social Psychology, 68*, 901–916.

Wills, T.A., Gibbons, F.X., Gerrard, M. & Brody, G.H. (2000). Protective and vulnerability processes for early onset of substance use: A test among African-American children. *Health Psychology, 19*, 253–263.

Wills, T.A., Gibbons, F.X., Gerrard, M., Murry, V.M. & Brody, G.H. (2003). Family communication and religiosity related to substance use and sexual behavior in early adolescence: A test for pathways through self-control and prototype perceptions. *Psychology of Addictive Behaviors, 17*, 312–323.

Wills, T.A., Murry, V.M., Brody, G.H., Gibbons, F.X., Gerrard, M. & Walker, C. (2006). *Ethnic pride and self-control related to protective and risk factors: Test of the model for the theoretical Strong African-American Families Program.* Unpublished manuscript.

Wills, T.A., Sandy, J.M. & Yeager, A. (2000). Temperament and adolescent substance use: An epigenetic approach to risk and protection, *Journal of Personality, 68*, 1127–1151.

Wills, T.A. & Stoolmiller, M. (2002). The role of self-control in early escalation of substance use: A time-varying analysis. *Journal of Consulting & Clinical Psychology, 70*, 986–997.

Wills, T. A, Windle, M. & Cleary, S.D. (1998). Temperament and novelty-seeking in adolescent substance use. *Journal of Personality and Social Psychology, 74*, 387–406.

Wills, T.A., Vaccaro, D. & McNamara, G. (1994). Novelty seeking, risk taking, and related constructs as predictors of adolescent substance use: An application of Cloninger's theory. *Journal of Substance Abuse, 6*, 1–20.

Windle, M. (1991). Alcohol use and abuse: Some findings from the national adolescent student health survey, special focus: Alcohol and youth. *Alcohol Health and Research World, 15*, 5–10.

Windle, M. & Lerner, R.M. (1986). The revised dimensions of temperament survey. *Journal of Adolescent Research, 1*, 213–229.

Goal Striving to Achieve Outcomes: Getting Started, Staying on Track, and Letting Go

CHAPTER 6

Implementation Intentions: Strategic Automatization of Goal Striving

Paschal Sheeran, Thomas L. Webb, and Peter M. Gollwitzer

Several theories that have been used to understand the self-regulation of behavior in pursuit of health goals, including the Theory of Planned Behavior (TPB; Ajzen, 1991), Protection Motivation Theory (PMT; Rogers, 1983), the Prototype/Willingness Model (PWM; Gibbons, Gerrard, Blanton & Russell, 1998), Control Theory (Carver & Scheier, 1982), and Social Cognitive Theory (Bandura, 1997), consider the formation of a goal intention as the key act of willing in promoting goal attainment. Goal intentions can be defined as the instructions that people give themselves to perform particular behaviors or to achieve certain desired outcomes (Triandis, 1980) and characteristically are measured by items of the form "I intend to achieve X!" Forming a goal intention serves to end deliberation about behaviors or outcomes and indicates the standard of performance that one has set oneself, one's commitment to the performance, and the amount of time and effort that will be expended during action (Ajzen, 1991; Gollwitzer, 1990; Webb & Sheeran, 2005a).

Although key health behavior theories construe goal intentions as the most important predictor of behavior and goal achievement, at least 3 lines of research indicate that there is often a substantial "gap" between intention and action. First, correlational studies indicate that much of the variance in behavior is not explained by measures of goal intentions. For instance, Sheeran (2002) meta-analyzed 10 previous meta-analyses of correlational research and found that intentions accounted for only 28% of the variance in behavior, on average, across 422 studies. Second, Fife-Schaw, Sheeran and Norman (in press) used statistical simulations to estimate the impact of maximally effective TPB interventions on the likelihood of performing 30 behaviors. Findings indicated that even if participants all had the maximum possible attitude, subjective norm, and perceived behavioral control scores, and thus the highest possible intention scores that could be

Self-regulation in Health Behavior. Edited by Denise T.D. de Ridder and John B.F. de Wit.
© 2006 John Wiley & Sons Ltd.

generated by a TPB intervention, the predicted probability was that 26% of the sample would still fail to translate their intentions into action. Finally, a meta-analysis of the experimental evidence indicates that intention change does not guarantee behavior change. Webb and Sheeran (in press) reviewed 47 intervention studies that generated statistically significant differences in intention scores between treatment versus control participants and subsequently followed up behavior. Findings indicated that the difference in behavior that accrued from successful intention-change interventions was only $d_+ = 0.36$ (equivalent to $R^2 = 0.03$). This is a modest effect size according to Cohen's (1992) criteria.

Evidence indicates that discrepancies between intentions and action arise because people find it difficult to translate their "good" intentions into action, that is, people often fail to do the things that they say they want to do, or fail to avoid doing things that they do not want to do (Orbell & Sheeran, 1998; Sheeran, 2002). A review of health behaviors (e.g., exercise, condom use, cancer screening) indicated that people were successful in enacting their goal intentions only 53% of the time (Sheeran, 2002). Thus, it is accurate to say that the "gap" between intention and action is substantial.

Gollwitzer and Sheeran (in press) pointed out that "good" intentions do not guarantee goal attainment because committing oneself to the pursuit of a particular goal (i.e., forming a respective goal intention) is only the starting point en route to goal completion. The person still must deal effectively with a series of self-regulatory problems in order to attain desired outcomes. Two particular problems that appear to plague strivings for health goals are failures to initiate action ("get started") or to shield an ongoing goal pursuit from unwanted influences ("stay on track") (Gollwitzer & Sheeran, in press; Sheeran, Milne, Webb & Gollwitzer, 2005). Clearly, it would benefit rates of attainment of health goals if there were some means of managing these self-regulatory problems, and thereby "bridging" the intention-behavior gap.

Gollwitzer (1993, 1996, 1999; Gollwitzer, Bayer & McCulloch, 2005; Gollwitzer & Schaal, 1998; Gollwitzer & Sheeran, in press) proposed the strategy of forming *implementation intentions* as a simple and effective tool for dealing with self-regulatory problems in goal striving. In the sections that follow, we define the concept of implementation intentions and describe how this type of planning promotes intention realization. Next, we review evidence concerning the effectiveness of implementation intention formation in promoting health behaviors and assess evidence about explanatory mechanisms. The final sections examine factors that determine the strength of implementation intention effects and offer suggestions for future research.

THE NATURE AND OPERATION OF IMPLEMENTATION INTENTIONS

Implementation intentions are if-then plans that connect good opportunities to act with responses that will be effective in accomplishing one's goals. Whereas goal intentions specify what one wants to do/achieve (i.e., "I intend to perform behavior W in order to obtain outcome X!"), implementation intentions specify the behavior that one will perform in the service of goal achievement and the situational context in which one will enact it (i.e., "If situation Y occurs, then I will initiate goal-directed behavior Z!").

Implementation intentions are subordinate to goal intentions because, whereas a goal intention specifies *what* one will do, an implementation intention spells out the *when*, *where*, and *how* of what one will do.

To form an implementation intention, the person must first identify a response that is instrumental for goal attainment and, second, anticipate a suitable occasion to initiate that response. For example, the person might specify the behavior "order the salad for lunch" and specify a suitable opportunity as "when the waiter takes my order at the café tomorrow" in order to enact the goal intention to eat healthily. Implementation intention formation is the mental act of linking an anticipated critical situation with an effective goal-directed response. An association is formed between mental representations of specified opportunities (situations) and means of attaining goals (cognitive or behavioral responses) in an act of will.

The mental links created by implementation intentions are expected to facilitate goal attainment on the basis of psychological processes that relate both to the anticipated situation (the if-component of the plan) and the intended behavior (the then-component of the plan). Because forming implementation intentions implies the selection of a critical future situation (i.e., a suitable opportunity), it is assumed that the mental representation of this situation becomes highly activated, and hence more accessible (Gollwitzer, 1999). This heightened accessibility should benefit information processing in relation to the specified situation. In particular, people should be in a good position to identify and take notice of the critical cue when they encounter it later.

Processes Related to the If-component

Several studies have tested the idea that the mental representation of the situation specified in the if-part of the implementation intention becomes highly accessible by examining how well participants holding implementation intentions detected and attended to the critical situation compared to participants who had only formed goal intentions (Gollwitzer, Bayer, Steller & Bargh, 2002; Webb & Sheeran, 2004). Evidence that implementation intentions improve detection of the critical situation was obtained in a study using the embedded figures test (Gottschaldt, 1926), where smaller a-figures were hidden within larger b-figures (Gollwitzer et al., 2002). Enhanced detection of the hidden a-figures was observed when participants had specified the a-figure in the if-part of an implementation intention (i.e., had made plans on how to create a traffic sign from the a-figure). Equivalent findings were obtained in a study that used a classic illusion from the psychology of language (Webb & Sheeran, 2004, Study 1). Participants who formed if-then plans in relation to the critical letter F showed superior letter detection compared to a variety of control conditions, even though detection was extremely difficult. Two additional experiments by Webb and Sheeran (2004) indicated that forming an if-then plan engendered faster and more accurate responses to critical cues without compromising responses to irrelevant or ambiguous cues.

In a study using a dichotic-listening paradigm, Gollwitzer et al. (2002) observed that words describing the anticipated critical situation attracted and focused attention among implementation intention participants. Participants who formed if-then plans seemed to find it difficult to overlook information about the critical situation presented in the unattended channel; the consequence was that their shadowing performance for the attended material decreased relative to goal intention participants. This finding implies that opportunities to act that are specified in implementation intentions will not easily escape people's attention, even when people are busy with other ongoing tasks.

Processes Related to the Then-component

The mental act of linking a critical situation and an intended goal-directed behavior in the form of an if-then plan parallels the formation of associations between situations and actions during the development of *habits*. Habits and if-plans both are characterized by strong links between (mental representations of) particular cues and responses. Moreover, in the same way that the operation of habits is automatic (Bargh, 1994) in the sense that action control becomes immediate, efficient, and needless of conscious intent (Aarts & Dijksterhuis, 2000a, b; Sheeran, Aarts et al., 2005; Verplanken & Aarts, 1999; Wood, Quinn & Kashy, 2002), there is evidence that action control by implementation intentions also exhibits these features of automaticity.

Gollwitzer and Brandstätter (1997, Study 3) showed the immediacy of action initiation by implementation intentions in a study where participants were asked to form plans that specified viable opportunities for presenting counterarguments to a series of racist remarks made by a confederate. Participants who formed implementation intentions initiated the relevant counterargument more quickly (i.e., closer to the intended time) than did participants who had only formed goal intentions to counter-argue (see Orbell & Sheeran, 2000; Webb & Sheeran, 2004 for similar findings). The efficiency of action initiation was tested by Brandstätter, Lengfelder and Gollwitzer (2001, Studies 3 and 4) using a Go/No-Go-task. Participants formed the goal intention to press a button as quickly as possible if numbers appeared on the computer screen, but not if letters appeared. Participants in the implementation intention condition also planned to press the button particularly fast if the number 3 was presented. This Go/No-Go task was then embedded as a secondary task in a dual task paradigm. Findings showed that implementation intention participants showed a substantial increase in speed of responding to the number 3 compared to the control group, regardless of whether the primary task that had to be performed simultaneously was easy or difficult. These findings support the idea that implementation intention effects are efficient; the operation of if-then plans cannot require much in the way of cognitive resources because they facilitated performance even when two tasks were undertaken at the same time.

The redundancy of conscious intent for implementation intention effects has also been demonstrated in several experiments. Bayer, Moskowitz and Gollwitzer (2002) tested whether implementation intentions lead to action initiation without conscious intent once the critical situation is encountered. In these experiments, the critical situation was presented subliminally and its impact on preparing to perform (Study 1) or performing (Study 2) respective goal-directed behaviors was assessed. For instance, participants in Study 2 were asked to classify a series of geometrical figures (e.g., circles, eclipses, triangles, squares) into rounded versus angular objects using left versus right button press responses. All participants formed the goal intention to classify the figures as quickly and accurately as possible. Implementation intention participants also made the following plan: "And if I see a triangle, then I press the respective button particularly fast!" Participants worked on a set of 240 figures, presented in succession on a computer screen. Some of the figures were preceded by the subliminal presentation of the critical figure (i.e., a triangle), whereas others were preceded by a control prime (i.e., the % symbol). Findings indicated that participants in the implementation intention condition had faster classification responses for angular figures when the triangle instead of the % symbol was presented as a subliminal prime; no such speed-up effect was observed among goal intention participants.

In another study, Sheeran, Webb and Gollwitzer (2005, Study 2) gave participants the conscious goal to solve a series of puzzles as accurately as possible. One half of the participants also formed an implementation intention in relation to another dimension of performance, namely, to answer the puzzles as quickly as possible. This implementation intention manipulation was then crossed with a situational priming manipulation that was designed to activate the goal of responding quickly. Speed and accuracy of responses to the puzzles was measured subsequently. Even though participants indicated no awareness that the puzzle task activated a task-relevant goal during debriefing (participants all reported that their only goal was to solve the puzzles accurately), the results showed that the puzzles were solved fastest when participants were primed with the goal of responding quickly and had formed an if-then plan. These findings indicate that people's conscious intent is not required for implementation intentions to affect performance—people need not be aware that they have encountered the critical cue specified in their plan (Bayer et al., 2002) or even be aware of the goal driving their behavior (Sheeran, Webb et al., 2005).

Both implementation intentions and habits engender swift, effortless responses that do not require conscious instigation or guidance. In addition, these effects of if-then plans and habits both are underpinned by strong associations between cues and responses. However, there is an important difference between implementation intentions and habits that accrues from the fact that the respective cue-response links have different origins. In the case of habits, frequent and consistent execution of a response in the presence of a particular stimulus leads to the development of the relevant associations. In the case of implementation intentions, the same linkage can be fashioned *in situ* by an act of will. Implementation intention effects thus represent an important sub-type of automaticity that differs from the automaticity in habits (Gollwitzer & Schaal, 1998; Sheeran, Webb et al., 2005). Implementation intentions allow people to choose, consciously and in advance, what goal-directed responses will be elicited automatically, and what situational cues will elicit them. By making an if-then plan, people decide to delegate control of their behavior to pre-selected situational features with the express purpose of reaching their goals. This is what is meant by the idea that forming an implementation intention entails *strategic automatization of goal striving*.

Implementation Intentions and Other Conceptions of Planning

Strategic automaticity distinguishes implementation intentions from other conceptions of planning. For instance, seminal research by Leventhal showed that giving participants action plans (e.g., instructions on how to stop smoking) enhanced the behavioral impact of fear appeals in relation to both smoking (Leventhal, Singer & Jones, 1965) and tetanus (Leventhal, Watts & Pagano, 1967). Similarly, the Health Action Process Approach (HAPA; Schwarzer, 1992) points to the importance of planning in helping people to translate intentions into action, and empirical studies have shown that plan formation improved prediction of health behaviors after goal intentions have been taken into account (e.g., Abraham et al., 1999; Jones, Abraham, Harris, Schulz & Chrispin, 2001). In the field of safer sex, Sheeran, Abraham and Orbell (1999) proposed that engaging in preparatory behaviors such as buying and carrying condoms and discussing their use with a sexual partner were prerequisites for condom use. Bryan, Fisher and Fisher (2002) tested this idea and found that performance of these preparatory behaviors mediated the relationship between intentions to use condoms and condom use. Action plans and preparatory behaviors are similar to implementation intentions in that these concepts all suggest that people benefit from working out a method of acting in some detail before getting started on goal striving (i.e., from having a plan). However, the literature on action plans and preparatory behaviors does not specify what components must be included in the plan (i.e., what details need to be spelled out), what the structure of the plan should be, or what are the mechanisms by which planning promotes goal achievement. Each of these features of plans is specified by implementation intention theory, on the other hand (Gollwitzer, 1993, 1996, 1999; Gollwitzer & Schaal, 1998; Gollwitzer & Sheeran, in press).

The components that should be specified in an implementation intention are a good opportunity to act (the if-component) and an instrumental goal-directed response (the then-component). Furthermore, the plan should have a conditional if-then structure ("If situation Y occurs, then I will initiate goal-directed behavior $Z!$"). This structure is important to ensure that the if-component of the plan becomes highly activated, and a strong link is forged between the if-component and then-component of the plan. Heightened accessibility of critical cues and strong cue-response links, in turn, are responsible for enhanced detection of situational cues and automation of responding; the processes that account for implementation intention effects on performance and goal attainment.

A study by Oettingen, Hönig and Gollwitzer (2000, Study 3) provided evidence that specifying the opportunity and goal-directed response in the format of an if-then plan has greater impact on performance compared to merely specifying the respective opportunity and goal-directed response. As part of the procedure, participants were provided with diskettes containing four concentration tasks and were asked to perform these tasks on their computers each Wednesday morning for the next four weeks. Participants in the control condition were asked to indicate what time they would perform the task by responding to the statement "I will perform as many arithmetic tasks as possible each Wednesday at _____ (self-chosen time before noon)." Participants in the implementation intention condition, on the other hand, indicated their chosen time by responding to the statement "If it is Wednesday at _____ (self-chosen time before noon), then I will perform as many arithmetic tasks as possible!" The program on the diskette recorded the time that participants started to work on the task from the clock on participants' computers.

Even though the implementation intention and control instructions involved the same components (i.e., specifying the performance of a particular behavior at a particular time on a particular day), the conditional structure of the implementation intention had an important effect on whether participants performed the task at the time they intended to perform it. The mean deviation from the intended start time was five times greater in the control condition (8 hours) compared to the implementation intention condition (1.5 hours). These findings suggest that respective opportunities and goal-directed responses should be specified in an if-then format to engender strategic automatization of goal striving (see also Jaudas & Gollwitzer, 2004, cited in Gollwitzer et al., in press).

IMPLEMENTATION INTENTIONS AND ATTAINMENT OF HEALTH GOALS

Accumulated evidence indicates that forming an implementation intention increases the likelihood of performing behaviors in the service of health goals compared to the formation of a goal intention on its own. Gollwitzer and Sheeran (in press) reviewed 23 studies of health goals as part of a larger meta-analysis of implementation intention effects. Table 6.1 describes the samples, behaviors, and effect sizes in these studies. The sample-weighted average effect size obtained from the 23 studies was $d_+ = 0.59$ (95% $CI = 0.52$ to 0.67) which was similar to the effect size obtained for the 94 studies included in the overall meta-analysis ($d_+ = 0.65$). According to Cohen's (1992) power primer, $d_+ = 0.20$ should be considered a "small" effect size, $d_+ = 0.50$ is a "medium" effect size, whereas $d_+ = 0.80$ is a "large" effect size. Thus, the effect of implementation intention formation on the attainment of health goals is of medium-to-large magnitude.

Types of Health Behavior

Several distinctions are worth making in relation to the reviewed health behaviors that serve to clarify the impact of implementation intention formation on attainment of health goals. The first concerns whether obtaining a wanted response or controlling an unwanted response was at issue (Gollwitzer et al., 2005). Findings indicate that implementation intentions were effective in promoting wanted responses such as exercise participation (Milne, Orbell & Sheeran, 2002; Prestwich, Lawton & Conner, 2003; Sniehotta, Scholz & Schwarzer, 2002b), healthy eating (Armitage, 2004; Verplanken & Faes, 1999) and various types of cancer screening (e.g., Orbell, Hodgkins & Sheeran, 1997; Sheeran & Orbell, 2000; Steadman & Quine, 2004). Although there were fewer studies concerned with controlling unwanted responses, implementation intention formation also proved beneficial in reducing consumption of snack foods (Orbell & Sheeran, 1999; Sheeran & Milne, 2003), regulating alcohol-related cognitions and behavior (Gollwitzer, Sheeran, Trötschel & Webb, 2005, Study 2; Murgraff, White & Phillips, 1996), and resisting smoking (Stephens & Conner, 1999; see also Higgins & Conner, 2004).

A second distinction concerns the frequency of performance of respective health behaviors. Wood and colleagues showed that behaviors that are performed frequently in stable situational contexts are controlled more by habits than by goal intentions (Ouellette & Wood, 1998; Wood, Kashy & Kenny, 2002). Given the parallels between habits and implementation intentions described earlier, this might suggest that if-then plans are

Table 6.1 Effects of implementation intention formation on the attainment of health goals

Author(s)	Sample	Goal	N	d
Wanted behaviours				
Armitage (2004)	Company employees	Eating a low-fat diet	126	0.30
Lippke & Ziegelmann (2002)	Myocardial infarction patients	Exercise	88	0.18
Milne, Orbell & Sheeran (2002)	University students	Exercise	248	1.25
Milne & Sheeran (2002a)	University students	Testicular self-examination	432	0.43
Orbell, Hodgkins & Sheeran (1997)	University Students and Staff	Breast self-examination	155	1.22
Orbell & Sheeran (2000)	Joint replacement patients	Recovery of functional activities	64	0.70
Prestwich, Lawton & Conner (2003b)	University students	Exercise	58	0.68
Sheeran & Orbell (1999) Study 1	University students	Vitamin supplement use	78	0.35
Sheeran & Orbell (1999) Study 2	University students	Vitamin supplement use	37	0.59
Sheeran & Orbell (2000)	Patients attending GP	Cervical cancer screening	104	0.58
Sheeran & Silverman (2003)	University employees	Workplace safety training attendance	271	0.52
Sniehotta, Scholz & Schwarzer (2002a)	Myocardial infarction patients	Cardiac rehabilitation training	74	0.61
Sniehotta, Scholz & Schwarzer (2002b)	Myocardial infarction patients	Physical activity	65	0.70
Steadman & Quine (2000)	University students	Vitamin supplement use	174	0.32
Steadman & Quine (2004)	University students	Testicular self-examination	75	0.54
Verplanken & Faes (1999)	University students	Healthy eating	102	0.47
Unwanted behaviours				
Orbell & Sheeran (1999) Study 3	University students	Reduce snack food consumption	111	0.61
Orbell & Sheeran (1999) Study 4	University students	Reduce snack food consumption	93	0.45
Sheeran & Milne (2003)	University students	Reduce snack food consumption	129	0.49
Murgraff, White & Phillips (1996)	University students	Reduce binge drinking	102	0.68
Gollwitzer, Sheeran et al. (2005) Study 3	University students	Reduced accessibility of drinking	72	0.49
Gollwitzer, Sheeran et al. (2005) Study 6	University students	Avoiding errors in driving simulator	72	0.49
Stephens & Conner (1999)	School children	Resist taking up smoking	124	0.37

mainly effective in promoting frequently performed behaviors. Implementation intention formation proved beneficial in promoting frequently performed behaviors (i.e., behaviors that are performed daily such as vitamin supplement use; e.g., Sheeran & Orbell, 1999; Steadman & Quine, 2000). Health behaviors that generally are performed with moderate frequency (i.e., monthly) such as breast and testicular self-examinations also benefited from implementation intention formation (Milne & Sheeran, 2002a; Orbell et al., 1997), as did behaviors that generally are performed infrequently (annually or biannually) including cervical cancer screening (Sheeran & Orbell, 2000) and workplace health and safety training (Sheeran & Silverman, 2003). These findings are consistent with the idea that implementation intentions involve a different sub-type of automaticity compared to habits. The automaticity in implementation intentions is strategic and does not appear to be affected by frequency of performance; unlike habits whose operation demands that respective responses were executed repeatedly and consistently in the presence of the same stimuli in the past.

A third important distinction concerns whether the initiation or maintenance of a health behavior was at issue. Orbell and Sheeran's (2000) study of patients undergoing joint replacement surgery provides a good example of behavioral initiation. This is because in the immediate wake of surgery, patients must try to resume activities of daily living (e.g., bathe, make a cup of tea) from scratch. Findings indicated that even though there were no differences between the groups on relevant clinical variables (type of surgery, pain, etc.), participants who formed implementation intentions initiated 18 out of 32 activities sooner than did participants who did not form if-then plans. On average, the implementation intention group was functionally active 2.5 weeks earlier than the control group. Several other studies that either examined behaviors that were novel for participants (e.g., testicular self-examinations; Milne & Sheeran, 2002a; Sheeran & Orbell, 1999) or explicitly asked participants to alter their usual behavior patterns (e.g., halve one's consumption of a favorite snack food; Sheeran & Milne, 2003) also speak to the utility of implementation intentions in promoting initiation of behavior.

It is important to note that when initiation of behavior is easy, positive goal intentions may satisfactorily promote performance, and forming an if-then plan may not confer any additional benefit. For instance, Sheeran and Orbell (1999, Study 1) found that participants who formed implementation intentions to take a vitamin pill each day fared no better in their pill intake over 10 days compared to participants who only formed goal intentions. A recent meta-analysis supports the idea that interventions that increase participants' goal intentions sometimes lead to initiation of behavior (Webb & Sheeran, in press). However, the findings also indicate that the impact of goal intention-change interventions declines rapidly over time (see also McCaul, Glasgow & O'Neill, 1992; Sheeran & Orbell, 1998), which suggests that appropriate motivation is not generally enough to maintain behavioral performance. In contrast, implementation intention effects are not characterized by such temporal decline. Sheeran and Orbell (1999) found that differences in vitamin pill intake between implementation intention and goal intention participants emerged after 3 weeks (but not 10 days). Moreover, Sheeran and Silverman (2003) showed that if-then planning increased attendance at health and safety training regardless of whether the training session specified by participants was in the near (0–3 weeks) or distant future (5–9 weeks). Perhaps the best evidence that if-then plans engender maintenance of behavior change comes from a longitudinal study of testicular self-examination (Milne & Sheeran, 2002a; see also Sheeran, Milne et al., 2005). Findings showed that implementation intention formation not only enhanced the rate of initiation of behavior over 1 month (rates were 44% versus 22% for implementation intention and control groups, respectively), but also enhanced the rate of behavioral maintenance over 1 year. Participants who formed implementation intentions were more than twice as likely to report routine performance of testicular self-examination each month during the preceding 12 months compared to controls (37% versus 15%). In sum, implementation intentions appear to be effective in promoting health behaviors no matter whether relevant performances are wanted or unwanted, frequent or infrequent, or novel, familiar, or persistent.

Types of Self-regulatory Problem

It is also the case that different self-regulatory problems are likely to characterize the reviewed health behaviors. Two key problems that can undermine behavioral performance and goal attainment are failing to get started with goal striving and failing to keep goal striving on track (Gollwitzer and Sheeran, in press). People may fail to start striving for health goals for at least three reasons. First, people might forget to act. Einstein, McDaniel, Williford, Pagan and Dismukes (2003) showed that when participants are preoccupied with other tasks, they generally fail to initiate intended behaviors, even when the time interval to performance is as short as 15 seconds. Retrospective reports from participants who did not act on their positive intentions to engage in breast self-examinations or exercise (Milne et al., 2002; Orbell et al., 1997) also confirm that remembering to act is a big problem in getting started. Second, even when they remember to act, people may fail to seize good opportunities to initiate goal striving. For example, participants in Sheeran and Silverman's (2003) study had to act within particular windows of opportunity in order to attend health and safety training (training courses were only available at particular dates, times, and locations). Failing to grasp available opportunities meant missing the course that semester. Similarly, people can miss out on opportune moments to move towards their goal because they do not know how to act at the critical juncture (e.g., how to reduce their cravings for snack food; e.g., Orbell & Sheeran, 1999).

A third problem in getting started with goal striving is overcoming initial reluctance to act. Decisions to perform health behaviors such as monthly testicular self-examinations often are based on the longer-term benefits of the action (e.g., the exam will prevent the development of serious cancer). However, short-term affective costs (e.g., embarrassment, discomfort) that perhaps were not anticipated at the time of deciding may loom large at the moment of acting, and lead to non-performance of the behavior. Initial reluctance to act can be a serious impediment to the achievement of health goals; for example, when the goal intention to halve one's consumption of a favorite snack (Sheeran & Milne, 2003) is faced with the reality of Italian ice cream, people might be inclined to deliberate anew about the desirability and feasibility of their original decision, and revise their goal intention in line with short-term considerations. However, the findings presented in Table 6.1 indicate that implementation intention formation helps people to overcome these various self-regulatory problems in initiating goal striving. Participants who furnished their goal intentions with if-then plans were unlikely to forget to act (e.g., Milne et al., 2002; Orbell et al., 1997; Sheeran & Orbell, 1999), and generally did not miss viable opportunities for acting (e.g., Sheeran & Orbell, 2000; Sheeran & Silverman, 2003) or become swayed by short-term costs at the moment of action (e.g., Milne & Sheeran, 2002a; Sheeran & Milne, 2003).

Forming implementation intentions can also help people deal effectively with the second major self-regulatory problem in goal striving, staying on track. Shielding ongoing activities from unwanted influences is important because most health behaviors require repeated and persistent performance in order to prevent illness and enhance longevity (e.g., vigorous exercise, good diet).

The reviewed health behaviors are likely to involve at least two factors that could derail ongoing goal pursuit, namely, adverse contextual influences and unwanted habitual responses (Gollwitzer & Sheeran, in press). Social pressure from other people to perform health-risk behaviors is one such adverse contextual influence. Behaviors such as smoking or binge drinking generally are performed in social contexts, and peers are likely to provide a good deal of verbal or non-verbal feedback about appropriate ways of behaving in that setting. When situational norms favor risk-taking, young people need to deal effectively with such unwanted social influences in order to resist smoking initiation and avoid binge drinking. Forming if-then plans about how to manage these interactions and withstand social pressure clearly benefited people who intended not to engage in these behaviors (e.g., Murgraff et al., 1996; Higgins & Conner, 2004; Stephens & Conner, 1999). For instance, Murgraff et al. (1996) asked participants to specify how they would respond if someone invited them to have another drink (e.g., "No thanks. I have to get up early tomorrow!"). Findings showed that student participants who formed this implementation intention significantly reduced their alcohol consumption over a two-week period compared to control participants who did not form a plan.

Whereas people may be aware of social pressure from others about how they should behave, there is another adverse contextual influence that could derail an ongoing goal pursuit of which people are unaware, namely, situational priming of behavior. Accumulated research indicates that activating stereotypes, traits, or goals outside of awareness (i.e., priming) has predictable effects on behavior (reviews by Bargh & Ferguson, 2000; Dijksterhuis & Bargh, 2001; Gollwitzer & Bargh, in press). Evidence that priming affects health-related behavior came from an experiment by Sheeran, Aarts, et al. (2005, Experiment 1). Participants who were habitual or non-habitual drinkers answered to a series of questions designed to activate the concept of socializing or they answered questions about a neutral concept. Subsequently, participants completed a lexical decision task where they responded to the verb "drinking" among other words. Findings indicated that activating the concept of socializing increased habitual drinkers' readiness to drink, as was shown by increased accessibility of the action concept *drinking*. Moreover, these effects occurred outside of awareness (automatically); participants reported no insight into the operation of the goal or its effects on behavioral readiness during debriefing.

Behavior priming effects cannot easily be controlled by goal intentions because people are not aware of the concepts (traits, goals) activated by the situation or of the effects of concept activation on their behavior. However, spelling out how the focal goal will be pursued in the format of an if-then plan can be used to shield the ongoing goal pursuit from the effects of antagonistic behavior primes (Gollwitzer, Sheeran, Trötschel & Webb, 2005). For instance, Gollwitzer et al. (2005, Study 3) replicated key features of the socializing-drinking experiment presented above. Participants were exposed to the socializing prime or neutral prime and undertook a lexical decision task as before. Prior to both of these tasks, however, participants formed an implementation intention about how they would suppress thoughts related to drinking or a neutral behavior (snacking) as part of an ostensibly unrelated first study. Among the irrelevant-plan participants, findings again showed that the socializing prime increased the accessibility of drinking behavior. Participants who formed relevant if-then plans, on the other hand, were protected against the impact of priming. Activation of the concept of socializing made no difference to these participants' readiness to drink. Thus, implementation intentions can be used to shield ongoing goal pursuit from adverse contextual influences, no matter whether these influences originate within, or outside of, people's awareness.

Unwanted habitual responding is the second problem that could derail ongoing pursuit of the health goals reviewed in Table 6.1. When relevant situational stimuli remain constant and the behavior is executed frequently, then the habitual mode of action control is more powerful than is the intentional mode (e.g., Ouellette & Wood, 1998). Findings from several studies that used frequency of past behavior to index habit bear out this idea; habits consistently offered better prediction of subsequent behavior compared to goal intentions (e.g., Orbell et al., 1997; Sheeran & Milne, 2003; Sheeran & Orbell, 2000). However, implementation intention formation appears to provide an effective defense against habitual responding. For instance, although previous delay behavior was the most important determinant of attendance for cervical cancer screening among the sample as a whole (Sheeran & Orbell, 2000), forming an if-then plan enhanced prediction of attendance even after delay behavior and motivational variables had been taken into account. In fact, having a plan significantly attenuated the relationship between previous delay and subsequent attendance among participants who planned (rs were -0.29 and -0.70, for the implementation intention and control groups, respectively).

A more compelling test is afforded by examining the impact of counter-intentional habits on subsequent performance. When respective goal intentions involve changing an established behavior pattern (e.g., halving consumption of a favorite snack food), situational contexts are likely to activate representations of previously performed behaviors and make it especially difficult to maintain goal striving. However, Sheeran (2004) found that even though snack consumption during the previous week was the best predictor of snack intake during the following week, implementation intention formation helped motivated individuals to reduce consumption. Conceptually equivalent findings were obtained by Verplanken and Faes (1999) using a response-frequency measure of dietary habits.

These findings for health behaviors parallel the results of social psychological research on implementation intentions and the control of unwanted habits. Implementation intentions proved effective in promoting goal attainment in the face of a wide variety of antagonistic habits including overlearned responding (Webb, Sheeran & Luszczynska, 2005) the Simon effect (Brüwer, Bayer & Gollwitzer, 2002), spider phobia (Schweiger-Gallo, McCulloch & Gollwitzer, 2002), and automatic stereotype activation (Gollwitzer, Achtziger, Schaal & Hammelbeck, 2002; see Gollwitzer, Jaudas, Parks & Sheeran, in press, for a review). Overall, the presented findings indicate that forming implementation intentions is an effective means of handling self-regulatory problems in initiating and maintaining goal striving, and can bridge the intention-behavior gap.

MECHANISMS OF IMPLEMENTATION INTENTION EFFECTS

Because implementation intention inductions ask participants to specify a behavior that will be instrumental for goal attainment and a good opportunity to initiate that behavior, it is possible that plan formation might enhance people's intentions or self-efficacy in relation to the focal goal. If this analysis is accurate, then implementation intention effects should be explained by motivational factors. However, at least two lines of research contradict this position. First, studies that measured goal intentions or self-efficacy both before and after respective implementation intention inductions found no evidence that plan formation increased scores on these variables in either within-participants analyses (differences within the intervention group over time) or between-participants analyses (differences between the intervention and control group at either time point) (e.g., Milne et al., 2002; Orbell et al., 1997; Sheeran & Orbell, 1999; Sheeran, Webb et al., 2005). Second, implementation intention formation enhanced rates of goal attainment even when participants already had extremely high scores on relevant motivational variables. For instance, Sheeran & Orbell (2000) found that if-then planning increased attendance for cervical cancer screening even though the pre-intervention means for intention and self-efficacy among the planning group were 4.60 and 4.63, respectively, on 1–5 scales. Clearly, it is implausible to attribute the observed 33% improvement in attendance behavior among implementation intention participants to post-manipulation increases in goal intentions or self-efficacy (see Sheeran & Orbell, 1999; Verplanken & Faes, 1999 for equivalent findings). These results, together with findings that show that implementation intention effects do not exhibit the temporal trajectory of motivational interventions (e.g., Sheeran & Silverman, 2003) and actually show stronger effects for difficult-to-implement goals as compared to easy-to-implement goals (Gollwitzer & Brandstätter, 1997), indicate that goal intentions and self-efficacy are not the mechanisms by which implementation intentions promote goal achievement.

Gollwitzer (1993, 1999; Gollwitzer & Schaal, 1998; Gollwitzer & Sheeran, in press) proposed that two mechanisms that correspond to features of the if- and then-components of the plan explain action control by implementation intentions. Figure 6.1 presents a model delineating the components, mechanisms, and outcomes of implementation intention formation. Forming an if-then plan involves specifying a then-component (an instrumental response or "goal-directed behavior Z") and an if-component (a viable future opportunity or "situation Y"), and creating mental links between these two components in an if-then format ("If situation Y occurs, then I will initiate goal-directed behavior Z!"). Specifying a good opportunity to act means that the critical situation becomes highly activated and hence more accessible. Enhanced accessibility of the critical situation in turn facilitates subsequent detection of that situation. Forging strong links between the if-component and then-component of the plan, on the other hand, means that the person does not have to deliberate about what to do once the critical situation is encountered. Instead, execution of the goal-directed response follows immediately, efficiently, and without needing conscious intent; responding is automatized.

Empirical studies presented earlier indicate that participants who furnish their goal intentions with respective implementation intentions: (a) exhibit superior detection of specified cues (see *Processes related to the if-component*), (b) respond swiftly, effortlessly, and without need for conscious intent (see *Processes related to the then-component*),

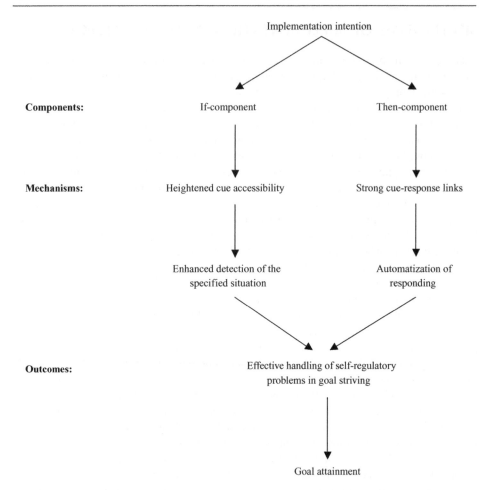

Figure 6.1   Components, mechanisms, and outcomes of implementation intention formation

(c) overcome self-regulatory problems to do with initiating goal striving and shielding ongoing goal pursuit from unwanted influences (see *Types of self-regulatory problem*), and (d) are likely to achieve their goals (see *Implementation intentions and attainment of health goals*). However, we have not so far demonstrated that enhanced cue accessibility and strong cue-response links mediate the relationship between implementation intention formation and goal attainment. Recent research by Webb and Sheeran (2005b) provided this evidence.

Participants' goal was to press a key as quickly as possible to indicate whether or not word search puzzles contained words or non-words that they had been shown at the beginning of the experiment (Webb & Sheeran, 2005b, Experiment 2). One-half of the participants formed an if-then plan to respond to one of the non-words (*avenda*) especially quickly. The other half of the participants were asked to familiarize themselves with this item in order to speed up their responses (goal intention condition). Prior to undertaking the main puzzle task, participants undertook a lexical decision task that ostensibly was designed to provide a baseline measure of their linguistic ability. In actual fact, the lexical decision task involved a priming procedure that had the following sequence: (a) presentation of a fixation dot for 1,500ms, (b) presentation of a prime word for 17ms, (c) presentation of a row of consonants the same length as the prime (postmask) for 225ms, and (d) presentation of the target word until the participant responded. There were 96 trials, and participants indicated whether each item presented was a word or a nonword.

Among the target and prime items was the cue specified in the implementation intention *(avenda)* and a word representing the target behavior *(press)* as well as matched neutral words for the prime and target, and filler words. *Accessibility of the critical cue* was measured by participants' responses to *avenda* after priming by neutral cues. The *strength of the cue-response link* was measured by participants' response latencies to the word *press* after priming by the critical cue *(avenda)*. Measures of the accessibility of the matched neutral cue, the accessibility of matched neutral behavior, and all other cue-target combinations were also taken.

The main puzzle task was undertaken immediately after the lexical decision task. Participants were presented with a series of 10 x 10 matrices of letters that either contained a word from the original memory set, a non-word from the original memory set, or a new word. Participants had to respond as quickly as possible by pressing one of three designated keys. The dependent variable was speed of response to the puzzle containing the non-word *avenda*.

Findings indicated that implementation intention formation promoted goal attainment. Participants who formed an if-then plan found the *avenda* item significantly faster than did goal intention participants. Importantly, this improvement in response times did not come at the cost of accuracy, or compromise responses to the other puzzles. Implementation intention participants were just as accurate responding to critical and non-critical puzzle items, and were just as fast in responding to non-critical items, compared to controls.

Findings for cue accessibility and the strength of cue-response links indexed via the lexical decision task also supported predictions. Participants who formed implementation intentions exhibited enhanced accessibility of the critical cue *(avenda)* compared to goal intention participants; the critical cue was also more accessible than was the matched cue word among participants who planned. Priming of the target behavior by the critical cue also produced faster responses among implementation intention compared to control participants, indicating that the cue-response association *(avenda-press)* was stronger among participants who planned. The difference between the groups was not significant, however, when the target behavior was primed by the matched neutral cue. The implementation intention and control conditions also did not differ on accessibility of the target behavior, accessibility of the critical cue following priming by the target behavior (response-cue association), or speed of performance in general. Thus, implementation intention formation heightened the accessibility of the critical cue and strengthened the link between the critical cue and the specified response but did not affect the accessibility of other concepts.

Accessibility of the critical cue and the strength of the cue-response link had significant correlations with goal attainment. Increased cue accessibility and stronger associations between the critical cue and the target behavior both were associated with faster responses to the *avenda* puzzle. To test mediation, goal attainment was regressed on cue accessibility, strength of the cue-response link, and condition (implementation intention: formed versus not formed). Findings showed that cue accessibility and strength of the cue-response links remained significant predictors of goal attainment whereas condition was no longer significant. Sobel's (1982) test confirmed that the mediating variables significantly attenuated the relationship between condition and the dependent variable.

These findings support the postulated mechanisms of implementation intention effects. Forming an if-then plan enhances accessibility of the critical situation and forges strong associations between that situation and the goal-directed response. Detection of the specified opportunity to act is facilitated by heightened cue accessibility, whereas strong cue-response links means that the person knows exactly how to act when the opportunity presents itself and so action initiation is automatized. In sum, if-then plans improve the likelihood of goal attainment because the person strategically switches goal striving from a conscious, effortful mode (action control by goal intentions) to a mode involving automatic initiation of behavior by situational cues (action control by implementation intentions).

It is worth noting that Webb and Sheeran's (2005b) findings are consistent with certain accounts of prospective memory (i.e., remembering intentions to perform future actions; reviews by Einstein & McDaniel, 1996; Ellis & Kvavilashvili, 2000). McDaniel and Einstein (2000) proposed a multiple-process account of prospective memory that includes both conscious and automatic mechanisms. When the cue is distinctive and there is a strong association between the environmental cue and the to-be-remembered intention, then anticipated environmental conditions should automatically trigger recall of the intended action. This analysis of prospective memory parallels Webb and Sheeran's (2005b) test of mediation of implementation intention effects. However, McDaniel and Einstein also posit a second "conscious" mechanism involved in prospective memory. According to this view, people strategically monitor the environment for the presence of the target event and, once this cue is encountered, perform an effortful memory search for the intended response. Such effortful monitoring and retrieval processes seem quite different to action control by implementation intention. For instance, prospective remembering by this route appears to be highly vulnerable to the cognitive demands of an ongoing activity (e.g., Marsh, Hancock & Hicks, 2002; Smith, 2003) whereas mental load does not compromise the strength of implementation intention effects (e.g., Brandstätter et al., 2001). Further research, and especially mediation analysis, is required on prospective memory processes to determine whether the mechanisms that explain implementation effects—enhanced cue accessibility and strength of cue-response links— may also explain how intentions are remembered.

DETERMINANTS OF THE STRENGTH OF IMPLEMENTATION INTENTION EFFECTS

Several factors determine the impact of implementation intention formation on rates of goal achievement. The first concerns the presence of self-regulatory problems. When there are few obstacles to goal achievement, then favorable goal intentions and self-efficacy could suffice in promoting performance, and implementation intention formation might be superfluous (e.g., Gollwitzer & Brandstätter, 1997; Sheeran & Orbell, 1999, Study 1). However, when the respective goal striving is difficult, or when people have difficulties pursuing their goals (e.g., schizophrenic patients, opiate addicts; see Brandstätter et al., 2001; Lengfelder & Gollwitzer, 2001) then it is especially worthwhile to engage in if-then planning (Gollwitzer & Sheeran, in press).

A second determinant of the strength of implementation intention effects is the state of the respective goal intention. When people have no intention of pursuing a health goal, then they are unlikely to form an implementation intention that spells out adequately when, where, and how the goal will be pursued, even when asked to do so (Sheeran, Milne et al., 2005). Sheeran et al. (2005) showed that strong effects of implementation intentions were obtained only when the underlying goal intention was strong and activated (see also Seehausen, Bayer & Gollwitzer, 1994, cited in Gollwitzer, 1996). Similarly, Koestner, Lekes, Powers and Chicoine, 2002 showed that if-then plans benefited the completion of personal projects more when those projects were self-concordant (i.e., consistent with personal interests and values) than when projects were self-discordant (motivated by external reasons such as social pressure). The implication is that intervention studies may need to start out with a motivational initiative to promote requisite goal intentions before having participants complete an implementation intention induction to promote effective translation of their intentions into action.

In addition, several features of the respective if-then plan are important in determining the magnitude of the impact of plan formation on goal attainment. As the model presented in Figure 6.1 suggests, strong implementation intention effects can be anticipated only if the person has: (a) specified a response that is instrumental for completing the goal in the then-component of the plan, (b) specified a viable opportunity to initiate that response in the plan's if-component, and (c) forged strong links between the if-component and then-component of the plan.

The goal-directed behavior specified in an implementation intention needs to be tailored to the self-regulatory problem at hand to promote effective realization of the super-ordinate goal intention. Three studies that ostensibly are concerned with the same activity, attendance behavior, serve to illustrate the types of response that might prove useful in dealing with particular self-regulatory problems (Sheeran & Silverman, 2003; Sheeran & Orbell, 2000; Sheeran, Aubrey & Kellett, 2005). Sheeran and Silverman (2003) investigated attendance at health and safety training courses among university employees. Evidence indicated that staff generally failed to attend because they found attendance unpleasant, and because they tended to forget relevant details concerning the times and places of different courses. Thus, the self-regulatory problems that prevented attendance had to do with getting started on goal striving. Consequently, the if-then plan was geared towards the initiation of attendance behavior.

Implementation intention and control participants were provided with information about times and locations of six upcoming training courses at the front of the questionnaire. The implementation intention induction came at the end of the ques-tionnaire. Participants were told: "You are more likely to attend a university fire training course in the next three months if you decide now which course you will attend. Using the information provided on the cover, please fill in the following ..." Spaces were provided for participants to write in the time, date, and location of their chosen course. The type of then-component specified in the plan is an instigation response (Sheeran, Milne et al., 2005); participants specify which course they will attend. Doing so means that participants come to terms with the immediate affective costs of attending (Trope & Fishbach, 2005). Moreover, if-then planning heightens the accessibility of the chosen time and date thereby making it less likely that attendance will be forgotten. Spelling out the goal-directed response in this way appeared to be highly effective in dealing with the problem of getting started. Objective records indicated if-then plans doubled the rate of attendance at health and safety training courses (35% versus 14%).

The same self-regulatory problems to do with forgetting to act and dealing with initial reluctance also explain non-attendance for cervical cancer screening (review by Orbell & Sheeran, 1993). However, it was not feasible simply to ask participants to specify when and where they would attend in this study (Sheeran & Orbell, 2000). This is because all participants received an invitation letter that merely informed them that they should obtain screening within the next three months. In order to be screened, the women had to contact their General Practitioner to arrange a suitable appointment. Thus, it was necessary to perform a behavior in the service of goal attainment (i.e., make an appointment) to achieve the desired outcome (i.e., screening attendance). The then-component of the implementation intention therefore specified instigation of the behavioral means of achieving the goal (rather than the goal per se).

Implementation intention participants received the following passage at the end of a questionnaire concerning their views about cervical cancer screening: "You are more likely to go for a cervical smear if you decide when and where you will go. Please write in below when, where, and how you will make an appointment." Participants wrote their answers under each of three headings using the spaces provided. Specifying the instigation of the behavioral means of achieving the goal appears to have been highly effective in promoting goal attainment. Medical records indicated that, whereas only 69% of the control group subsequently attended for screening, 92% of participants who formed implementation intentions did so. Post hoc analyses indicated that making an appointment was an effectual means of ensuring attendance—100% of participants who made an appointment subsequently attended for cervical cancer screening. This finding underlines the role of instrumentality of the goal-directed response in determining the strength of implementation intention effects.

The final attendance behavior concerned appointments for psychotherapy (Sheeran, Aubrey & Kellett, 2005). Here, the relevant self-regulatory problem has less to do with the initiation of goal striving than with shielding goal striving from unwanted influences during the lengthy interval between seeking help and obtaining treatment. There are long waiting lists for psychotherapy in the UK, and people generally wait at least 6 months to see a clinical psychologist or psychotherapist. During this time, people are likely to have to deal with a variety of negative thoughts and feelings that could undermine attendance for psychotherapy. For instance, people may ruminate about the self-evaluative implications of seeking psychological help, or they may feel ashamed, embarrassed, or stigmatized about needing therapy. Not surprisingly, therefore, 30–60% of people who are offered psychotherapy fail to attend their appointment (Hughes, 1995).

The then-component specified in this study was therefore geared at dealing effectively with unwanted influences that might derail goal striving, and in particular, negative affective experiences that could prevent attendance. The goal-directed behavior involved the suppression of responses that could hinder goal attainment. The following imple-mentation intention induction was included at the end of a questionnaire concerning perceptions of therapy:

> People can sometimes feel concerned about attending their appointment. To help you manage these concerns, please read the statement below 3 times and then repeat the statement silently to yourself one more time:
>
> *As soon as I feel concerned about attending my appointment, I will ignore that feeling and tell myself this is perfectly understandable!*
>
> Now please tick the box below if you have read the statement three times and said it to yourself once (please be honest; do not tick the box until you have read and repeated the statement)

Implementation intention formation again proved effective in promoting attendance behavior. Whereas only 57% of control participants attended their psychotherapy appointment, 83% of participants who formed an if-then plan did so. These findings demonstrate the importance of: (a) identifying the key self-regulatory problems that undermine people's ability to translate a focal intention into action, and (b) specifying a response that is effective in dealing with these self-regulatory problems in the then-component of the implementation intention. Implementation intentions can be targeted at instigating a response that leads to goal attainment or at suppressing a response that prevents goal attainment. Clearly, in order to observe the greatest benefits for goal completion, it is important to specify the response that has the greatest instrumentality with respect to reaching the goal.

Gollwitzer and Sheeran (in press) pointed out that features of the if-then component of the plan also can have an important influence on the extent to which implementation intention formation promotes goal achievement. In particular, the specified opportunity needs to be both viable and precise to obtain strong implementation intention effects. For instance, if the specified situation is not viable (e.g., because the situation hardly ever arises, or presents urgent competing goals) then goal-directed behavior might never be initiated. Similarly, if the critical situation is spelled out only vaguely in the plan (e.g., "next week"), then the person may fail to detect relevant cues or may have to deliberate *in situ* about whether or not this is a good time to act. As a result, crucial chances to pursue the goal might be missed. Of course, the opportunities specified in the if-component of the plan can refer either to environmental circumstances (e.g., a particular time and place) or internal states (e.g., feelings of concern about attending for psychotherapy). The issue of precision is not to do with specifying internal versus external cues, but rather whether the person is forced to reflect on whether the critical situation has arrived. In the same way that implementation intentions benefit rates of goal attainment because the person does not have to deliberate *in situ* about action to perform (because the action was specified in advance in the then-component of the plan), the person also should not need to deliberate *in situ* about when and where to act.

The final feature of implementation intention formation that is important in determin-ing how much planning benefits goal attainment concerns the strength of the association between the if-component and then-component of the plan (cue-response linkage). Webb and Sheeran's (2005b) findings indicate that strong links between the specified opportunity and goal-directed behavior mediate the relationship between if-then planning and action initiation. However, this analysis also implies that procedures that serve to strengthen or weaken cue-response associations should fortify or attenuate implementation intention effects, respectively. For instance, if participants pay little attention to the link between the cue and response during implementation intention formation then modest implementation intention effects would be anticipated. Conversely, instructing participants to concentrate on this link should enhance the impact of the plan. Consistent with this idea, Milne and Sheeran (2002b) found that participants who rehearsed the link between their specified opportunity and specified action were much more likely to visit a target website than were participants who specified these components on a reminder note and put it in a prominent place at home (rates were 87% versus 40%, respectively). In sum, the presence of a self-regulatory problem, the state (activation, strength) of the underlying goal intention and features of the plan (instrumentality of the response, viability and precision of the opportunity, cue-response linkage) all are important determinants of the strength of implementation intention effects.

CONCLUSION

Models of health behavior predominantly are concerned with the factors that determine strong goal intentions. However, accumulated evidence indicates that people often fail to convert even strong goal intentions into successful attainment of health goals. This is because of self-regulatory problems to do with initiating goal striving or shielding an ongoing goal pursuit from unwanted influences which undermine goal progress. Forming implementation intentions in the service of goal intentions engenders strategic automatization of goal striving and thus helps people to deal effectively with these self-regulatory problems. The consequence is that if-then plan formation enhances rates of attainment of health goals compared to the formation of a goal intention on its own.

Although progress in implementation intention research has been substantial, there is considerable scope for further research. For instance, relatively few studies have examined the control of unwanted, health-risk behaviors (e.g., smoking, over-eating), and further tests are warranted. Comparisons of the effectiveness of different goal-directed responses (e.g., instigation versus ignore responses) in dealing with particular self-regulatory problems would be valuable, as would tests of the utility of combining these different goal-directed responses. Characteristics of implementation intention inductions that ensure optimal specification of opportunities and responses in people's plans, and optimize the strength of cue-response links also deserve rigorous analysis. Finally, people typically hold manifold, complex health goals (e.g., to eat a low-fat diet and avoid smoking) and future studies will need to assess to what extent people benefit from forming multiple implementation intentions (with respect to both one or more different behaviors). Provided that there is no conflict between the opportunities and responses specified in respective if-then plans, then implementation intention formation should promote the attainment of both complex and various goals. However, these are all empirical issues that can, and should be, tested by health psychologists in future research.

REFERENCES

Aarts, H. & Dijksterhuis, A. (2000a). Habits as knowledge structures: Automaticity in goal-directed behavior. *Journal of Personality and Social Psychology, 78*, 53–63.

Aarts, H. & Dijksterhuis, A. (2000b). On the automatic activation of goal-directed behavior: The case of travel habit. *Journal of Environmental Psychology, 20*, 75–82.

Aarts, H., Dijksterhuis, A. & Midden, C. (1999). To plan or not to plan? Goal achievement or interrupting the performance of mundane behaviors. *European Journal of Social Psychology, 29*, 971–979.

Ajzen, I. (1991). The theory of planned behavior. *Organizational Behavior and Human Decision Processes, 50*, 179–211.

Armitage, C.J. (2004). Implementation intentions and eating a low-fat diet: A randomized controlled trial. *Health Psychology, 23*, 319–323.

Bandura, A. (1997). *Self-efficacy: The exercise of control*. New York: W.H. Freeman.

Bargh, J.A. (1994). The four horsemen of automaticity: Awareness, efficiency, intention, and control in social interaction. In R.S. Wyer, Jr. & T.K. Srull (Eds), *Handbook of Social Cognition* (2nd edn, pp. 1–40). Hillsdale, NJ: Erlbaum.

Bayer, U.C., Moskowitz, G.B. & Gollwitzer, P.M. (2002). *Implementation Intentions and Action Initiation Without Conscious Intent*. Unpublished manuscript, University of Konstanz, Germany.

Brandstätter, V., Lengfelder, A. & Gollwitzer, P.M. (2001). Implementation intentions and efficient action initiation. *Journal of Personality and Social Psychology, 81*, 946–960.

Bryan, A., Fisher, J.D. & Fisher, W.A. (2002). Tests of the mediational role of preparatory safer sexual behavior in the context of the theory of planned behavior. *Health Psychology, 21*, 71–80.

Brüwer, J., Bayer, U.C. & Gollwitzer, P.M. (2002, July). *Intentional Control of the Simon Effect*. Poster presented at the International Conference on Executive Functions, Konstanz, Germany.

Carver, C.S. & Scheier, M.F. (1982). Control theory: A useful conceptual framework for personality-social, clinical, and health psychology. *Psychological Bulletin, 92*, 111–135.

Cohen, J. (1992). A power primer. *Psychological Bulletin, 112*, 155–159.

Einstein, G.O. & McDaniel, M.A. (1996). Retrieval processes in prospective memory: Theoretical approaches and some new empirical findings. In M. Bradimonte, G.O. Einstein & M.A. McDaniel (Eds), *Prospective Memory: Theory and applications*. Mahwah, NJ: Erlbaum.

Einstein, G.O., McDaniel, M.A., Williford, C.L., Pagan, J.L. & Dismukes, R.K. (2003). Forgetting of intentions in demanding situations is rapid. *Journal of Experimental Psychology: Applied, 9*, 147–162.

Ellis, J. & Kvavilashvili, L. (2000). Prospective memory in 2000: Past, present, and future directions. *Applied Cognitive Psychology, 14 (Suppl.)*, 1–9.

Fife-Schaw, C., Sheeran, P. & Norman, P. (in press). *Simulating Behaviour Change Interventions Based on the Theory of Planned Behaviour: Impacts on intentions and behaviour. British Journal of Social Psychology*.

Gibbons, F.X., Gerrard, M., Blanton, H. & Russell, D.W. (1998). Reasoned action and social reaction: Willingness and intention as independent predictors of health risk. *Journal of Personality and Social Psychology, 74*, 1164–1180.

Gollwitzer, P.M. (1990). Action phases and mindsets. In E.T. Higgins & J.R.M. Sorrentino (Eds), *The Handbook of Motivation and Cognition* (Vol. 2, pp. 53–92). New York: Guilford.

Gollwitzer, P.M. (1993). Goal achievement: The role of intentions. In W. Stroebe & M. Hewstone (Eds), *European Review of Social Psychology* (Vol. 4, pp. 141–185). Chichester: John Wiley & Sons, Ltd.

Gollwitzer, P.M. (1996). The volitional benefits of planning. In P.M. Gollwitzer & J.A. Bargh (Eds), *The Psychology of Action: Linking cognition and motivation to behavior* (pp. 287–312). New York: Guilford.

Gollwitzer, P.M. (1999). Implementation intentions: Strong effects of simple plans. *American Psychologist, 54*, 493–503.

Gollwitzer, P.M., Achtziger, A., Schaal, B. & Hammelbeck, J.P. (2002). *Intentional Control of Stereotypical Beliefs and Prejudicial Feelings.* Unpublished manuscript, University of Konstanz, Germany.

Gollwitzer, P.M., Bayer, U.C. & McCulloch, K.C. (2005). The control of the unwanted. In R.R. Hassin, J.S. Uleman & J.A. Bargh (Eds), *The New Unconscious* (pp. 485–515). New York: Oxford University Press.

Gollwitzer, P.M., Bayer, U.C., Steller, B. & Bargh, J.A. (2002). *Delegating Control to the Environment: Perception, attention, and memory for pre-selected behavioral cues.* Unpublished manuscript, University of Konstanz, Germany.

Gollwitzer, P.M. & Brandstätter, V. (1997). Implementation intentions and effective goal pursuit. *Journal of Personality and Social Psychology, 73*, 186–199.

Gollwitzer, P.M., Jaudas, A., Parks, E. & Sheeran, P. (in press). Flexibility tenacity in goal pursuit. In J. Shah & W. Gardner (Eds), *Handbook of Motivation Science.* New York: Guilford.

Gollwitzer, P.M. & Schaal, B. (1998). Metacognition in action: The importance of implementation intentions. *Personality and Social Psychology Review, 2*, 124–136.

Gollwitzer, P.M. & Sheeran, P. (in press). Implementation intentions and goal achievement: A meta-analysis of effects and processes. *Advances in Experimental Social Psychology.*

Gollwitzer, P.M., Sheeran, P., Trötschel, R. & Webb, T.L. (2005). *The Control of Behavior Priming Effects by Implementation Intentions.* Manuscript submitted for publication.

Gottschaldt, K. (1926). Über den Einfluß der Erfahrung auf die Wahrnehmung von Figuren (On the effects of familiarity on the perception of figures). *Psychologische Forschung, 8*, 261–317.

Higgins, A. & Conner, M. (2004). *Preventing Adolescent Smoking Using Implementation Intentions.* Manuscript submitted for publication.

Hughes, I. (1995). Why do they stop coming? Reasons for therapy termination by adult clinical psychology clients. *Clinical Psychology Forum, 81*, 7–12.

Jones, F., Abraham, C., Harris, P., Schulz, J. & Chrispin, C. (2001). From knowledge to action regulation: Modeling the cognitive prerequisites of sun screen use in Australian and UK samples. *Psychology and Health, 16*, 191–206.

Koestner, R., Lekes, N., Powers, T.A. & Chicoine, E. (2002). Attaining personal goals: Self-concordance plus implementation intentions equals success. *Journal of Personality and Social Psychology, 83*, 231–244.

Lengfelder, A. & Gollwitzer, P.M. (2001). Reflective and reflexive action control in patients with frontal brain lesions. *Neuropsychology, 15*, 80–100.

Leventhal, H., Singer, R. & Jones, S. (1965). Effects of fear and specificity of recommendation upon attitudes and behaviour. *Journal of Personality and Social Psychology, 2*, 20–29.

Leventhal, H., Watts, J.C., Pagano, F. (1967). Effects of fear and instructions on how to cope with danger. *Journal of Personality and Social Psychology, 6*, 313–321.

Lippke, S. & Ziegelmann, J.P. (2002). *Self-regulation and exercise: A Study on Stages of Change and Successful Ageing.* Unpublished manuscript, Free University of Berlin, Germany.

Marsh, R.L., Hancock, T.W. & Hicks, J.L. (2002). The demands of an ongoing activity influence the success of event-based prospective memory. *Psychonomic Bulletin and Review, 9*, 604–610.

Marsh, R.L., Hicks, J.L. & Watson, V. (2002). The dynamics of intention retrieval and coordination of action in event-based prospective memory. *Journal of Experimental Psychology: Learning, Memory, and Cognition, 28*, 652–659.

McCaul, K.D., Glasgow, R.E. & O'Neill, H.K. (1992). The problem of creating habits: Establishing health-protective dental behaviors. *Health Psychology, 11*, 101–110.

McDaniel, M.A. & Einstein, G.O. (2000). Strategic and automatic processes in prospective memory retrieval: A multiprocess framework. *Applied Cognitive Psychology, 14*, S127–S144.

Milne, S., Orbell, S. & Sheeran, P. (2002). Combining motivational and volitional interventions to promote exercise participation: Protection motivation theory and implementation intentions. *British Journal of Health Psychology, 7*, 163–184.

Milne, S. & Sheeran, P. (2002a, June). *Combining motivational and volitional interventions to prevent testicular cancer.* Paper presented to the 13th General Meeting of the European Association of Experimental Social Psychology, San Sebastian, Spain.

Milne, S. & Sheeran, P. (2002b, October). *Making Good Implementation Intentions: Comparing Associative Learning and Prospective Memory in Remembering Intentions.* Paper presented to the 16th Conference of the European Health Psychology Society, Lisbon, Portugal.

Murgraff, V., White, D. & Phillips, K. (1996). Moderating binge drinking: It is possible to change behaviour if you plan it in advance. *Alcohol and Alcoholism, 6*, 577–582.

Oettingen, G., Hönig, G. & Gollwitzer, P.M. (2002). Effective self-regulation of goal attainment. *International Journal of Educational Research, 33*, 705–732.

Oettingen, G. & Gollwitzer, P.M. (2001). Goal setting and goal striving. In A. Tesser & N. Schwarz (Eds), *Intraindividual Processes (Volume 1 of the Blackwell Handbook in Social Psychology,* pp. 329–347). Oxford, UK: Blackwell.

Orbell, S., Hodgkins, S. & Sheeran, P. (1997). Implementation intentions and the theory of planned behavior. *Personality and Social Psychology Bulletin, 23*, 945–954.

Orbell, S. & Sheeran, P. (1993). Health Psychology and the uptake of preventive health services: A review of thirty years' research on cervical screening. *Psychology and Health, 8*, 417–433.

Orbell, S. & Sheeran, P. (1998). 'Inclined abstainers': A problem for predicting health-related behavior. *British Journal of Social Psychology, 37*, 151–165.

Orbell, S. & Sheeran, P. (1999). *Volitional Strategies and the Theory of Planned Behavior.* Unpublished manuscript, University of Sheffield, UK.

Orbell, S. & Sheeran, P. (2000). Motivational and volitional processes in action initiation: A field study of the role of implementation intentions. *Journal of Applied Social Psychology, 30*, 780–797.

Ouellette, J.A. & Wood, W. (1998). Habit and intention in everyday life: The multiple processes by which past behavior predicts future behavior. *Psychological Bulletin, 124*, 54–74.

Prestwich, A., Lawton, R. & Conner, M. (2003a). Use of implementation intentions and the decision balance sheet in promoting exercise behaviour. *Psychology and Health, 18*, 707–721.

Prestwich, A., Lawton, R. & Conner, M. (2003b). *Increasing the Impact of Implementation Intentions: The impact of environmental cues, rehearsal and sufficient plans.* Unpublished manuscript, University of Leeds, UK.

Rise, J., Thompson, M. & Verplanken, B. (2003). Measuring implementation intentions in the context of the theory of planned behavior. *Scandinavian Journal of Psychology, 44*, 87–95.

Rogers, R.W. (1983). Cognitive and physiological processes in fear appeals and attitude change: a revised theory of protection motivation. In B.L. Cacioppo & L.L. Petty (Eds), *Social Psychophysiology: A sourcebook* (pp. 153–176). London: Guildford.

Schwarzer, R. (1992). Self-efficacy in the adoption and maintenance of health behaviours: Theoretical approaches and a new model. In R. Schwarzer (Ed.), *Self-efficacy: Thought control of action.* Washington, DC: Hemisphere.

Schweiger Gallo, I., McCulloch, K.C. & Gollwitzer, P.M. (2005, January). *"Don't Get So Emotional!" Volitional Control of Emotions Via Implementation Intentions.* Poster presented at the Society for Personality and Social Psychology Annual Meeting, New Orleans, Louisiana.

Sheeran, P. (2002). Intention-behavior relations: A conceptual and empirical review. In W. Stroebe & M. Hewstone (Eds), *European Review of Social Psychology* (Vol. 12., pp. 1–30). Chichester: John Wiley & Sons, Ltd.

Sheeran, P. (2004). Unpublished raw data, University of Sheffield, UK.

Sheeran, P., Aarts, H., Custers, R., Rivis, A., Webb, T.L. & Cooke, R. (2005). The goal-dependent automaticity of drinking habits. *British Journal of Social Psychology, 44*, 47–64.

Sheeran, P., Abraham, C. & Orbell, S. (1999). Psychosocial correlates of heterosexual condom use: A meta-analysis. *Psychological Bulletin, 125*, 90–132.

Sheeran, P. & Armitage, C.J. (2003). Unpublished raw data, University of Sheffield, UK.

Sheeran, P., Aubrey, R. & Kellett, S. (2003). Unpublished raw data, University of Sheffield, UK.

Sheeran, P. & Milne, S. (2003). Unpublished raw data, University of Sheffield, UK.

Sheeran, P., Milne, S.E., Webb, T.L. & Gollwitzer, P.M. (2005). Implementation intentions. In M. Conner & P. Norman (Eds), *Predicting Health Behaviour* (pp. 276–323). Buckingham, UK: Open University Press.

Sheeran, P. & Orbell, S. (1998). Do intentions predict condom use? A meta-analysis and examination of six moderator variables. *British Journal of Social Psychology, 37*, 231–250.

Sheeran, P. & Orbell, S. (1999). Implementation intentions and repeated behavior: Augmenting the predictive validity of the theory of planned behavior. *European Journal of Social Psychology, 29*, 349–369.

Sheeran, P. & Orbell, S. (2000). Using implementation intentions to increase attendance for cervical cancer screening. *Health Psychology, 19*, 283–289.

Sheeran, P. & Silverman, M. (2003). Evaluation of three interventions to promote workplace health and safety: Evidence for the utility of implementation intentions. *Social Science and Medicine, 56*, 2153–2163.

Sheeran, P., Webb, T.L. & Gollwitzer, P.M. (2005). The interplay between goal intentions and implementation intentions. *Personality and Social Psychology Bulletin, 31*, 87–98.

Smith, R.E. (2003). The cost of remembering to remember in event-based prospective memory: Investigating the capacity demands of delayed intention performance. *Journal of Experimental Psychology: Learning, Memory, and Cognition, 29*, 347–361.

Sniehotta, F.F., Scholtz, U. & Schwarzer, R. (2002a). *The Effects of Planning on Initiation and Maintenance of Physical Activity in Cardiac Rehabilitation Patients.* Unpublished manuscript, Free University, Berlin, Germany.

Sniehotta, F.F., Scholtz, U. & Schwarzer, R. (2002b). *Implementation Intentions and Coping Intentions.* Unpublished manuscript, Free University, Berlin, Germany.

Steadman, L. & Quine, L. (2000). *Are Implementation Intentions Useful for Bridging the Intention-behavior Gap in Adhering to Long-term Medication Regimens? An Attempt to Replicate Sheeran and Orbell's (1999) Intervention to Enhance Adherence to Daily Vitamin C Intake.* Paper presented to the British Psychological Society Division of Health Psychology Annual Conference, University of Kent at Canterbury, UK.

Steadman, L. & Quine, L. (2004). Encouraging males to perform testicular self-examination: A simple, but effective, implementation intention intervention. *British Journal of Health Psychology, 9*, 479–487.

Stephens, A. & Conner, M. (1999, September). *A Smoking Prevention Intervention in Adolescents.* Paper presented at the British Psychological Society Division of Health Psychology Annual Conference, University of Leeds, UK.

Triandis, H.C. (1980). Values, attitudes, and interpersonal behavior. In H. Howe & M. Page (Eds), *Nebraska Symposium on Motivation* (Vol. 27, pp. 195–259). Lincoln, NE: University of Nebraska Press.

Trope, Y. & Fishbach, Y. (2005). Going beyond the motivation given: Self-control and situational control over behavior. In R.R. Hassin, J.S. Uleman & J.A. Bargh (Eds), *The New Unconscious* (pp. 537–566). New York: Oxford University Press.

Verplanken, B. & Faes, S. (1999). Good intentions, bad habits, and effects of forming implementation intentions on healthy eating. *European Journal of Social Psychology, 29*, 591–604.

Webb, T.L. & Sheeran, P. (2004). Identifying good opportunities to act: Implementation intentions and cue discrimination. *European Journal of Social Psychology, 34*, 407–419.

Webb, T.L. & Sheeran, P. (2005a). Integrating concepts from goal theories to understand the achievement of personal goals. *European Journal of Social Psychology, 35*, 69–96.

Webb, T.L. & Sheeran, P. (in press). *Does Changing Behavioral Intentions Engender Behavior Change? A Meta-analysis of the Experimental Evidence.* Psychologica Bulletin.

Webb, T.L. & Sheeran, P. (2005b). *How Do Implementation Intentions Promote Goal Attainment? Tests of Component Processes.* Manuscript submitted for publication.

Webb, T.L., Sheeran, P. & Luszczynska, A. (2005). Unpublished raw data, University of Sheffield, UK.

Wood, W., Quinn, J.M. & Kashy, D. (2002). Habits in everyday life: The thought and feel of action. *Journal of Personality and Social Psychology, 83*, 1281–1297.

CHAPTER 7

Managing Immediate Needs in the Pursuit of Health Goals: The Role of Coping in Self-regulation

Denise T.D. de Ridder and Roeline G. Kuijer

Suppose that you have a goal of weight loss and you are trying to diet to lose some pounds. Once you have started to restrict your caloric intake it seems that your mind becomes occupied with thinking of delicious forbidden foods—much like the white bears that occupied the minds of the subjects in Wegner's experiments who were instructed *not* to think of these bears (Wegner, Schneider, Carter & White, 1987). Of course, thinking of delicious foods makes dieting more difficult—and often dieters eventually succumb to these temptations and give up on their goal of weight loss (Polivy, 1998). Food and food deprivation are emphasized by the diet and therefore the intent to ignore food is subverted (Heatherton, Mahamedi, Striepe, Field & Keel, 1997). Indeed, not being able to maintain a diet is often regarded as the prototypical case of self-regulation failure (Herman & Polivy, 2003). Take another example of a health goal that seems rather difficult to attain even though many people consider it worth while striving for: quit smoking. Many people who smoke have become aware of the risks that smoking poses to their health and have adopted the goal of quitting. Those who make an initial attempt do so then all of a sudden seem to be surrounded by people who are enjoying smoking and they are thus continuously reminded of the pleasures of their bad habit (Waters et al., 2003). Like in dieting, the frustrations that accompany quitting efforts make it very difficult to resist the temptation to take up smoking again. Not being able to deal with this frustration many quitters give in and fail in their self-regulatory efforts. These examples show that attempts at self-change often prove false (Polivy & Herman, 2002) and suggest that self-regulation failure seems to be far more common than successful self-regulation (Baumeister & Heatherton, 1996), especially in the health domain. No doubt these failures are related to the fact that many health goals (dieting, quit smoking, compliance with medication, sun protection, or dental care—to name just a few) require making trade-offs between short-term costs (e.g., bypass desert, not smoke) in exchange for long-term benefits

Self-regulation in Health Behavior.   Edited by Denise T.D. de Ridder and John B.F. de Wit.
© 2006 John Wiley & Sons Ltd.

(e.g. weight goal, good health). Sometimes these benefits do not occur until decades into the future. Research in the field of time preference (i.e., the value that people assign to future outcomes relative to immediate ones) has shown that people tend to discount future outcomes as a function of, among other things, the delay of that outcome. That is, the more delayed a future outcome is, the less it will be worth relative to the immediate reward (e.g., Chapman, 1996, 2005). To make matters worse, delayed outcomes such as good health are also more uncertain than are immediate outcomes. Hence, the more difficult it will be to resist temptations.

Many of the self-regulation failures in the health domain are not primarily related to problems in goal-setting or in initiating goal pursuit—illustrated, for example, by the high numbers of people who make New Year's resolutions to change their health behavior (Norcross, Mrykalo & Blagys, 2002)—but to maintain goal pursuit over an extended period of time (Rothman, 2000; see also De Wit, this volume). Whilst acting upon one's good intentions is an important self-regulatory problem, as exemplified in the so-called intention-behavior gap (Sheeran, Webb & Gollwitzer, this volume), figures show that many people are eager (perhaps too eager) to adopt health goals and engage in initial attempts to change their behavior without giving much thought to the long-term investment behavioral change requires. An important issue then is how people deal with frustrations and distractions once they have made initial efforts to achieve a health goal important to them.

Like other goals, health goals are difficult to attain. By definition, goals are characterized by a discrepancy between a current state and a desired one (Carver & Scheier, 1998). It is obvious, then, that some frustration is inherent in trying to achieve an ambitious goal. If goals were easy to attain, they would not be regarded as goals in the first place but rather as ordinary tasks that do not require much consideration. Yet, most self-regulation approaches are rather indifferent about the frustrations that characterize goal striving, generally acknowledging that these frustrations exist but rarely bothering about what people should do about them. To date, many self-regulation approaches acknowledge frustrations as serious obstacles that make it more difficult to stay on track and continue engagement in goal striving but they also show a tendency for denying the importance of dealing with frustration as an important self-regulatory task (Leith & Baumeister, 1996; Tice & Bratslavsky, 2000). It is assumed that some individuals will be able to deny distractions and forego temptations and thus prove to be successful self-regulators, whereas those who are not capable of doing so will eventually fail—thereby neglecting this aspect of successfully striving for goals. However, if frustrations are more or less inherent in goal striving, it makes sense that the way people deal with frustration in some way or another should affect self-regulation. Indeed, it has been argued that the simultaneous task of tenacious goal pursuit while at the same time dealing with frustrations and distractions is in fact the most important component of self-regulation (Brandtstädter & Renner, 1990; Mischel, Cantor & Feldman, 1996).

In this chapter, we will highlight this specific task and address the question how people manage to deal with the frustrations, distractions, and temptations that seem to impose a threat to goal striving, and still remain involved in goal pursuit. Whereas the dominant self-regulation view suggests that these tasks are in conflict, implying that people are either successful in striving for their long-term goals or give in to their immediate needs (e.g., Tice, Bratslavsky & Baumeister, 2001), we will consider an alternative view and examine to what extent these needs are always interfering with goal pursuit. Indeed, attractive opportunities that are at odds with one's goal may compromise goal striving as many accounts of self-regulation failure seem to suggest, but given that people rarely have the luxury of attending to one goal at a time unless one is a single-minded and rigid person, it seems worthwhile to consider the possibility that both aspects of self-regulation—dealing with long-term goals and dealing with immediate distractions—are not necessarily competitive but may actually facilitate each other. That is, striving for goals may benefit from having taken good care of immediate frustration whereas dealing with frustration may be easier in the perspective of some long-term goal.

The main idea we propose is that in order to be able to continue striving for ambitious goals people must in one way or another manage to deal with frustrations instead of simply denying them. In elaborating this idea, we will rely on notions derived from the stress and coping literature as this approach offers a conceptual framework for explaining how people deal with the demands that are perceived as taxing their resources, albeit with an emphasis on how people react to frustration in an attempt for short-term relief—that is, without considering long-term goals. Although it seems relevant to apply the theoretical framework of coping to this particular aspect of self-regulation, few attempts have been made to employ stress and coping concepts in self-regulation research (e.g., Brandstädter & Renner, 1990; Carver & Scheier, 1999; Leventhal, Brisette & Leventhal, 2003) and both literatures have largely developed in isolation (Aspinwall, 2004). Only recently, an explicit attempt was made to explore the possibilities for integrating both perspectives, highlighting how research on dealing with adversity may benefit from these complementary perspectives (Aspinwall, 2004). Yet, the full potential of the stress and coping literature for understanding self-regulatory processes remains to be determined.

In the remainder of this chapter we will first examine to what extent an integration of stress-coping concepts in the self-regulation literature may benefit our understanding of how dealing with frustration affects self-regulation. Next, we will discuss in detail the role of distress in goal striving as well as the role of affect regulation in continued goal effort. We will use the terms emotional distress and affect interchangeably. Affect is a broad category comprising the subcategories of both emotions as a label for strong feelings with a clear action component and moods as a label for mild feelings without a clear cause and no action component (Larsen, 2000), whereas emotional distress is generally used to refer to strong feelings accompanied by physiological arousal but without a clear content (Lazarus, 1991). Despite these differences, many authors make no distinction between these concepts (e.g., Tice, et al., 2001) or regard (negative) affect as synonymous with emotional distress (Carver & Scheier, 1998). Hence, we regard affect and emotional distress (but not mood) to have similar properties regarding their implications for action-readiness. We also assume that frustrations, distractions, or any other obstacles to goal pursuit represent immediate needs that create emotional distress or, for that matter, affect and thus require coping efforts.

COPING IN THE SERVICE OF SELF-REGULATION

Dealing with emotional distress is the central topic of emotional-motivational theories of stress and coping (Lazarus, 1991; Lazarus & Folkman, 1984). Generally, these theories view coping as a response to immediate threats or stressors and pay far less attention—or perhaps more accurate, no attention at all—to the role of coping with distress in long-term goal striving. To increase our understanding of the way people manage distress and at the same time remain involved in goal pursuit, an integration of emotional-motivational concepts into self-regulation approaches seems worth examining, however. In this section, we will evaluate the stress and coping literature from a self-regulation perspective, highlighting the way responding to distress might reconcile the conflict between immediate needs and long-term goals that often precedes self-regulation failure. In doing so, we will pay special attention to what extent the emotional-motivational system is different from the system engaged in long-term goal striving.

Coping in Response to Goal Threat

Although large portions of the coping literature have been devoted to developing a decent taxonomy of coping strategies (for an overview, see Skinner, Edge, Altman & Sherwood, 2003) or have addressed problems associated with operationalizing and measuring coping strategies (e.g., Coyne & Gottlieb, 1996; De Ridder, 1997; De Ridder & Kerssens, 2003; Stone, Kennedy-Moore, Newman, Greenberg & Neale, 1992; Van Heck & De Ridder, 2001), the basic premise of emotional-motivational theories of stress and coping has remained unchallenged. This premise states that coping, defined as the efforts in response to demands that are perceived as taxing the resources (Lazarus & Folkman, 1984), is elicited by the experience of emotional distress. More important, the transactional view on coping holds that the experience of distress results from an appraisal of threats to goals that are important to the person (Lazarus & Folkman, 1984). That is, distress is experienced as such because goals that represent important personal strivings are at stake. For example, someone who has adopted the goal of healthy diet may become emotionally upset when he or she is confronted with fatty foods because the possibility of giving in to this temptation is a threat to the goal of healthy diet or a slim waist. Likewise, a person who has the goal of regular exercise may feel distressed when a favorite television show challenges one's intention to go to the gym. The Lazarus and Folkman perspective on distress also implies that distress creates action-preparedness to solve the goal-threatening conditions, generally referred to as problem-focused coping, or to decrease negative feelings resulting from distress, referred to as emotion-focused coping. Put in those terms, there is a close resemblance between stress coping theory and self-regulation theory as both highlight the role of distress as goal-related.[1] Indeed, Carver and Scheier consider stress and coping basically an alternative vocabulary for the concepts that are central in self-regulation: "Stress is the condition that exists when something interferes with movement toward desired goals . . . Coping is what people do in response to that perception." (Carver & Scheier, 1998, p. 214). According to Carver and Scheier, then, coping equals goal striving as it is an attempt to decrease the discrepancy between a

---

[1] The similarities between stress coping theory and self-regulation theory in their conceptualization of distress hold in particular for the self-regulation approach adopted by Carver and Scheier (1998) and are absent in the self-regulation approach by Baumeister and colleagues (1996) that emphasizes the role of distress as interfering with self-regulation.

current and a desired state. A similar proposition has been made in Brandtstädter's dual process theory of assimilative persistence and accommodative flexibility, which identifies two main coping strategies that may be used in response to the perception of progress toward goals (Brandtstädter, 1989; Brandtstädter & Renner, 1990; see also Rothermund, this volume): Assimilative coping is used as a strategy to change circumstances and make increased efforts to attain a goal whereas accommodative coping is employed as a strategy to adjust a goal in response to situational constraints and neutralize goal discrepancies by, for example, downgrading aspirations. The conceptualization of coping merely in terms of strategies of goal pursuit, allows for a smooth integration of coping into the self-regulation framework but may neglect, however, special properties of coping defined as a response to emotional distress. We will discuss this issue in more detail after presenting another model that examines coping in the context of self-regulation.

Proactive Coping

The proactive coping model, developed by Aspinwall and Taylor (1997), also considers coping as a self-regulatory strategy and proposes that in order to offset or reduce potential stressors, people need to engage in coping before these potential stressors develop into real threats to personal goals. The model distinguishes five stages: accumulation of (for instance, financial or social) resources, screening the environment for potential stressors, appraisal of such potential stressors, preliminary coping to offset the potential stressor, and evaluating to what extent preliminary coping efforts had an effect. According to Aspinwall and Taylor (1997), an important advantage of proactive coping over reactive coping (coping with actual threats or stressors) is that proactive coping reduces distress resulting from the potential threat while there are still sufficient coping resources. In addition, proactive coping would allow for choosing the best option from a broader coping repertoire because at an early stage many coping options are still available. However, the model remains somewhat obscure about the extent to which potential threats may create sufficient distress to engage in coping efforts. Our own studies on proactive coping in middle-aged and older adults demonstrated that potential threats to important goals like, for instance, maintaining social relationships or staying healthy, did not elicit any feelings of emotional discomfort unless they were more or less experienced as real and actual threats (Ouwehand, De Ridder & Bensing, 2005). In addition, the model emphasizes the role of active, problem-focused coping strategies as the superior way of dealing with potential stressors as emotion-focused coping would prevent people from taking appropriate measures to offset the potential stressor—thereby neglecting one particularly important strategy of dealing with (potential) distress (i.e., emotion-focused coping). Another issue that deserves attention is to what extent proactive coping may not only prevent actual stressors but also benefit goal striving as the concept of goals is absent in the model. In a slightly different version of the proactive coping model it is emphasized that engagement in proactive coping would also increase the chances of realizing goals (Bode, De Ridder & Bensing, in press; Greenglass, 2002; Schwarzer, 2001; Schwarzer, 2002; Schwarzer & Taubert, 2002; cf. Aspinwall, 1997). Overall, the interesting thing about the proactive coping model is that it goes beyond coping as a response to distress and examines the way in which coping might affect future states. Because the emphasis is on preventing the development of potential stressors into full stressors, the model does not provide an answer to the important question of what ways of coping may benefit goal striving once an individual is confronted with a stressful situation.

Coping: Taking Advantage from Adversity

In a recent chapter, Aspinwall (2004) pointed out in which way the coping literature may be informative for a better understanding of self-regulation processes.[2] She argues that the way people deal with adversity such as serious illness and other negative life events may provide a window on crucial self-regulatory processes in a way that the study of deliberate and planful striving for goals—emphasized in self-regulation approaches— cannot. In adapting to adversity, people may make changes in their daily activities, personal priorities, and comparison standards. People not only withstand adversity, but they learn from it as well: They may find new ways to deal with frustrations or other negative feelings by extending their repertoire of emotion-focused and problem-focused strategies. This line of reasoning suggests that the self-regulation literature may benefit from greater attention to how people manage these changes in a creative and adaptive manner.

Extending the arguments given by Aspinwall for integrating the coping concept into self-regulation frameworks, we propose especially that more attention to emotion-focused coping will increase our understanding of self-regulation because problem-focused strategies may come close to the strategies used for goal striving that are already addressed in the self-regulation literature. Moreover, with the notable exception of Kuhl's (1984, 2000) action control theory that emphasizes the role of "non-cognitive" strategies in goal-directed action (e.g., emotion control and coping with failure) dealing with emotions is a topic that is typically not explicitly addressed in self-regulation theories. It must be noted, however, that also in the coping literature the processes underlying emotion-focused coping are not well understood—although this may be an artefact of the way emotion-focused coping is usually assessed, with an emphasis on venting emotions instead of confronting and understanding them (Austenfeld & Stanton, 2004). We will address the topic of emotion-focused coping and emotion regulation in goal pursuit in more detail later in this chapter. For now, we conclude that the coping literature may broaden the perspective of self-regulation as it provides a framework for examining how people react in meaningful ways to the experience of emotional distress when easy solutions are not available.

Coping and Self-regulation: One or Two Systems?

Stress and coping theory emphasizes that emotional distress cannot be neglected because of the strong action-tendencies distress creates. This means that engaging in coping

---

[2] It should be noted that in a similar vein research on coping might benefit from the self-regulation literature, especially insofar as it relates to issues like the way goals influence the experience of distress and the way people deal with stress (Aspinwall, 2004).

efforts is often not planful, thought out, or premeditated but an immediate response to a stressful situation; and this is exactly the reason why it has proven difficult to integrate the concept of coping into self-regulation frameworks that deal primarily with rational decision making about acting upon one's goals. Recently, it has been argued, however, that there may not be just one self-regulation system but two systems with two sorts of operating characteristics: One dealing with the restraint of unwanted impulses and urges, called the "hot" system; and one dealing with planful behavior regarding long-term goals, labeled as the "cool" system (Metcalfe & Mischel, 1999; Mischel, Ayduk & Mendoza-Denton, 2003; cf. Chaiken & Trope, 1999).[3] The hot/cool distinction does not explicitly address the role of stress and coping, but it does allow for a somewhat different framing of the role of coping with immediate distress in the process of long-term goal pursuit. That is, whereas most self-regulation approaches (with the exception of Carver and Scheier's control theory; see next section) consider emotional distress created by immediate needs as interfering with goal pursuit because it takes attention away from the long-term goal and thus needs to be controlled (even if it involves large costs with the possibility of depletion of resources; cf. Baumeister, Bratslavsky, Muraven & Tice, 1998; Muraven & Baumeister, 2000), a two systems approach implies that stoic denial of immediate needs is not always possible or even adaptive (Metcalfe & Mischel, 1999). Short-term needs represent goals in their own right: Indeed, eating fatty foods or watching a television show are not merely interfering with the long-term goals of healthy diet or regular exercise but also serve the immediate goals of pleasure or relaxation (see Gebhardt, this volume).

Framed in this way, the tempting situations that may create distress are short-term goals that are in conflict with long-term goals. Treating them as goals in their own right implies that these situations cannot be simply neglected. Metcalfe and Mischel (1999) emphasize the employment of smart cooling down strategies (such as distracting and distancing, and other strategies that remind of emotion-focused coping) to avert attention from the immediate need and to attenuate the hot system but the mere experience of distress may make it difficult to do so because distress activates the hot system. This suggests that attention should be paid to the immediate source of distress to allow (continued) engagement in the pursuit of temporally distal goals. Suggestive evidence for this counterintuitive idea was provided in a series of provocative experiments by Fischbach, Friedman and Kruglanski (2003; see also Trope & Fischbach, 2000), which demonstrated that temptations do not necessarily interfere with goal striving but may actually remind individuals of their long-term goals and have an adaptive function in goal striving. These studies did not include concepts of stress and coping or emotion regulation. However, arguing that temptations may create a considerable amount of distress because they confront individuals with the regulatory dilemma of either giving in to immediate needs or continuing goal pursuit implies that effective self-regulation does not require the sacrifice of immediate needs but, in contrast, benefits from attending to immediate needs—thus giving credit to the counterintuitive hypothesis that under conditions of distress goal-striving is harnessed by taking care of one's momentary allurements.

---

[3] This distinction reminds us of what Wills (Wills, Sandy & Yaeger, 2001) has labeled "good" and "poor" self-control (see Gibbons and colleagues, this volume, for a discussion of good and poor self-control).

Implications

The foregoing suggests that situations that create distress because they form a threat to long-term goals need to be taken care of in a careful way. Whereas most research has either addressed emotional distress as an important source of self-regulatory failure (e.g. Baumeister et al., 1998) or, in contrast, assumes that the mere experience of distress will promote striving for long-term goals (e.g., Carver & Scheier, 1998), we take a somewhat different approach to the role of distress in self-regulation. Our view on the role of coping with emotional distress in goal striving holds two central assumptions: First, we believe that emotional distress is adaptive because it is a signal that important goals are threatened and activates a system to act upon those threats (coping)—this assumption comes close to the role of distress in Carver and Scheier's control theory of self-regulation but puts more emphasis on stress and coping as a system that is governed by its own rules and not just works in service of long-term goal striving. Second, we assume that the mere experience of emotional distress will not automatically lead to greater efforts for goal pursuit because distress signifies that there is some unfinished business that needs to be taken care of before people can continue goal striving. We will address both issues in the next sections.

NEGATIVE AND POSITIVE AFFECT FROM A SELF-REGULATION PERSPECTIVE

Although the emphasis in self-regulation theories lies on the ways people control and direct their own actions in the pursuit of their long-term goals (Carver & Scheier, 1998), some of these theories hold explicit views about the role of frustration during goal attainment. It is generally acknowledged that frustrations and distractions may be quite upsetting and lead to emotional distress (Baumeister, Heatherton & Tice, 1994) or negative affect (Carver & Scheier, 1998). Indeed, a number of empirical studies have shown that goal frustrations, or even doubts about the attainability or the importance of (health) goals may create considerable distress (Brunstein, 1993; De Ridder, Kuijer & Ouwehand, 2005; Kuijer & De Ridder, 2003). That said, there appear to exist two opposing views on the role of negative affect as the result of goal frustration in self-regulation: One in which emotional distress is the villain and regarded as the main cause of self-regulatory failure (Baumeister et al. 1994; Tice et al., 2001); and another in which the adaptive nature of distress in self-regulation is emphasized (Carver & Scheier, 1998).

Is Negative Affect Good or Bad?

In their authoritative account of a broad range of self-regulation failures, including many related to health behavior, Baumeister and colleagues (e.g., Baumeister, et al., 1994) propose emotional distress as the main reason of why so many people give up on striving for their long-term goals. For example, negative moods or other types of emotional distress have been linked to relapses in addictive behaviors such as smoking, drinking, and gambling (see Tice et al., 2001, for a review).[4] In a similar vein, studies in the eating domain have shown that emotional distress triggers relapses among dieters and causes restrained eaters to eat more (e.g., Herman & Polivy, 1975; Heatherton, Striepe & Wittenberg, 1998; Van der Heijden, De Ridder & De Wit, 2005; Wallis & Hetherington, 2004).

Baumeister and colleagues argue that people's capacity for self-regulation depends on a limited resource akin to a strength or energy (Baumeister et al., 1998; Muraven & Baumeister, 2000). As the capacity for self-regulation is limited, long-term goal striving will be compromised when people use precious resources to regulate their negative emotions. In this view, negative mood predisposes people to fail at self-regulation. In laboratory studies, especially bad moods characterized by high arousal, such as anger and embarrassment, have been shown to inflict self-defeating patterns of behavior, whereas bad moods with low arousal, such as sadness, do not seem to have such detrimental effects on self-control (Leith & Baumeister, 1996). One particularly important, albeit controversial (e.g., Freitas & Salovey, 2000; Hirt & McCrae, 2000) aspect of the approach adopted by Baumeister and colleagues is that losing control and acting impulsively under conditions of distress is caused by the hedonistic motive of wanting to feel good in the short run (Tice & Bratslavsky, 2000; Tice et al., 2001). In this view, distress makes individuals more vulnerable to temptations that they would otherwise be able to with-stand, and as a result feeling good takes precedence over self-control. This line of reasoning thus states that emotional distress creates a need for immediate solutions (mood repair) that are regarded to be in conflict with long-term goals.

The Baumeister approach to self-regulation provides a good account of why so many people fail to act upon their good intentions to behave healthily or otherwise rationally when they are faced with distress, but it cannot explain how people would ever be able to maintain their efforts to invest in long-term goals under difficult conditions—except for individuals with extremely high levels of self-control who may neglect temptations and deny frustrations even under the most adverse circumstances. Theoretically, that may be an attractive explanation for the high numbers of self-regulation failure. However, given that goal commitment is a choice under uncertainty (Mischel et al., 1996), distractions and frustrations during goal pursuit are more the rule than the exception. Hence, two important questions are the following: First, to what extent is distress always at odds with goal pursuit? And second, if distress compromises self-regulation, what can people do to repair their moods in order to continue goal striving?

Distress and Goal Pursuit

Whereas in the Baumeister approach to self-regulation distress is considered to be in conflict with one's long-term interests, the self-regulation approach by Carver and Scheier (1998) considers negative affect or, for that matter, distress to be an important and even functional ingredient of self-regulation and goal striving. Their theory states that negative

---

[4] Remember that in the limited resource approach by Baumeister and colleagues (1996) no distinction is made between distress, mood, and affect.

affect results from an evaluation of how good one is doing in trying to attain a goal. That is, negative affect is a signal that one is proceeding towards the goal slower than expected or hoped for and therefore will promote increased efforts to attain the goal or, if increased effort does not result in progress, will eventually lead to disengagement from the goal. This so-called "cruise control model" thus holds that the experience of discrepancy between a current state and a desired state produces negative affect, implying that negative affect is adaptive in goal-striving as it leads to continued engagement. This view is in line with approaches that emphasize the informational properties of (negative) affect such as the safety-signal approach (Frijda, 1988), the affect-as-information approach (Schwartz & Clore, 1988; 1996), and of course also the stress-coping approach (Lazarus & Folkman, 1984). A large body of literature emphasizes the benefits of negative affect in self-regulation, highlighting that negative affect triggers a more effortful, analytic, and vigilant processing style (see Forgas, 2000 for a review), and that negative affect alerts people to potential threats of their goals and motivates them to take appropriate action (Aspinwall, 1998).

In evaluating the effects of negative affect on self-regulation it is important to distinguish between negative affect that is related to a particular goal and more general-ized negative affect that is unrelated to a particular goal. In Baumeister's research where negative affect leads to self-regulatory failure, the negative mood is typically unrelated to the self-regulatory goal (Baumeister et al., 1998; Leith & Baumeister, 1996; Tice et al., 2001). For example, Tice and colleagues (Tice et al., 2001) induced a sad and depressed mood by having participants read a story about a driver causing an accident that resulted in the death of a child. In a series of three experiments, participants responded to these bad moods by increasing impulsive behaviors (i.e., eating, immediate gratification, and procrastination). When participants were made to believe that their mood was frozen for a certain amount of time, the negative effects on self-control disappeared. In contrast, in Carver and Scheier's (1998) approach, negative affect originates when midcourse evaluations of progress is slower than expected or hoped for. In their approach negative affect is goal-related and as such functions as a source of information. This line of reasoning resembles the distinction that is often made between "moods" and "emotions" (Forgas, 2000; Gross, 1998a; Larsen, 2000). Emotions are thought to have a definite cause and a clear cognitive content. Moods on the other hand do not have a salient antecedent cause and have therefore little cognitive content. Thus, emotions contain much more information about the external environment than do moods.

To conclude, it seems that negative affect is not necessarily conflicting with long-term goals but may be interpreted as a signal that something needs to be done about the goal— a view that is also prominent in theories of stress and coping that we discussed previously.

Repair of Negative Affect

What about the repair of negative affect? Whereas negative affect is supposed to facilitate goal striving because it motivates individuals to increase their efforts, positive affect is often considered to be at odds with goal striving as it may lead to feeling satisfied and not doing anything about one's goals. In a more general view, positive affect is believed to be related to biased information processing, underestimation of risk, and decreased goal-directed behavior (see for a review on the role of positive affect in self-regulation Aspinwall, 1998). In Carver and Scheier's approach people who exceed the criterion rate of progress will experience positive feelings that elicit a tendency to "coast" with respect to the particular goal that elicited the positive affect in the first place (Carver, 2003). This position would strongly argue against a beneficial role of positive affect in self-regulation, and thus also against a need for the repair of negative affect in the service of long-term goal striving. However, a growing literature suggests that positive affect may not necessarily compromise goal-striving but instead benefit self-regulation (e.g., Forgas, 2002). Although this seems to be contradicting the literature on the role of negative affect in self-regulation, this is not necessarily true. That is, whereas positive affect may reflect satisfaction about progress toward a goal and thus result in decreased effort with regard to that specific goal, this also means that there is an opportunity for attending to other goals which may be in need of repair and, more generally, that there is an opportunity to be more open to alternative goals (Carver, 2003). Indeed, it appears that the experience of feeling good about oneself does not necessarily mean that individuals are only interested in maintaining their positive affect, rather they may be more attentive to threatening self-relevant information—as if they can afford it when feeling good (Frederickson, 1998; Diamond & Aspinwall, 2003; Trope & Pomerantz, 1998; see Aspinwall, 1998 for a review). An experimental study by Reed and Aspinwall (1998) demonstrated that participants who had an opportunity to affirm their kindness made these persons more open to information revealing how caffeine poses a health threat compared to individuals who had not been exposed to such information; the effects were even larger for caffeine users who had the greatest reason to feel threatened by the information. In a similar vein, other research has shown that people experiencing positive affect tend to adopt a more open, constructive, and creative thinking style (see Forgas, 2002, for a review). A number of authors have now argued that positive and negative affect trigger different, but not necessarily better or worse, processing styles. Fiedler (2000; Fiedler, 2001) distinguishes between an accommodative and an assimilative processing style of information.[5] An accommodative processing style is stimulus-driven and requires careful, exhaustive perception and conservation of stimulus information. An assimilative processing style is knowledge-driven and involves active cognitive elaboration and transformation of information using internal knowledge structures. Central to Fiedler's dual process model is the assumption that negative affect promotes an accommodative bottom-up processing style, whereas positive affect facilitates a more assimilative, creative and top-down processing style. It depends upon the situation or goal at hand whether an accommodative or assimilative processing style is more beneficial. For example, when one has to finish a task that requires one to be accurate and precise, a bottom-up processing style aimed at avoiding mistakes might work better than a creative and exploring processing style.

In a recent study in our lab we found evidence for an opposite effect of positive affect on self-regulation depending on the particular task (Kuijer, De Ridder & Ouwehand, 2005). In this study, female undergraduates who were concerned about their weight

---

[5] Note that the terms assimilative and accommodative in Fiedler's model are used in a different way than in the Brandtstädter model of assimilative and accommodative coping and bear more resemblance to the Piagetian conceptualization of assimilation and accommodation (see also Rothermund, this volume, footnote 1).

completed a decision-making task. Before they completed the task they were asked about their current mood. After they had finished the task they were asked to write a plan on how they would try to attain their weight goal. The decision making task that was used was a computerized version of the Iowa Gambling Task (Bechera, Damasio, Damasio & Anderson, 1994) which simulates real-life decision making under uncertain conditions. This task requires participants to choose from four decks of cards that provide losses and gains in money: Two decks have high gains but even higher losses, and two decks have low gains but lower losses. In total, they make 100 choices. In the long run, the high gain—high loss decks are disadvantageous, whereas the low gain—low loss decks are advantageous. This task was originally developed to test patients with damage to the ventromedial region of the brain (Bechera et al., 1994). More recently, the Iowa Gambling Task has been used with participants from the general population as well (e.g., Crone, Vendel & Van der Molen, 2003; Peters & Slovic, 2000) and it is generally found that as the task proceeds participants learn to choose from the "good" decks and avoid the "bad" decks. In our study we indeed found that, in general, participants made more advantageous choices as the task progressed. Interestingly, by the end of the game participants in a more positive mood made fewer advantageous choices than did participants in a less positive mood ($r = -0.29$, $p < 0.05$). This was not the case in the beginning of the task. In Carver's terminology it seems like participants experiencing positive affect tended to "coast" toward the end of the gambling task. In contrast, there was a tendency for participants in a positive mood to spend more time on writing down plans on how to attain their weight goal ($r = 0.21$, $p = 0.09$). These findings suggest that positive affect may have a negative effect on self-regulation when the task involves accurate and conscientious decision making, but a positive effect when the task requires one to be creative in making up plans (see Taylor & Gollwitzer, 1995 for similar results regarding the effects of positive outcome expectancies on self-regulation).

Our findings have important implications for the role of mood repair in self-regulation. As emotional distress is characterized by negative feelings and thus may decrease the willingness to engage in making plans for long-term goal pursuit, strategies that help to repair mood will promote reengagement in goal striving.

AFFECT REGULATION IN SELF-REGULATION

Thus, if positive affect may promote self-regulation, it follows that repairing negative affect may decrease the risk of self-regulation failure instead of increasing it. Indeed, there is some evidence for the benefits of affect regulation, especially for individuals experiencing heightened distress. For example, Goldman, Kraemer and Salovey (1996) found that college students who reported that they generally tried to repair bad moods were less likely to complain of illness. This effect was much more pronounced for students who experienced heightened distress in response to impending exams. A recent study by Hamilton, Zautra and Reich (2005) among women with rheumatoid arthritis suggests that recovery from pain is faster for women who possess good affect regulation skills. They found that pain prospectively predicted negative affect one week later only among women who scored below average on affect regulation skills.

Taking this line of reasoning one step further one may argue that there is little benefit in the stoic denial of bad moods, contrary to what is suggested in the studies by Tice and colleagues (Tice & Bratslavsky, 2000; Tice et al., 2001). In fact, it may even be more adaptive to take care of immediate needs and engage in the repair of negative affect in the best long-term interest. Is this view incompatible with the literature on distress as a promoter of goal-striving? We think not. Both the literatures on distress as a signal that one needs to spend more effort to attain goals and the literature on the role of positive affect in self-regulation consider emotional distress to be basically adaptive. Crucial in both literatures is that distress is not something arbitrary that distracts people from higher goals and keeps the mind captured in fixing immediate needs. Both literatures emphasize the role of distress as a warning that action is required—either action aimed at the realization of goals or action to alleviate emotional distress. However, in addition to the important signaling function of affect, affective states may have an impact on subsequent behavior and experience (Larsen & Prizmic, 2004). For example, if a woman with a weight goal feels sad after finding out that she has not lost weight that week, this feeling should signal to her that the weight goal is important to her (otherwise she would not feel sad) and that she did not make progress. However, we also know that emotional distress often triggers relapses among dieters (e.g., Heatherton et al., 1998; Wallis & Hetherington, 2004). This suggests that the woman needs to somehow regulate her sadness to avoid residual negative impact on her behavior.

Adaptive Emotion-focused Coping

How do people regulate affect? As mentioned earlier in this chapter, in the coping literature, a major distinction is generally made between problem-focused and emotion-focused coping. The latter is defined as the efforts of people to regulate emotions associated with a stressor (Lazarus & Folkman, 1984). Examples of emotion-focused coping strategies measured with the most commonly used coping inventories are strategies such as wishful thinking, distancing, emphasizing the positive (Ways of Coping Questionnaire; Lazarus & Folkman, 1985), seeking emotional support, reinterpretation, acceptance (the COPE: Carver, Scheier & Weintraub, 1989), and reducing stress through emotional responses, pre-occupation with self and fantasizing (Coping Inventory for Stressful Situations; Endler & Parker, 1990). Research has rather consistently shown that the employment of emotion-focused coping strategies is associated with maladaptive outcomes (Austenfeld & Stanton, 2004). This led many researchers to conclude that problem-focused coping is more adaptive than emotion-focused coping. This conclusion may be a little premature, however. A major problem with a lot of the emotion-focused coping scales is that many items are confounded with expressions of distress or self-deprecation (Stanton, Danoff-Burg, Cameron & Ellis, 1994; Austenfeld & Stanton, 2004). For example, coping strategies that are supposed to measure emotion-focused coping have included items like "become very tense," "focus on my general inadequacies" (both in the Coping Inventory for Stressful Situations; Endler & Parker, 1990). Another issue addressed by Stanton and colleagues (Stanton et al., 1994) that is particularly important for the present discussion is that most of these emotion-oriented strategies focus on avoiding negative emotions without actively confronting or processing of these emotions.

Lazarus and Folkman (1984) did not originally conceptualize emotion-focused coping as dysfunctional or less adaptive than problem-focused coping. Moreover, these robust negative findings are inconsistent with theory and research based on functionalist views of emotion in which recognition, processing, and expression of emotion is seen as functional (e.g. Gross, 1999; Larsen, 2000; Smyth & Pennebaker, 1999). Stanton and colleagues (Austenfeld & Stanton, 2004; Stanton et al., 1994; Stanton, Kirk, Cameron & Danoff-Burg, 2000) have attempted to reconcile the two literatures by examining coping through emotional approach (i.e., coping through emotional processing by actively acknowledging, exploring, and identifying one's emotions and coping through emotional expression). They found evidence that these strategies are adaptive, but not for everyone or under all circumstances. Adaptiveness was found to be a function of the environmental context, nature of the stressor, and characteristics of the individual (e.g., gender and personality) (Austenfeld & Stanton, 2004).

Our own studies on coping by confronting emotions with health-related stressors have demonstrated that people may find it difficult to engage in this type of strategy even when they are faced with stressful situations that seem beyond repair and thus would benefit from understanding one's emotions about these situations. For example, in a vignette study among patients with asthma or diabetes we gave these patients the option to choose their preferred way of coping, either a problem solving strategy or a confronting emotions strategy (Stanton, et al., 2000), in dealing with a number of stressful situations that differed in personal evaluations of feasibility. Results indicated a clear preference for problem solving, regardless of the personal feasibility appraisal of the stressful situation (De Ridder, Kuijer, Sprangers & Hox, 2005). Moreover, these preferences for problem-focused coping remained stable for a period of three months after the original assessment, suggesting that people may find it difficult to adjust their favorite or familiar coping strategies (De Ridder & Kuijer, in press). These findings show that even though confronting emotions may be an adaptive strategy, people may not easily recognize it as such, which makes sense given the social norms that exist upon fixing problems instead of acknowledging that some problems are beyond repair (Weber, 2000). Combining the finding that people may have a preference for problem-focused coping with research that has demonstrated that people become less flexible in determining their strategies once they experience emotional distress (Cheng, 2003; De Ridder, Leseman & De Rijk, 2004), it seems that turning to adaptive emotion regulation is quite a challenge for people in a state of distress.

Dealing with Emotions before They Actually Occur

In addition to the literature on emotion-focused coping, there is a growing literature on the topic of emotion regulation (or affect regulation) that is concerned with how individuals influence "which emotions they have, when they have them, and how they experience and express these emotions" (Gross, 1998a, p. 275). Whereas emotion-focused coping is focused exclusively on decreasing negative emotions, emotion regulation refers to the attempt to regulate negative as well as positive emotions (Gross, 1998a).

Moreover, the goal of emotion regulation is to change an affective state, which may or may not be related to a stressor (Gross, 1998a; Larsen, 2000), whereas emotion-focused coping is always a response to a stressor. Because of its focus on the affective state itself, emotion regulation theories allow for a more fine-grained analysis of affect regulation processes. In the process model of emotion regulation (Gross, 1998a; Gross & John, 2003) it is assumed that emotions unfold over time and that different regulation strategies can be employed during the process. Gross (1998a) distinguishes between antecedent-focused emotion regulation strategies, that is, the things we do before the emotion is generated (four stages: situation selection, situation modification, attention deployment, cognitive change) and response-focused emotion regulation strategies, that is, the things we do once the emotion is already generated (one stage: response modulation). Research by Gross and colleagues focused on two particular strategies, that is, cognitive reappraisal or "construing a potentially emotion-eliciting situation in a way that changes its emotional impact" (John & Gross, 2004, p. 1304) as a form of cognitive change (an antecedent-focused strategy) and expressive suppression or "inhibiting ongoing emotion-expressive behavior" (John & Gross, 2004, p. 1304) as a form of response modulation (a response-focused strategy) (Gross, 1998b; Gross & John, 2003). A number of studies conducted by Gross showed that the antecedent strategy of reappraisal had more adaptive consequences for affect and well-being than did the response-focused strategy of suppression (John & Gross, 2004; Gross, 1998b; Gross & John, 2003). These findings suggest that regulating emotions before they are experienced in full may benefit the individual. It should be noted that the strategies identified by Gross are conceptually related to two strategies that are also studied in the stress and coping literature (John & Gross, 2004): Cognitive reappraisal is conceptually similar to "positive reappraisal" (both in the COPE, Carver et al., 1989; and the Ways of Coping Questionnaire, Lazarus & Folkman, 1985) whereas expressive suppression resembles the (opposite of) "venting emotions" (COPE; Carver et al., 1989). However, in sharp contrast with process models of emotion regulation the coping research rarely addresses issues related to the timing of coping efforts.

The importance of timely emotion regulation, that is, dealing with emotions before they result in a state of complete emotional distress, is also addressed in research on so called "coping plans," albeit from a different perspective. Elaborating on the work of Gollwitzer on implementation intentions (Gollwitzer, 1999; see also Sheeran et al., this volume), Sniehotta and colleagues (Sniehotta, Scholz & Schwarzer, 2005; Sniehotta, Schwarzer, Scholz & Schüz, 2005) have proposed that determining one's coping strategies before one is experiencing actual frustration and distress allows for a more careful deliberation of what one will do when the going gets tough. Although the concept of coping plans reminds of related constructs like proactive coping (engaging in coping to offset a potential stressor; Aspinwall & Taylor, 1997) or preventive coping (engaging in coping to offset an identified stressor; Aspinwall & Taylor, 1997), coping plans are different insofar as they refer to the anticipation of a stressful situation that will probably happen and thus allow the individual to determine a course of action before one is overwhelmed by feelings of distress.

In a recent study in our lab, we found evidence that determining a strategy for dealing with frustration and distress at an early stage may have a beneficial effect on long-term goal striving (De Ridder, Kuijer & Ouwehand, 2005). In this study we confronted undergraduate female students who were concerned about their weight (although all of them had normal weight or were only slightly overweight) with the possibility that they might fail in their attempts to lose weight. As expected, the possibility of goal failure was a stressful experience for these young women, although of a mild nature (they were more annoyed than having strong feelings of distress, although effects depended on how important the goal of weight loss was to them). We also found that the women who had experienced goal frustration performed better at two self-regulation tasks: They spent more time on making a plan of action to attain their goal of weight loss and they also showed better self-control in withstanding a temptation that would violate their goal (that is, consumption of chocolate cookies). Interestingly, we did not find any evidence that feelings of distress affected self-regulation efforts. That is, even though the women who had experienced goal frustration performed better on both self-regulation measures as they spent more time on planning and they were better able to resist the temptation of cookies, the experience of emotional distress could not explain their greater involvement in self-regulation (see Baumeister, DeWall, Ciarocco & Twenge, 2005 for similar results regarding the role of distress in self-regulation). The absence of a mediating role of distress in self-regulation makes sense from the perspective of a two systems approach (Metcalfe & Mischel, 1999), which states that the hot stress system reacts independently from the cool system that is engaged in planning and goal striving. Still, we wondered what it was that made these girls better at self-regulation. It may be that the mere experience of goal frustration was responsible, which reminds of a series of studies by Gabrielle Oettingen who found that individuals who were asked to consider a future goal from the perspective of the present negative reality (referred to as "mental contrasting') identified better strategies for goal achievement and increased their efforts to achieve the goal (Oettingen & Mayer, 2002; Oettingen, Pak & Schnetter, 2001). The concept of coping plans, however, allows for another interpretation of our findings. By encouraging the young women in our study to think about their strategies for goal pursuit we may have given them the opportunity to consider their strategies for dealing with difficulties during goal striving and we may thus unintentionally have provided them with a chance to confront their emotions about goal pursuit, thus decreasing their feelings of mild distress at an early stage—which may, in turn, have affected self-regulatory effort.

These findings strongly suggest that dealing with (anticipated) emotions and feelings of distress are not necessarily at odds with attempts for continued goal striving and may actually benefit goal striving, especially when individuals are in a stage that they can still control feelings of emotional distress. Moreover, our findings show that attending to one's immediate needs may also boost self-control (as exemplified in being able to resist the temptation of chocolate cookies) and thus promote strategies for goal pursuit.

CONCLUSION

In the foregoing, we argued that frustrations and distractions are more or less inherent in the pursuit of ambitious health goals. These frustrations and distractions may create considerable feelings of emotional discomfort. Whereas large portions of the self-regulation literature tend to view emotional distress as interfering with goal pursuit, we have argued that feelings of distress may be adaptive in a sense that distress signals goal threat and thus may promote efforts for continued goal pursuit. However, only when there is an opportunity for dealing with emotional distress, such as when one can determine a course of action before emotional distress takes precedence, it is likely that dealing with distress and goal striving will mutually benefit each other.

The implications of this line of reasoning for the promotion of health behavior are obvious. Whereas many health promotion efforts tend to emphasize the benefits of health behavior in the long run (longevity, absence of disease) and encourage people to deny the frustrations that accompany the efforts to attain these health goals, they typically do not provide individuals with smart strategies to take care of their frustrations but instead require them to focus on their long-term goals. From the perspective that we have described in this chapter, asking individuals to deny their short-term needs may have counterproductive results as is, for example, demonstrated in the prototypical case of failure to continue attempts for weight loss. The failure to maintain diet presents a typical case of "misregulation" (Baumeister & Heatherton, 1996), as exemplified in a zero-tolerance diet in which one denies oneself even the smallest food reward. Whereas in reality small lapses do not pose a serious threat to the dieter's goal of weight loss, a zero-tolerance regimen is prone to total breakdown in case of small lapses, often leading to the "what the hell effect" (Cochran & Tesser, 1996) causing dieters to give up totally on their diet. If dieters would be allowed to take care of their immediate needs by, for example, eating high-caloric foods once in a while they would probably experience less distress, experience more positive affect, and eventually be more prepared to continue their long-term goal striving. In a similar vein, those why try to quit smoking, exercise more, or pursue any other ambitious health goal, may benefit from attending to their immediate needs at an early stage before emotional distress rises to a level at which temporally distal goals do not seem to matter anymore—with a complete abandonment of the goal as a result.

REFERENCES

Aspinwall, L.G. (1997). Where planning meets coping: Proactive coping and the detection and management of potential stressors. In S.L. Friedman & E.K. Scholnick (Eds), *The Developmental Psychology of Planning: Why, how, and when do we plan?* (pp. 285–320). London: Erlbaum.

Aspinwall, L.G. (1998). Rethinking the positive affect in self-regulation. *Motivation and Emotion*, 22, 1–32.

Aspinwall, L.G. (2004). Dealing with adversity: Self-regulation, coping, adaptation, and health. In M. Hewstone & M.B. Brewer (Eds), *Applied Social Psychology* (pp. 3–27). Malden, MA: Blackwell.

Aspinwall, L.G. & Taylor, S.E. (1997). A stitch in time: Self-regulation and proactive coping. *Psychological Bulletin, 121*, 417–436.

Austenfeld, J.L. & Stanton, A.L. (2004). Coping through emotional approach: A new look at emotion, coping, and health-related outcomes. *Journal of Personality, 72*, 1335–1363.

Baumeister, R.F., Bratslavsky, E., Muraven, M. & Tice, D.M. (1998). Ego depletion: Is the active self a limited resource? *Journal of Personality and Social Psychology, 74*, 1252–1265.

Baumeister, R.F., DeWall, C.N., Ciarocco, N.J. & Twenge, J.M. (2005). Social exclusion impairs self-regulation. *Journal of Personality and Social Psychology, 88*, 589–604.

Baumeister, R.F. & Heatherton, T.F. (1996). Self-regulation failure: An overview. *Psychological Inquiry, 7*, 1–15.

Baumeister, R.F., Heatherton, T.F. & Tice, D.M. (1994). *Losing Control: How and why people fail at self-regulation*. San Diego, CA: Academic Press.

Bechera, A., Damasio, A.R., Damasio, H., & Anderson, S.W. (1994). Insensitivity to future consequences following damage to human prefrontal cortex. *Cognition, 50*, 7–15.

Bode, C., De Ridder, D. & Bensing, J. (in press). Preparing for aging: Development, feasibility and preliminary results of an educational program for midlife and older based on proactive coping theory. *Patient Education and Counseling*.

Brandstädter, J. (1989). Personal self-regulation of development: Cross-sequential analyses of development-related control beliefs and emotions. *Developmental Psychology, 25*, 96–108.

Brandtstädter, J. & Renner, G. (1990). Tenacious goal pursuit and flexible goal adjustment: Explication and age-related analysis of assimilative and accommodative strategies of coping. *Psychology and Aging, 5*, 58–67.

Brunstein, J.C. (1993). Personal goals and subjective well-being: A longitudinal study. *Journal of Personality and Social Psychology, 65*, 1061–1070.

Carver, C.S. (2003). Pleasure as a sign that you can attend to something else: Placing positive feelings within a general model of affect. *Cognition and Emotion, 17*, 241–261.

Carver, C.S., Scheier, M.F. & Weintraub, J.K. (1989). Assessing coping strategies: A theoretically based approach. *Journal of Personality and Social Psychology, 56*, 267–283.

Carver, C.S. & Scheier, M.F. (1998). *On the Self-regulation of Behavior*. New York: Cambridge University Press.

Carver, C.S. & Scheier, M.F. (1999). Stress, coping, and self-regulatory processes. In L.A. Pervin & J.P. Oliver (Eds), *Handbook of Personality Theory and Research* (pp. 553–575). New York: Guilford.

Chaiken, S.L. & Trope, Y. (Eds). (1999). *Dual Process Theories in Social Psychology*. New York: Guilford.

Chapman, G.B. (1996). Temporal discounting and utility for health and money. *Journal of Experimental and Psychology: Learning, Memory and Cognition, 22*, 771–791.

Chapman, G.B. (2005). Short-term costs for long-term benefit: Time preference and cancer control. *Health Psychology, 24*, S41–S48.

Cheng, C. (2003). Cognitive and motivational processes underlying coping flexibility: A dual-process model. *Journal of Personality and Social Psychology, 84*, 425–438.

Cochran, W. & Tesser, A. (1996). The "What the hell effect": Some effects of goal proximity and goal framing on performance. In L. Martin & A. Tesser (Eds), *Striving and Feeling: Interactions among goals, affect, and self-regulation* (pp. 99–120). Hillsdale, NJ: Erlbaum.

Coyne, J.C. & Gottlieb, B.H. (1996). The mismeasure of coping by checklist. *Journal of Personality, 61*, 959–991.

Crone, E.A., Vendel, I. & Van der Molen, M.W. (2003). Decision making in disinhibited adolescents and adults: Insensitivity to future consequences or driven by immediate reward? *Personality and Individual Differences, 35*, 1625–1641.

De Ridder, D. (1997). What is wrong with coping assessment? A review of conceptual and methodological issues. *Psychology and Health, 12*, 311–324.

De Ridder, D. & Kerssens, J. (2003). Owing to the force of circumstances? The impact of situational features and personal characteristics on coping patterns across situations. *Psychology and Health, 18*, 217–236.

De Ridder, D., Leseman, P. & De Rijk, A. (2004). Predicting the short-term course of fatigue symptoms: Does adjustment of habitual coping strategies matter? *British Journal of Health Psychology, 9*, 67–80.

De Ridder, D. & Kuijer, R.G. (in press). *Reconsidering Illness-related Goals: Is discrepancy resolved by confronting emotions?* Psychology of Health.

De Ridder, D., Kuijer, R.G. & Ouwehand, C. (2005). *Does Confrontation with Potential Goal Failure Promote Self-regulation? Examining the Role of Emotional Distress in the Pursuit of Weight Goals* Manuscript under review.

De Ridder, D., Kuijer, R.G., Sprangers, M. & Hox, J. (2005). *Keep Striving at All Costs: Coping preferences in dealing with illness-related goals.* Unpublished data.

Diamond, L.M. & Aspinwall, L.G. (2003). Emotion regulation across the life span: An integrative perspective emphasizing self-regulation, positive affect, and dyadic processes. *Motivation and Emotion, 27,* 125–156.

Endler, N.S. & Parker, J.D.A. (1994). Assessment of multidimensional coping: Task, emotion and avoidance strategies. *Psychological Assessment, 6,* 50–60.

Fiedler, K. (2000). Towards an integrative account of affect and cognition phenomena using the BIAS computer algorithm. In J.P. Forgas (Ed.), *Feeling and Thinking: The role of affect and social cognition* (pp. 163–185). Mahwah, NJ: Erlbaum.

Fiedler, K. (2001). Affective influences on social information processing. In J.P. Forgas (Ed), *The Handbook of Affect and Social Cognition* (pp. 163–185). Mahwah, NJ: Erlbaum.

Fischbach, A., Friedman, R.S. & Kruglanski, A. (2003). Leading us not unto temptation: Momentary allurements elicit overriding goal activation. *Journal of Personality and Social Psychology, 84,* 296–309.

Forgas, J.P. (Ed.). (2000). *Feeling and Thinking: The role of affect in social cognition.* New York: Cambridge University Press.

Forgas, J.P. (2002). Feeling and doing: Affective influences on interpersonal behavior. *Psychological Inquiry, 13,* 1–28.

Fredrickson, B.L. (1998). What good are positive emotions? *Review of General Psychology, 2,* 300–319.

Freitas, A. & Salovey, P. (2000). Regulating emotion in the short term and long term. *Psychological Inquiry, 11,* 178–179.

Frijda, N. (1988). The laws of emotion. *American Psychologist, 43,* 349–358.

Goldman, S.L., Kraemer, D.T. & Salovey, P. (1996). Beliefs about mood moderate the relationship of stress to illness and symptom reporting. *Journal of Psychosomatic Research, 41,* 115–128.

Gollwitzer, P.M. (1999). Implementation intentions: Strong effects of simple plans. *American Psychologist, 54,* 493–503.

Greenglass, E.R. (2002). Proactive coping and quality of life management. In E. Frydenberg (Ed.), *Beyond Coping: Meeting goals, visions, and challenges* (pp. 37–62). Oxford: Oxford University Press.

Gross, J.J. (1998a). The emerging field of emotion regulation: An integrative review. *Review of General Psychology, 2,* 271–299.

Gross. J.J. (1998b). Antecedent- and response-focused emotion regulation: Divergent consequences for experience, expression, and physiology. *Journal of Personality and Social Psychology, 74,* 224–237.

Gross, J.J. (1999). Emotion regulation: Past, present, and future. *Cognition and Emotion, 13,* 551–573.

Gross, J.J. & John, O.P. (2003). Individual differences in two emotion regulation processes: Implications for affect, relationships, and well-being. *Journal of Personality and Social Psychology, 85,* 348–362.

Hamilton, N.A., Zautra, A.J. & Reich, J.W. (2005). Affect and pain in rheumatoid arthritis: Do individual differences in affect regulation and affect intensity predict emotional recovery from pain? *Annals of Behavioral Medicine, 29,* 216–224.

Heatherton, T.F., Mahamedi, F., Striepe, M., Field, A.E. & Keel, P. (1997). A 10-year longitudinal study of body weight, dieting, and eating disorder symptoms. *Journal of Abnormal Psychology, 106,* 117–125.

Heatherton, T.F., Striepe, M. & Wittenberg, L. (1998). Emotional distress and disinhibited eating: The role of self. *Personality and Social Psychology Bulletin*, *24*, 301–313.

Herman, C.P. & Polivy, J. (1975). Anxiety, restraint, and eating behaviour. *Journal of Abnormal Psychology*, *84*, 666–672.

Herman, C.P. & Polivy, J. (2003). Dieting as an exercise in behavioral economics. In G. Loewenstein, D. Reed, & R.F. Baumeister (Eds), *Time and Decision. Economic and Psychological Perspectives on Intertemporal Choice* (pp. 459–489). New York: Russell Sage Foundation.

Hirt, E.R. & McCrea, S.M. (2000). Beyond hedonism: Broadening the scope of affect regulation. *Psychological Inquiry*, *11*, 180–183.

John, O.P. & Gross, J.J. (2004). Healthy and unhealthy emotion regulation: Personality processes, individual differences, and life span development. *Journal of Personality*, *72*, 1301–1333.

Kuijer, R.G. & De Ridder, D. (2003). Discrepancy in illness-related goals and quality of life in chronically ill patients: The role of self-efficacy. *Psychology and Health*, *18*, 313–330.

Kuijer, R.G., De Ridder, D. & Ouwehand, C. (2005). Self control in the short term and the long term: Examining dieters' strategies for self-regulation. [Manuscript in preparation].

Kuhl, J. (1984). Volitional aspects of achievement motivation and learned helplessness: Toward a comprehensive theory of action control. In B.A. Maher (Ed.), *Progress in Experimental Personality Research* (Vol .13, pp .99–171). New York: Academic Press.

Kuhl, J. (2000). A functional-design approach to motivation and self-regulation: The dynamics of personality systems and interactions. In M. Boekaerts, P.R. Pintrich & M. Zeidner (Eds), *Handbook of Self-regulation* (pp. 111–169). San Diego, CA: Academic Press.

Larsen, R.J. (2000). Toward a science of mood regulation. *Psychological Inquiry*, *11*, 129–141.

Larsen, R.F. & Prizmic, Z. (2004). Affect regulation. In R.F. Baumeister & K.D. Vohs (Eds). *Handbook of Self-regulation: Research, theory, and applications* (pp. 40–61). New York: Guilford.

Lazarus, R.S. (1991). *Emotion and Adaptation*. Oxford: Oxford University Press.

Lazarus, R.S. & Folkman, S. (1984). *Stress, Appraisal, and Coping*. New York: Springer.

Lazarus, R.S. & Folkman, S. (1985). If it changes it must be a process: Study of emotion and coping during three stages of a college examination. *Journal of Personality and Social Psychology*, *70*, 271–282.

Leith, K.P. & Baumeister, R.F. (1996). Why do bad moods increase self-defeating behavior? Emotion, risk taking, and self-regulation. *Journal of Personality and Social Psychology*, *71*, 1250–1267.

Leventhal, H., Brisette, I. & Leventhal, E.A. (2003). The common-sense model of self-regulation of health and illness. In L.D. Cameron & H. Leventhal (Eds), *The Self-regulation of Health and Illness Behavior* (pp. 42–65). London: Routledge.

Metcalfe, J. & Mischel, W. (1999). A hot/cool system analysis of delay of gratification: Dynamics of willpower. *Psychological Review*, *106*, 3–19.

Mischel, W., Ayduk, O. & Mendoza-Denton, R. (2003). Sustaining delay of gratification over time: A hot-cool systems perspective. In G. Loewenstein, D. Reed, & R.F. Baumeister (Eds), *Time and Decision. Economic and Psychological Perspectives on Intertemporal Choice* (pp. 175–200). New York: Russell Sage Foundation.

Mischel, W., Cantor, N. & Feldman, S. (1996). Principles of self-regulation: The nature of willpower and self-control. In E. Higgins & A. Kruglanski (Eds), *Social Psychology: Handbook of basic principles* (pp. 329–360). New York: Guilford.

Muraven, M., & Baumeister, R.F. (2000). Self-regulation and depletion of limited resources: Does self-control resemble a muscle? *Psychological Bulletin*, *126*, 247–259.

Norcross, J.C., Mrykalo, M.S. & Blagys, M.D. (2002). *Auld Lang Syne*: Success predictors, change processes, and self-reported outcomes of New Year's resolvers and non-resolvers. *Journal of Clinical Psychology*, *58*, 397–405.

Oettingen, G. & Mayer, D. (2002). The motivating function of thinking about the future: Expectations versus fantasies. *Journal of Personality and Social Psychology, 83*, 1198–1212.

Oettingen, G., Pak, H. & Schnetter, K. (2001). Self-regulation of goal setting: Turning free fantasies about the future into binding goals. *Journal of Personality and Social Psychology, 80*, 736–753.

Ouwehand, C., De Ridder, D. & Bensing, J. (2005). Unpublished data.

Peters, E., & Slovic, P. (2000). The springs of action: Affective and analytical information processing in choice. *Personality and Social Psychology Bulletin, 26*, 1465–1475.

Polivy, J. (1998). The effect of behavioral inhibition: Integrating internal cues, cognition, behavior, and affect. *Psychological Inquiry, 9*, 181–204.

Polivy, J. & Herman, C.P. (2002). If at first you don't succeed: False hopes of self-change. *American Psychologist, 57*, 677–689.

Reed, M.B. & Aspinwall, L.G. (1998). Self-affirmation reduces biased processing of health-risk information. *Motivation and Emotion, 22*, 99–132.

Rothman, A. (2000). Toward a theory-based analysis of behavioral maintenance. *Health Psychology, 19*, 64–69.

Schwartz, N. & Clore, G.L. (1988) How do I feel about it? Informative functions of affective states. In K. Fiedler & J. Forgas (Eds), *Affect, Cognition, and Social Behaviour* (pp. 44–62). Toronto: Hogrefe.

Schwartz, N. & Clore, G.L. (1996). Feelings and phenomenal experiences. In E.T. Higgins & A.W. Kruglanski (Eds), *Social Psychology: Handbook of basic principles*, (pp. 433–465). New York: Guilford.

Schwarzer, R. (2001). Stress, resources, and proactive coping. *Applied Psychology: An International Review, 50*, 400–407.

Schwarzer, R. (2002). Tenacious goal pursuits and striving toward personal growth: Proactive coping. In E. Frydenberg (Ed.), *Beyond Coping: Meeting goals, visions, and challenges* (pp. 19–35). Oxford: Oxford University Press.

Schwarzer, R. & Taubert, S. (2002). Tenacious goal pursuits and striving toward personal growth: Proactive coping. In E. Frydenberg (Ed.), *Beyond Coping: Meeting goals, visions and challenges* (pp. 19–35). New York: Oxford University Press.

Skinner, E.A., Edge, K., Altman, J. & Sherwood, H. (2003). Searching for the structure of coping: A review and critique of category systems for classifying ways of coping. *Psychological Bulletin, 129*, 216–269.

Smyth, J.M. & Pennebaker, J.W. (1999). Sharing one's story: Translating emotional experiences into words as a coping tool. In C.R. Snyder (Ed.), *Coping: The psychology of what works* (pp. 70–89). New York: Oxford University Press.

Sniehotta, F.F., Scholz, U. & Schwarzer, R. (2005). Bridging the intention-behavior gap: Planning, self-efficacy, and action control in the adoption and maintenance of physical exercise. *Psychology and Health, 20*, 143–160.

Sniehotta, F.F., Schwarzer, R., Scholz, U. & Schüz, B. (2005). Action plans and coping plans for long-term lifestyle change: Theory and assessment. *European Journal of Social Psychology, 35*, 565–576.

Stanton, A.L., Danoff-Burg, S., Cameron, C.L. & Ellis, A.P. (1994). Coping through emotional approach: Problems of conceptualization and confounding. *Journal of Personality and Social Psychology, 66*, 350–362.

Stanton, A.L., Kirk, S.B., Cameron, C.L. & Danoff-Burg, S. (2000). Coping through emotional approach: Scale construction and validation. *Journal of Personality and Social Psychology, 78*, 1150–1169.

Stone, A.A., Kennedy-Moore, E., Newman, M.G., Greenberg, M. & Neale, J.M. (1992). Conceptual and methodological issues in current coping assessments. In B.N. Carpenter (Ed.), *Personal Coping: Theory, research, and applications* (pp. 15–29). Westport, CT: Praeger.

Taylor, S.E. & Gollwitzer, P.M. (1995). Effects of mindset on positive illusions. *Journal of Personality and Social Psychology, 69*, 213–226.

Tice, D.M. & Bratslavsky, E. (2000). Giving in to feel good: The place of emotion regulation in the context of general self-control. *Psychological Inquiry, 11*, 149–159.

Tice, D.M., Bratslavsky, E. & Baumeister, R.F. (2001). Emotional distress regulation takes precedence over impulse control: If you feel bad, do it! *Journal of Personality and Social Psychology, 80*, 53–67.

Trope, Y. & Fischbach, A. (2000). Counteractive self-control in overcoming temptation. *Journal of Personality and Social Psychology, 79*, 493–506.

Trope, Y. & Pomerantz, E.M. (1998). Resolving conflicts among self-evaluative motives: Positive experiences as a resource for overcoming defensiveness. *Motivation and Emotion, 22*, 53–72.

Van der Heijden, P., De Ridder, D. & De Wit, J. (2005). Emotional eating as an attempt to compensate for lack of action orientation. Paper presented at the *19th Conference of the European Health Psychology Society*, 31 August–3 September. Dublin, Ireland.

Van Heck, G. & De Ridder, D. (2001). Dimensions and measurement of coping with loss. In M. Stroebe, W. Stroebe, R. Hansson, & H. Schut (Eds), *New Handbook of Bereavement: Consequences, coping, and care* (pp. 449–469). Washington, DC: American Psychological Association.

Wallis, D.J. & Hetherington, M.M. (2004). Stress and eating: The effects of ego-threat and cognitive demand on food intake in restrained and emotional eaters. *Appetite, 43*, 39–46.

Waters, A.J., Shiffman, S., Sayette, M.A., Paty, J.A., Gwaltney, C.J. & Balabanis, M.H. (2003). Attentional bias predicts outcome in smoking cessation. *Health Psychology, 22*, 378–387.

Weber, H. (2000). Breaking all the rules: Impact of social norms on coping. Paper presented at the *14th Conference of the European Health Psychology Society*, 16–19 August. Leiden, The Netherlands.

Wegner, D.M., Schneider, D.J., Carter, S.R. & White, T.L. (1987). Paradoxical effects of thought suppression. *Journal of Personality and Social Psychology, 53*, 5–13.

Wills, T.A., Sandy, J.M. & Yaeger, A.M. (2001). Time perspective and early-onset substance use: A model based on stress-coping theory. *Psychology of Addictive Behaviors, 15*, 118–125.

CHAPTER 8

Maintaining Self-control: The Role of Expectancies

Carolien Martijn, Hugo J.E.M. Alberts, and Nanne K. de Vries

If people try to exchange their bad habits for better ones, this typically involves self-regulation. Giving up smoking or controlling your weight implies that you have to say "no" to yourself instead of giving in to craving or appetite. For example, when non-smoking or a low calorie diet are not a habit yet, people need to control their urge for a cigarette or fattening snack not only once, but on occasion after occasion. Researchers have recently theorized that self-regulation is dependent on a limited resource that allows people to manage their impulses and desires. According to the limited resources model, the resource available to manage self-regulatory effort can be exhausted or depleted by self-regulatory demands (Baumeister & Heatherton, 1996; Baumeister, Heatherton & Tice, 1994). The work of Baumeister and Muraven and their colleagues showed that self-control efforts often fail when people attempt to control themselves repeatedly within a relatively short period of time. Because people only have a limited supply of energy for active self-control, controlling behavior at one occasion leaves less capacity to manage their behavior at a next occasion (Baumeister, Bratslavsky, Muraven & Tice, 1998; Muraven, Tice & Baumeister, 1998).

In this chapter, we provide a critical discussion of the assumption that self-control primarily depends on energy and that loss of self-control should be first and foremost attributed to depletion of energy. Before starting this discussion, we would like to emphasize that we do not disagree with the idea that people may be left with fatigue when they repeatedly resist tempting but fattening snacks, control their anger when arguing with their rebellious teenage son or daughter, or become more irritable during the first days of cigarette abstinence. Feelings of fatigue, or the urge to let "it all go" after active attempts to control oneself are probably a widely shared experience (see for example Tice, Bratslavsky & Baumeister, 2001). However, we do wish to argue the assumption that loss of self-control should be first and foremost attributed to loss of energy and the related proposition that impaired self-control is almost inevitable when preceded by

Self-regulation in Health Behavior. Edited by Denise T.D. de Ridder and John B.F. de Wit.
© 2006 John Wiley & Sons Ltd.

another self-control effort. In this chapter, we will compare the conceptualization of self-control as energy resource with the view that self-control performance, and especially continuous attempts of active self-control, are strongly guided by people's expectations and cognitions about how self-control operates. We will discuss research, including our own recent research findings that show that self-control failure largely depends on the fact that most people *expect* that actively controlling themselves requires effort and is tiring. This expectation may serve as a self-fulfilling prophecy: Because we expect that self-control depletes our resources, we will encounter a next self-control activity as if we are tired, go a bit easier on things, and consequently perform less well. For example, most individuals who recently quit smoking know that resisting cigarettes involves self-control and that it is hard to keep on track. Likewise, they expect their resources for control in other behavioral domains to be diminished. Whether this is true or not, this expectation alone may be enough to visit the refrigerator more often, to drink a few extra glasses of wine, or to act grumpier towards spouses and children.

A while ago, Ellen Langer described the expectation that our energy or limits are fixed as follows: "To a large extent, mental and physical exhaustion may be determined by premature cognitive commitments; in other words, unquestioned expectations dictate when our energy will run out" (Langer, 1989, p. 135). The question then is whether a change of expectations may help people to manage their self-control efforts more effectively. Thus, are people more successful in self-control if they think that self-control primarily depends on their motivation and perseverance, or if their self regulatory capacity is governed by a limited resource?

The purpose of the present chapter is to review the existing evidence on self-control being dependent on some limited resource and to confront this with recent findings that imply that self-control depends on people's expectations about the operation of self-control.

SELF-REGULATION AND SELF-CONTROL

Although terms such as "self-control" and "self-regulation" are often treated as synonyms, we will try to define them for further use in this chapter. We will use "self-regulation" to refer to a more general, regulatory cycle of comparing the self against a relevant standard, operating the self to reduce a possible discrepancy, testing again and continuing the process until a test reveals that the standard has been reached, whereupon the person exits the cycle (conform TOTE: Test, Operate, Test, Exit; Carver & Scheier, 1982). Self-control is often defined as the overriding or inhibition of competing urges, behaviors, or desires (Barkley, 1997; Baumeister et al., 1994; Shallice & Burgess, 1993). Therefore, we will reserve "self-control" for the operate phase in which the self alters itself in order to move closer to the desired standard (Baumeister & Excline, 2000). In practice, this often means the overruling of one incipient pattern of response and replacing it with another (Baumeister, 2002). Thus, one suppresses an unwanted thought and tries to think of something else, or one ignores the elevator and takes the stairs instead. This active control process serves to reduce the risk that any thought, feeling, or behavior that is incompatible with the desired standard could take over.

SELF-CONTROL AND REGULATORY RESOURCES

Self-control as Energy

The first empirical demonstration of the assumption that self-control depends on available energy comes from Baumeister et al. (1998) who reported a series of four experiments on the so-called ego depletion phenomenon. In the most appealing experiment, Baumeister and colleagues invited three-hour food-deprived participants to a laboratory room that was filled with the aroma of freshly baked chocolate cookies (Experiment 1). Participants were confronted with two displays of food: a stack of fresh chocolate cookies and a bowl of radishes. Next, some participants were instructed to eat only from the radishes (high self-control) whereas other participants were instructed to eat the cookies (low self-control). In each condition, participants were instructed to eat at least some of the food item they were allowed to eat (some radishes in the radish condition or a cookie in the chocolate condition). This manipulation intended to manipulate participants' self-control; participants in the radish condition were hungry, and then confronted with deliciously smelling food. However, they were only permitted to eat the radishes and not allowed to touch the cookies. After that, all participants took part in a "problem-solving task" that consisted of a series of geometrical figure-tracing puzzles. What participants did not know was that these puzzles were in fact unsolvable and that the time they spent on this frustrating task served as a measure of their self-control. A group of control participants was not subjected to the food part of the experiment but started directly with the puzzle task. The exertion of self-control, that is, resisting chocolate cookies, was found to undermine subsequent persistence with unsolvable puzzles. Participants who refrained from eating cookies spent relatively less time and made fewer attempts to solve the puzzles than participants who were allowed to eat chocolate cookies and control participants who were neither hungry or exposed to food. Thus, initial exercise of self-control (refraining from eating attractive food when hungry), hampered participants' behavior on a second, unrelated self-control task (persisting on a frustrating task). According to the researchers, initial exercise of self-control consumed energy from some limited resource and left participants in a state that was labeled as *ego depletion*. Because of depletion of resources, impaired performance on a next self-control activity will follow. Hence, as Baumeister and colleagues see it, the capacity to control ourselves is defined by our own restrictions (Muraven et al., 1998; Baumeister, Muraven & Tice, 2000). These restrictions are a direct consequence of self-control drawing on a fixed and limited resource, akin to strength or energy. After an act of self-control, the resource becomes temporarily depleted leaving the individual in a state of ego depletion. Therefore, performance on a subsequent self-control act will be impaired because of a lack of resources.

The literature on ego depletion identifies a number of features of the energy resource. First, the source is non-specific and is used for a broad variety of self-control operations such as overriding or inhibiting impulses, thought suppression, regulating emotions, making choices, and so on. Second, the resource is limited, that is, the energy spent on resisting a fattening snack is no longer available to suppress a negative emotion. Third, self-control operates like a muscle. Like a muscle, self-control becomes tired after use and needs rest and relaxation to recover. Baumeister and colleagues assume that suboptimal performance may be a sign of ego depletion (complete exhaustion) but is more likely to reflect an individual's desire to spare some energy in case an emergency will arise (i.e., conservation). This so-called conservation hypothesis states that if people's resources are diminished because of an initial act of self-control, they will slow down on a subsequent task to rebuild their energy again (Baumeister et al., 2000; pp. 138–139).

Demonstrations of Ego Depletion

Experiments designed to study manifestations of limited resources and the related ego depletion phenomenon, usually consist of two tasks that both appeal to participants' self-control. The first task is always used to manipulate initial self-control and therefore varies in the amount of self-control required (high versus low self-control demand). Next, all participants engage in a second task which, again, appeals to their self-control. The typical finding is that participants who exercised high self-control at the first task show impaired performance at the second task. The difference in self-control performance between participants who employed high or low initial self-control is treated as evidence of the existence of a common resource for self-control. Participants, who exercised self-control twice in a row, will see their performance drop because both activities required energy from a shared resource. By now, the phenomenon of ego depletion is a well-researched phenomenon and empirical tests have shown that self-regulatory resources underlie a wide range of domains. Examples of findings are that the regulation of thoughts (i.e., suppressing a specific thought), altering one's emotional state (i.e., suppressing or exaggerating happy or sad emotions) and decision making involve self-control, and that each of these activities results in impaired performance on a second self-control activity (see for an overview, Schmeichel & Baumeister, 2004). For example, Muraven, Collins and Nienhaus (2002) manipulated initial self-control by instructing half of their participants to suppress a forbidden thought (high self-control) whereas the other half worked on simple arithmetic problems (low self-control). Next, all participants were invited for a 20 minute beer drinking session in which they were asked to rate the qualities of different beers. Although participants were allowed to drink as much beer as they liked, they were also provided a reason to limit their alcohol intake, so as to perform well on a subsequent driving test. In spite of the prospect of the driving test, participants who were instructed to suppress a forbidden thought consumed more beer than participants who employed low initial self-control. Interestingly, increased alcohol intake in the suppression condition was especially high for those participants who scored high on an earlier assessed alcohol preoccupation measure. Thus, particularly those people who already experience self-control difficulties in a specific domain are likely to break down when their resources are low. In similar vein, Vohs and Heatherton (2000) showed that chronic dieters who controlled their impulse to eat from easily available tempting food (bowls of snacks and sweets within arm's reach) consumed more on a subsequent ice-tasting session than non-dieters who were exposed to the same variety of snacks. Thus, the dieter who visits a birthday party is probably capable of resisting the cake and snacks offered by the friendly host ("Thanks, your cake looks delicious, but I really shouldn't") but only at great self-regulatory costs. When the dieter arrives at home, he or she is likely to break loose and eat more for supper that he or she normally does.

Other demonstrations of ego depletion are related to emotion regulation and show that participants who suppressed or exaggerated their feelings performed less well on a next self-control task than participants who were allowed to act naturally (Muraven et al., 1998). Also, initial depletion affects consumer behavior in the sense that ego depleted individuals are more likely to engage in impulse purchases (i.e., buying items that one did not intend to buy) than non-depleted individuals (Baumeister, 2002; Faber & Vohs, 2004).

Although most of the empirical evidence for self-control as limited strength was obtained by Baumeister, Muraven and their co-workers, we managed to replicate the ego depletion phenomenon in our own laboratory. In one of our first experiments (Tenbült, Dreezens & Martijn, 2002), we tried to demonstrate the ego depletion phenomenon in a decision-making domain because active involvement in decisions is also expected to deplete regulatory resources (see Baumeister et al., 1998). Participants were presented with a series of eight moral dilemmas about societal issues such as euthanasia, xeno-transplantation (transplantation of animal organs into humans), or personal dilemma's. One of the personal dilemmas we used was formulated as follows:

Friends.

You go out with your friends to a discotheque. Your best friend did not join you because she had a row with her boyfriend and did not feel like going out. Late in the evening, when you take a walk through the discotheque you suddenly see this boyfriend and catch him kissing with another girl who is obviously not your best friend. The day after, you meet your best friend. She tells you that she has been thinking a lot about her relationship and that she has decided to make up with her boyfriend. They have been quarrelling a lot lately, and she has not been very nice to him. She thinks that all this is going to change: They love each other and their relationship deserves a new chance.

Each dilemma was described in about 150 words and after reading a description all participants were required to answer a series of questions, such as whether the dilemma appeared to them as credible, true to life, or difficult, etc. Additionally, participants in the "active choice" condition were asked to make a choice between two options. For example, in the case of the "friends" dilemma participants were presented with option A: *I would tell my best friend what I saw,* or option B: *I would not tell my best friend what I saw.* In the no choice condition participants were not confronted with these two options. Next, all participants received a rather thick booklet with extremely difficult and frustrating puzzles (anagrams and mathematical problems). The experimenter explained that it was not necessary to solve all puzzles but that she would be grateful if they would solve as many puzzles as they could. She stressed that participants were free to decide when they wanted to quit and that they could press a button in order to let her know that they wanted to stop. The time that participants spent on puzzling was unobtrusively registered. Figure 8.1 displays the minutes that participants spent on the puzzle task. In the active choice condition, participants gave up puzzling after about 15 minutes whereas participants in the no choice condition persisted much longer and kept on puzzling for a generous 25 minutes. In sum, our results replicated the ego depletion phenomenon and

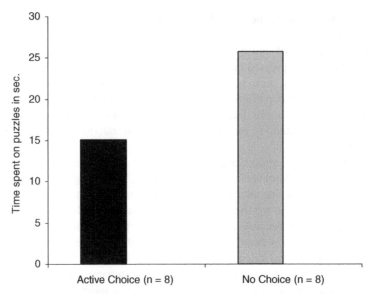

Figure 8.1 Minutes spent on puzzle task as a function of decision making (active choice versus no choice)
Data from Tenbült, Dreezens & Martijn (2002, Experiment 1, p. 231).

demonstrated that an initial exercise of self-control (such as making an active, difficult decision) reverberated negatively on a second act of self-control (forcing oneself to go on with a difficult and boring task).

Avoiding Ego Depletion

Most suggestions to improve self-regulatory strength and, hence, to avoid ego depletion are primarily inspired by the "self-control as muscle" analogy (Baumeister et al., 2000). Just as muscles profit from a balanced mix of training and recovery, self-control may also be strengthened by a regime of training and rest. Some evidence for this was provided by Muraven, Baumeister and Tice (1999), who instructed students to engage in self-control training (such as keeping food diaries or improving posture) for a two-week period. After that period, students showed improved performance on a physical self-control measurement when compared to a control group.

According to the limited strength model, it does not matter much whether people *think* they are good or bad at a specific self-control activity. Wallace and Baumeister (2002) provided half of their participants with positive feedback on a Stroop task (fewer errors and faster reaction times than 95% of prior participants) and the other half with negative feedback (more errors and reaction times in the lower twenty-fifth percentile of previous participant times). Subsequent persistence on an unsolvable figure-tracing puzzle showed no difference in persistence between participants who received positive or negative feedback. Consequently, the authors conclude that self-control failure should be primarily ascribed to depletion of a limited resource. That is, reduced performance due to ego depletion is not determined by self-perception mechanisms ("I am good/bad at this task") but rather by the amount of prior self-control effort exerted. However, a possible critique on this study is that feedback manipulations only affected participants' beliefs about their ability to solve a Stroop task. It is unclear whether Wallace and Baumeister's manipulation also affected participants' perceptions of how well (or badly) they perform on different kinds of self-control tasks, or their capacity for self-control in general. Obviously, changes in participants' perceptions of their self-control are essential if one wants to establish or exclude a feedback effect on a subsequent self-control task. Thus, the question whether self-control is affected by people's belief in their self-controlling abilities seems unresolved.

According to Baumeister and colleagues, self-control or ego-training may help to increase the energy resource for self-control, whereas rest may help to restore expended resources. Apart from rest and sleep, the preliminary results of Baumeister, Dale and Tice (1998 cited in Baumeister et al., 2000), imply that positive affect may also help to restore the depleted source. Participants who took part in an initial self-control task and then received a positive mood manipulation (watching a brief comic video), performed better on a subsequent self-control task than participants who received no mood manipulation.

A different approach comes from Webb and Sheeran (2003) who found that forming "implementation intentions" provided a helpful strategy to overcome ego depletion. Formation of implementation intentions seemed to bypass the need to exercise self-control because performance became largely automated (also see Sheeran, Webb & Gollwitzer, this volume).

In sum, some evidence exists that depletion of resources may be prevented or overridden in several ways. First, training the self may help to expand one's resources by which ego depletion effects will be less immediate. Interestingly, these "training methods" seem to develop one's capacity on activities on which one did not train. Second, it is suggested that rest and sleep may help to replenish the depleted self and preliminary evidence points at the possibility that positive affect may also have a restoring effect. Third, automation strategies such as implementation intentions may help to operate one's resources in a more economic way.

SELF-CONTROL AND EXPECTANCIES

The Flexibility of Limits

If we want to explain to our students the subjective nature of fatigue and flexible limits, a catching way to do so is to describe the so-called "Coolidge effect" (Bermant, 1976; Dewsbury, 1981). The phenomenon was identified by animal behaviorists who studied the effects of novelty on sexual activity. If a male rat is introduced to a female rat in a cage, he will immediately start copulating at a remarkably high rate. With time, the male will grow tired of that particular female and, even though there is no apparent change in her receptivity, he eventually reaches a point where he has little apparent libido. However, when a new female of the species is brought in, he will immediately resume mating with the same vigor and enthusiasm as before. This phenomenon clearly describes that experience of exhaustion is not fixed. A novel stimulus (bring on the (new) girls!), a change of context, can mobilize new energy. As a result, feelings of fatigue may vanish into thin air.

A more psychologically colored demonstration comes from Karsten (1928, cited in Langer, 1989) who studied situations that first feel good, but with repetition become uncomfortable. Participants were given tasks such as writing *ababab* as often as they could, or reading a short poem aloud over and over again. They were told that they could stop writing or reading when they were tired. From a self-control angle, reading a poem once or twice is probably fun, but after twenty-eight recitals it involves self-control to read it again. After seemingly endless repetitions, all participants felt mentally and physically exhausted: Participants reported numb hands or sore throats. However, when the participants who read the poems aloud complained to Karsten how much they hated the task, their voices were not croaky. Also, when Karsten asked the *ababab* participants to sign their names and addresses for another purpose, they did so quite easily. According to Karsten, this should not be interpreted as feigning: All participants genuinely felt exhausted. Rather, the change of context renewed their energy. Their mindset of fatigue was changed and lifted by a shift in context.

Therefore it seems likely that the fact that people *think* of their capacity for self-control as fixed and limited plays an important role in self-regulatory failure. After all, the thought that self-control is limited and self-control "eats up" your energy may be learned by experience or by internalizing folk wisdoms such as "you can't burn the candle both ends," or "a bow long bent at least waxes weak." Of interest then is the question if the notion of limited regulatory resources of Baumeister and others primarily reflects such a "naive" expectancy, rather than describing the invariant processes that underlies self-control. The relevance of naive expectancies on self-regulation was recently demonstrated by Tice, Bratslavsky and Baumeister (2001) who showed that sad people often indulge in fattening snacks because they believe that eating repairs your mood. However, when this expectancy was challenged, and people were informed that eating does nothing for your mood, they did not snack more than control participants who were in a neutral mood. Do note that, on closer consideration, the results of Tice, Bratslavsky and Baumeister, who all (co-) authored on many of the ego depletion articles discussed earlier in this chapter, seem at odds with the basic assumption that self-control primarily depends on limited energy. After all, the role of expectancies on subsequent self-control performance clearly demonstrates that such performances do not solely depend on strength but on what people expect and think.

Expectancies and Self-control

The influence of expectancies, (implicit) beliefs, and thoughts on judgments and behavior is a well-studied phenomenon in many domains of social psychology. Such expectancies are sometimes called "mindsets," premature cognitive commitments, or implicit or lay theory (Dweck, Chui & Hong, 1995; Furnham, 1988; Langer, 1989). For example, Dweck and colleagues distinguished two main implicit theories about personality. The so-called "incremental" theory of personality refers to the belief that personality characteristics such as intelligence or ability are malleable and can be improved by increasing effort. "Entity" theorists, on the other hand, believe that intelligence and ability are predetermined and fixed quantities. Advocates of this position are more ready to see behavior as stable, consistent, and diagnostic of underlying attributes than incremental theorists (McConnell, 2001). Thus, when faced with enduring self-control demands, incremental theorists will probably increase their efforts in order to succeed, whereas entity theorists are less likely to mobilize energy and will resign to failure: When it's gone, it's gone. A recent series of studies of Mukhopadhyay and Johar (2005) showed that persons who think that self-control is an unlimited and malleable ability tend to set more goals than persons who believe their capacity is finite.

In one of our studies, we tried to examine whether people hold different classes of beliefs about self-control (Martijn, Tenbült, Merckelbach, Dreezens & De Vries, 2002). We compared two different views about self-control. The first view was labeled as the "self-control as energy" expectancy. This refers to the expectancy that self-control draws on a limited and thus fixed amount of energy. This expectancy matches the manner in which Baumeister and co-workers conceptualize self-control. The second view was labeled as "self-control as motivation" and referred to the expectancy that self-control depends on perseverance, holding on and thus, motivation. As opposed to the "self-control as energy" expectancy, the motivation expectancy views self-control *not* as a fixed entity but as flexible, malleable and, in principle, unlimited: If you want to, and really try hard, you can always control yourself. A 20-item questionnaire was constructed that consisted of 10 questions intended to tap the "self-control as energy" view and 10 questions to measure participants agreement with the "self-control as motivation" view (see Table 8.1 for the exact phrasing of the items). A sample of undergraduate psychology students who indicated their agreement to the self-control scales (items were presented in a random order) tended to agree with both views on self-control, but showed relatively more agreement to the "self-control as energy" scale than with the "self-control as motivation" scale. The answers on the two scales were not correlated. This implies that (at least) two types of expectancies exist about the operation of self-control. The most prominent or "default" expectancy is that self-control is primarily a matter of energy; to succeed on a self-controlling activity you need to be well-rested, free of other self-control demands, and you feel pretty tired afterwards. However, people also endorse the view of "self-control as motivation"; with the "right" attitude you can control yourself, even if you are tired or busy with something else. Corroborating evidence comes from Muraven et al. (1998, Study 4) who asked their participants to write two autobiographical stories: one about a situation in which they successfully controlled their emotions and one about a situation in which they failed to control their emotions. Stories that described loss of control referred relatively more frequently to being tired, feeling stressed, or being drunk than stories that described successful emotional coping. The fact that such references are mentioned spontaneously in stories about self-regulatory failures, suggests that "conscious sensation of fatigue is associated with poorer self-regulation" (Muraven et al., 1998, p. 768).

Challenging Expectancies about Self-control

In one of our first studies, we tested whether expectancies about self-control influence performance on a task that requires self-control (Martijn, Tenbült, Merckelbach, Dreezens

Table 8.1 Item means and standard deviations for the "Self-control as Energy" subscale and the "Self-control as Motivation" subscale ($n = 47$)

"Self-control as energy" items	Mean	SD	"Self-control as motivation" items	Mean	SD
1. After putting my best foot forward, I need to replenish my reserves	2.63	0.74	1. I perform better when I am under pressure	2.49	0.65
2. After trying to control my emotions, I feel tired	2.65	0.51	2. I always manage to find the energy for the things I want to do	2.28	0.57
3. After finishing something I don't like to do, I feel like letting it all hang out	3.22	0.49	3. Sometimes, when I feel like I am finished, I can do a lot more than I thought	2.51	0.51
4. I get tired when I have to control myself	2.72	0.57	4. If things don't go my way, I add a little extra	3.03	0.79
5. I have difficulties to control myself when I am tired	3.17	0.79	5. If I am really motivated, I always manage to control myself	2.59	0.45
6. If I try hard my battery runs down: I need a break before I can go on	2.80	0.45	6. If you really want to, there are no limits to the extent to which you can control yourself	2.66	0.54
7. If I control myself, this costs me a lot of energy	2.68	0.61	7. If I manage to control myself, I feel more energetic	2.37	0.55
8. After completing an exacting task, I take some time to relax	3.29	0.57	8. If I feel tired, I try to compensate by trying extra hard	2.71	0.66
9. Controlling intense emotions wears me out	2.91	0.55	9. Successful control is a matter of the right mentality	2.77	0.49
10. If I plan to do something that involves self-control, I try to be well-rested	3.05	0.66	10. If I control myself, I feel strong	2.65	0.48
Total Subscale	2.92	0.37	**Total Subscale**	2.61	0.41

Data from Martijn, Tenbült, Dreezens, Merckelbach & De Vries (2002, Study 2, p. 456).

& De Vries, 2002, Exp. 1). In this experiment, we examined the effects of emotion regulation on a subsequent muscular endurance test. First, all participants performed a baseline assessment on a handgrip task and it was measured how long they could squeeze the handles together (this procedure was adapted from Muraven et al., 1998, Exp. 1). Next, all participants were asked to watch a highly disgusting video-excerpt that showed an Asian woman who causes herself to throw up and subsequently eats her own vomit. Prior to watching the video, in the *no suppression* condition participants received the following instructions:

> In a moment you will see a video. Before the video starts, the screen will turn blank for a while. It is important that you watch the video with attention. As I explained earlier, the video may evoke an emotional reaction so please be aware that you can signal me to stop the video at any time you wish.

In the *suppression* and the *suppression-expectancy challenge* condition, participants received the same instructions with the following addition:

> If you experience any emotions during watching the video, try not to show them. In other words, try to behave in such a way that other people cannot see what you are feeling.

Thus, all participants were required to watch the aversive video and probably all experienced the same negative emotions. In the no suppression condition participants could freely express such feelings whereas participants in the two suppression conditions were instructed to inhibit their emotions and thus exerted self-control. After watching the video, all participants filled out a short questionnaire to assess their mood and to check whether they complied with the suppression instructions (the latter for suppression conditions only). Then, the experimenter read the following text to the participants in the *suppression-expectancy challenge* condition:

> Often people believe that they have to rest after an effortful task. However, scientific investigations have proven that this is not the case after an emotional effort. It seems that people do not have to rest after emotional effort. In contrast to their expectations, people may actually perform better on a physical exertion task after an emotional effort.

Participants in the no suppression and the suppression only conditions received no such instructions. Next participants squeezed the handgrip for the second time. The main dependent variable was the difference in squeezing times between the base line handgrip measurement and the second handgrip measurement. Notably, squeezing times at the base line measurement did not significantly vary between the three conditions (no suppression, suppression only, and suppression-expectancy challenge).

The pattern of results was largely consistent with our expectancy hypothesis (see Figure 8.2). When participants exercised self-control by actively suppressing their feelings elicited through watching a highly aversive video episode, their persistence on

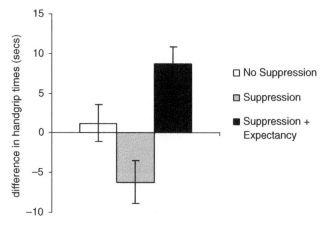

Figure 8.2 Mean difference (± 1 SE) in seconds of the two handgrip measurements of the three conditions (no suppression, suppression only, and suppression + expectancy challenge) Data from Martijn, Tenbült, Dreezens, Merckelbach & De Vries (2002, Experiment 1, p. 450).

an immediately following physical stamina task dropped dramatically as compared to control participants who did not control their emotional responses. This pattern replicates the classical ego depletion phenomenon: Exercising initial self-control impairs performance on a subsequent self-control task. However, the ego depletion phenomenon was completely eliminated and even reversed when people were told that inhibiting your emotions does not affect a next physical performance in a harmful manner. Thus, challenging people's expectancies about the limits to their control capacities seemed to eliminate the negative effects of ego depletion and resulted in even better performance on the physical self-control task than the performances of control participants who exercised no initial self-control effort.

Priming Self-control as Motivation

Simply telling people that they had no need of a break because of a prior effort, proved to be sufficient to counter-act the negative effects of ego depletion. In a further series of experiments we tried to change people's expectancy of self-control in a more subtle manner (Alberts, Martijn, Greb, Merckelbach & De Vries, 2005). Instead of offering explicit information on what to expect, we used different priming procedures to see whether people's expectations about self-control can be altered. Again, we departed from the assumption that people, when faced with a series of control-demanding operations, expect and act upon the belief that self-control consumes energy. This will result in a decrease of self-control performance. In these experiments, our approach was different in the sense that we did not refute participants' belief that self-control depends on energy but tried to activate the opposite belief that self-control depends on motivation. In the first experiment, we followed approximately the same procedure as in Martijn et al. (2002, Exp. 1). At the beginning of the experiment, participants' baseline performance on a handgrip task was assessed and their squeezing times were registered. Then the manipulation of initial self-control followed; participants tried to solve either easy labyrinths (low self-control) or extremely difficult labyrinths (high self-control). Next, participants supposedly took part in a language test and unscrambled 25 four-word sentences (scrambled sentence task, SST; see Srull & Wyer, 1979). Their task was to form grammatically correct sentences of three words; to form a correct sentence the order of the words had to be rearranged and the word that did not fit in had to be detected. Half of the participants received a set of scrambled sentences of which 15 were related to perseverance, holding on, etc. (e.g., holds Peter the on → Peter holds on the); the other 10 were neutral (e.g., bread Sam in buys → Sam buys bread in). Thus, by presenting these biased sentences we tried to activate self-control as motivation (see for a similar procedure Araya, Akrami, Ekehammar & Hedlund, 2002). In the neutral priming condition, participants unscrambled 25 neutral sentences. Directly after the SST, all participants took part in a self-control measurement and squeezed the handles of a handgrip as long as they could. Thus, the experiment consisted of a two (initial self-control: low versus high) by two (type of prime: perseverance SST versus neutral SST) between subjects design. The main dependent variable was again the difference in handgrip time between the second handgrip measurement and the baseline handgrip measurement. There were no a priori differences between conditions at the base line handgrip measurement.

The main outcomes were that participants who were initially depleted with difficult labyrinths kept their physical self-control performance at the same level when they were primed with perseverance (SST with perseverance related sentences). It is important to note that none of the participants was aware that the SST included sentences that were related to perseverance, nor did they make a connection between the SST and the earlier or subsequent self-control task. However, in the neutral SST condition, participants' handgrip performance went down, replicating a standard effect of ego depletion. Participants who solved easy labyrinths (low self-control) showed no difference between the first and second handgrip measurement and, as predicted, their performance was unaffected by type of SST.

The same outcomes were found in a similarly designed experiment (Alberts et al., 2005, Exp. 2). First, we assessed participants' base line self-control on a weight-lifting task. This task resembled the handgrip task, only this time participants were instructed to hold a 1.5 kg dumb-bell as long as possible with their arm stretched in a 90° angle to their torso while sitting on a chair in front of a computer screen. When they lost this position, the weight hit a bell that was placed beneath the dumb-bell. The experimenter started a stopwatch the moment the participant held the 1.5 kg dumb-bell in the described position and stopped timing when the dumb-bell hit the bell underneath. Figure 8.3 presents an image of the experimental situation.

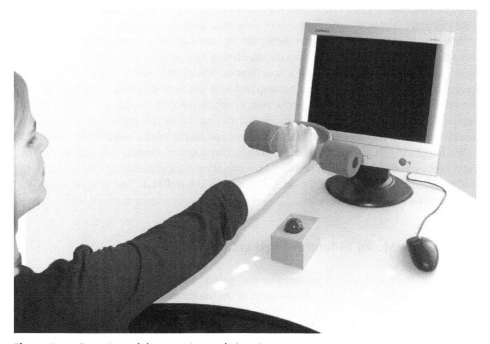

Figure 8.3 Overview of the experimental situation

Participants held a 1.5 kg weight with their arm stretched in a 90° angle to their torso while seated in front of a computer screen. When they no longer managed to lift the weight, their arm hit the bell beneath the weight, and the experimenter stopped timing. Reproduced by permission of Carolien Martijn.

After assessing participants' base line weight-lifting performance, participants underwent a low or high initial self-control manipulation by an attention control task. In the low initial self-control condition participants solved relatively easy 1- and 2-digit calculations that were presented on a computer screen. In the high initial control condition participants wore headphones and while solving fairly difficult 2-digit calculations they were simultaneously exposed to a voice randomly naming digits and thereby interfering with their calculations. Thus, self-control was needed to override the impulse to listen to the voice and to focus attention on the calculations on the screen (see for a similar procedure to elicit depletion Schmeichel, Vohs & Baumeister, 2003). Next, all participants were again instructed to hold the 1.5 kg weight as long as possible with their arm stretched in a 90° angle to their torso while sitting on a chair in front of a computer screen (see Figure 8.3). Again, the time they managed to lift the weight in the described position was registered.

When participants were lifting the weight for the second time, half of the participants were primed with perseverance. As described, they lifted the weight in front of a computer screen on which, suddenly, a screensaver appeared that depicted a young man in a business suit winning a hurdle race and a logo saying: "www.you-can-do-it.com, wallpapers and screensavers." In the neutral prime condition the screensaver showed a vase and a similar logo saying: "www.myscreensaver.com, wallpaper and screensavers."

Our main dependent variable was the difference between the second and baseline weight-lifting task. The results showed a pattern analogue to our first priming study. When initially depleted participants were presented with a perseverance-related prime (a screensaver that depicted a winner) their performances on the second weight-lifting task were equal to their performances on the baseline measurement. When initially depleted participants saw a neutral picture of a vase (neutral prime) their performance on the second weight-lifting task went down. The participants who were not depleted (easy calculations) showed the same weight-lifting performance on the second weight-lifting task as on baseline. Thus, for non-depleted participants, the nature of the prime (perseverance or neutral) did not affect their performances. These results are summarized in Figure 8.4.

We conclude that using different priming techniques to increase the salience of the expectancy of self-control as depending on motivation (i.e., persevering and holding on), enabled people to perform better on a second self-control task, and counter-acted the negative effects of ego depletion.

Using a Role Model to Improve Self-control

In the studies described in the previous paragraph, we used rather subtle techniques to increase the accessibility of self-control as motivation. But is it also possible to increase people's self-control performance by modeling and imitation? Therefore, in a next study, we examined the influence of a highly motivated and perseverant role model on self-control performances (Martijn et al., in press). We were particularly interested in the question whether a perseverant role model can help under circumstances in which people experience difficulties in controlling themselves (i.e., are "suffering" from ego depletion).

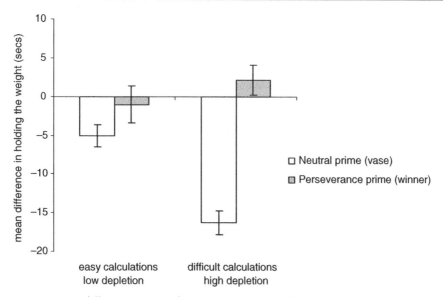

Figure 8.4 Mean difference ($\pm$ 1 SE) between two weight-lifting measurements in seconds as a function of depletion and type of prime

Data from Alberts, Martijn, Greb, Merckelbach & De Vries (2005, Exp. 2).

To study this, all participants performed the same sequence of tasks. First, participants' baseline handgrip performance was assessed in a baseline measurement. Then, the amount of initially exerted self-control was manipulated. Participants were required to solve for a 10 minute period a series of relatively easy labyrinths (low self-control condition), or a series of extremely difficult and frustrating labyrinths (high self-control condition). After that, participants engaged in a supposedly different study for which they read a text. Half of these participants received a text in which a well-known Dutch ice-skater describes his races and state of mind during the 2002 Olympic winter games in Salt Lake City (perseverance prime condition). The text was written in the form of a newspaper article and the core of the ice-skater's story was that, at a certain point, he felt like he had spent all his energy and reached his limits. Somehow, he got himself together again and he skated his best race ever, because: "I gave my best shot when I was out there. I kept telling myself: Don't give up, don't quit. At a certain moment I thought I gave it all. Strange enough, you can do more than you think. I have learned that I can do much more than I thought: You have to go for it." The other half of the participants read a neutral text about the International Olympic Committee (neutral prime condition). After reading one of the texts, participants' squeezing time on a handgrip was measured again. The difference between this second, and the baseline handgrip measurement was calculated and served as our main dependent variable. Thus, to summarize, our design consisted of a 2 (low versus high initial self-control) by 2 (text about a perseverant role model versus neutral text) between subjects design with the difference between the first and second handgrip measurement as main dependent variable.

Results replicated our earlier findings in which we tried to influence self-control expectations by means of an expectancy challenge, or by several priming procedures:

Initially depleted participants managed to keep their self-control performance at the same level after being presented with a perseverant role model. Their handgrip times did not go down and were equally well as good as the baseline measurement. Initially depleted participants who received a neutral prime instead, demonstrated a decline in their performance and thus showed the standard ego-depletion effect. Again, exit interviews revealed that participants did not suspect any relation between reading a text about a successful sportsperson and their own performances. This result corroborates Bargh's automotive model which states that the presence of a relevant situational feature may automatically activate a mindset that operates without any role played by conscious intention (Bargh, Chen & Burrows, 1996). Thus, reading about a perseverant role model, may have increased the accessibility of the expectancy of self-control as motivation which prevented a loss of control. Surprisingly, in the conditions in which participants exercised relatively low initial self-control, the opposite pattern of results was observed. If these low depleted participants were primed with a perseverant role model, subsequent self-control performance went down. A neutral prime did not affect their self-control performance. Thus, whereas depleted participants demonstrated an assimilation effect in the direction of the prime, relatively low depleted participants showed a contrast-effect and were less able to control themselves (see Figure 8.5).

At first sight, the results of participants who did not engage in a prior self-control task seem awkward. However, as argued by Dijksterhuis et al. (1998, p. 870) "automatic behavior is not a one-way street ending up in assimilation." These authors demonstrated that participants slowed down their pace when primed with the stereotype of the elderly but that they walked away faster when primed with a concrete and rather extreme

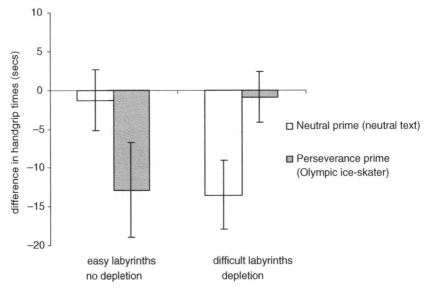

Figure 8.5 Mean difference (±1 SE) between the two handgrip measurements in seconds as a function of initial self-control and type of priming
Data from Martijn et al., (2005).

exemplar of an elderly person (the Dutch Queen Mother, then aged age 89). Dijksterhuis and colleagues proposed that traits and stereotypes elicit assimilation whereas priming exemplars of a category elicits contrast by evoking a social comparison (e.g., "I am much younger and fitter than the Queen Mother"). The same suggestion comes from Stapel and colleagues (Stapel & Blanton, 2004; Stapel, Koomen & Van der Pligt, 1996) who argued that in order to predict the direction of a priming effect one should always attend to the extremity and distinctiveness of primed information. The Dutch Olympic ice-skater we used as a role model in our study is very likely to have represented a rather extreme exemplar of self-control and perseverance. This may have evoked social comparison amongst low depleted participants who drew a negative conclusion: "I am not such a go-getter as that Olympic ice-skater." This corroborates the findings of Stapel and Koomen (2001) that showed that comparison mindsets typically result in contrast effects. More-over, the previously discussed studies in which the accessibility of perseverance was increased by means of a trait-priming procedure (i.e., a scrambled sentences task) did *not* result in contrast effects for low depleted participants (Alberts et al., 2005).

Thus, given the existing evidence, it is not so much a surprise that low depleted participants contrasted their behavior but rather that high depleted participants showed assimilation. It is possible that depleted participants did engage in social comparison but focused primarily on the similarities between themselves and the troubled, but never-theless successful ice-skater. As Lockwood and Kunda (1997) noted, a role model will only become a source of inspiration if one compares oneself to this person. This other person should be viewed as similar and relevant in terms of features and/or circumstances. Although comparison is more likely if a role model excels in the same domain (e.g., a university professor comparing to an academic superstar), a role model may affect one's self-view even if he or she excels in an irrelevant domain (Lockwood & Kunda, 1997) Depleted participants in our experiment may have perceived a relevant similarity between the state of mind in which the Olympic medalist found himself (experiencing fatigue and feeling the urge to give up) which inspired them to act in the same way (holding on despite fatigue): *What he can do, I can do too.*

Taken together then, our results suggest that self-control performances may benefit from unrelated thinking about a role model who as a consequence of his or her persistence and motivation managed to realize a goal. Whether such a role model results in assimilation or contrast, is likely to depend on one's depletion level. Especially if one's own resources are low, a successful role model may facilitate thinking about self-control as a state of mind and become a source of inspiration.

Perceptions of One's Own Self-controlling Abilities

In one of our recent studies, we examined whether people's self-control performance is influenced by the extent to which they believe they are good or bad at self-control (Martijn, Alberts & Goedegebuure, 2005). Thus, are self-control performances affected by whether people think of themselves as perseverant, self-controlled individuals and does this perception counteract the negative effects of ego depletion? The design of our study resembled the design of previous described studies. First, baseline performances on a physical handgrip task were assessed for all participants. Next, all participants filled out a computerized version of a self-control personality questionnaire (Tangney, Baumeister & Boone, 2004). Subsequently, half of the participants were depleted by means of extremely difficult labyrinths, whereas the other half exercised relatively low self-control and solved relatively easy labyrinths. Then half of the participants were told the computer calculated their "self-control" scores when they were solving labyrinths and that, if they wished, a short interpretation of these scores was available to them. All participants indicated that they wanted to see their feedback and the following text was printed on the screen:

> On the basis of your answers on the personality questionnaire, the computer calculated your personal self-control score. Your score indicates that you are a typical go-getter. When you start something, you will almost certainly finish. Giving up is no option to you. Setbacks or misfortune do not discourage you but instead motivate you to persist in order to reach your goal.

Thus, participants in the self-control feedback condition received information that they were rather good at self-control. Answers on additional questions at the end of the experiment indicated that participants considered the feedback as trustworthy and correct. The other half of the participants received no feedback. Finally, all participants squeezed the handgrip again and their handgrip times were compared to the baseline measurement. The most important finding was that initially depleted participants (difficult labyrinths) who were led to believe that they scored high on the self-control scale did not show any sign of ego depletion; they performed equally well as participants who exercised low self-control (easy labyrinths). When depleted participants received no feedback, their performance on the second physical self-control measurement went down. It is important to note that the effect of self-control feedback on subsequent self-control performance was not mediated by mood.

Thus, when people believe that they are high in self-control, they consequently perform better on self-control demanding tasks. This result implies again that successes or failures on a series of tasks that require self-control are not only determined by the amount of remaining energy but dependent on people's expectations of how they will perform on a self-control demanding task. Of course, the finding that whether people believe or not that they are able to perform a certain task affects their task performance, is not new and closely matches well-established behavioral mediators such as "self-efficacy" (Bandura, 1977) or perceived behavioral control (Ajzen & Madden, 1986). However, our finding does illustrate again that self-control performance does not solely draw on energy but strongly depends on people's expectations, i.e., whether you are good or bad at self-control.

Conservation of Energy

In the previous part of this chapter, we described a series of studies that showed that challenging self-control expectancies or activating "self-control as motivation" helped participants to overcome ego depletion. However, the question remains what exactly happens when such manipulations are applied. Do the findings of these studies imply that ego depletion is not a necessary consequence of enacting self-control? In other words, can ego depletion be diminished or even eliminated?

According to the so-called conservation hypothesis (Baumeister et al., 2000), our manipulations are not likely to eliminate or diminish the ego-depletion phenomenon. Instead, they simply postpone its effect. According to this hypothesis, an act of self-control only partly depletes the self. People are able to conserve their energy when, for example, the need to exert self-control is not great enough. In line with this, a series of experiments by Muraven and Slessareva (2003) demonstrated that ego depletion may be compensated by increasing people's motivation to perform well on a subsequent self-control task. Muraven and Slessareva explained the compensatory effect of motivation on ego depletion in terms of incentives that motivate people to use more of their energy resources. If such an incentive is absent, individuals who had already used up part of their resources tend to conserve their leftover energy, which is reflected in impaired self-control performance on a subsequent task. Yet, if breaking into one's reserves seems worthwhile (either for one's own benefit or that of others), the tendency to mobilize costly energy will dominate the tendency to conserve. Thus, Muraven and Slessareva concluded that the natural (not necessarily conscious) tendency of depleted individuals is to conserve their scarce resources, and what is left will only be brought to action in the presence of an important goal.

If people indeed conserve their energy, it seems likely that priming or using other strategies to enhance control, somehow causes people to invest more energy in a self-control demanding task. In terms of motivational factors, this would mean that participants only become more motivated to perform well at the specific task at hand which encourages them to mobilize their (last) energy resources (Muraven & Slessareva, 2003). If true, then making people invest more energy to keep their self-control performance stable after being depleted, should cause them to have less energy available for a subsequent, third task, since they spent (most of their) resources on the previous (second) task. In contrast, people who are not depleted or motivated to keep their performance stable should have conserved their energy and, accordingly, have more energy left to spend. Therefore, mobilization of energy should be reflected in a decreased performance on and willingness to invest in a subsequent self-control task. In a recent experiment we tested the conservation hypothesis (Alberts, Martijn & De Vries, 2005). In this study, all participants were exposed to a series of three computerized self-control tasks in a fixed order. However, the information that participants received about the number of tasks was manipulated. To the first group, the experimenter gave non-specific information about the number of tasks; these participants were told that "The present experiment consists of a series of exacting tasks that will require a lot of effort." The second group was falsely informed that "The present experiment consists of *two* exacting tasks that will require a lot of effort." Finally, the third group was correctly briefed that "The present experiment consists of *three* exacting tasks that will require a lot of effort." The conservation model predicts that people are sensitive to future self-control demands. In other words, if people expect exposure to a considerable number of self-control demanding tasks, they should be more inclined to conserve energy and deal with their available energy in a way that takes future self-control acts in to account. However, the results of the study failed to show any significant differences between groups. Performance did not suffer nor benefit from the information given by the experimenter. Participants who were correctly informed about the number of tasks did not make fewer mistakes and did not exhibit faster reaction times than the other groups. In sum, these findings show no evidence for the supposed tendency and capability of people to conserve energy when they engage in self-control demanding tasks.

CONCLUSION

This chapter started off with a discussion of recent theorizing and research findings that aim at demonstrating that self-controlled action is a heavy consumer of mental resources (Baumeister et al., 1998; Baumeister & Heatherton, 1996; Muraven & Baumeister, 2000). Admittedly, self-control attempts can feel as arduous and demanding. However, in our view the proposition that self-control first and foremost depends on limited energy and that subsequent acts of self-control are therefore destined to fail, is too rigid. To us, the idea that people rely on some mental petrol tank for self-controlled action has little appeal. What makes this picture especially unattractive is the assumption that the amount of mental strength or energy is a direct function of prior consumption and that after initial depletion not much can be done to boost one's energy again. Moreover, the precise nature of this strength or energy remains unclear and seems, as Metcalfe and Mischel have argued "... much in need of a theory that specifies how it comes about and operates and when it goes up and down, and who has it and who lacks it" (1999, p. 16). It looks as if recent studies on limited strength and the related ego depletion phenomenon are trying to meet this need. For example, self-controlled action appears to be related to biased time-perception (Vohs & Schmeichel, 2003). In a series of studies, it was demonstrated that participants who took part in a self-control demanding task, as compared to a control group, systematically overestimated the duration of that task. This belief may result in abandonment of further self-control. This points to the fact that subsequent self-control efforts are, at least in part, guided by subjective interpretations of prior efforts and not by the "objective" amount of energy invested per se.

Additionally, room is created for motivational factors to explain and predict self-control by the previously discussed work of Muraven and Slessareva (2003). Their work underlined the importance of goals for subsequent self-control effort. In our view, the consideration of such factors might be a worthwhile addition to the limited strength model because it leads to a better understanding of how self-control really works. Although the self-control as a muscle analogy seems powerful and appealing, the role of the athlete was put somehow out of action. After all, self-control does not only involve (mental) muscles but also a brain: It is the athlete who decides whether the game is important enough to give it all or to save some for the next. In other words, determining whether the stake is high enough and acting upon it is a consideration that requires a brain, and not only muscle.

The starting point of our own studies was that self-control performance might be guided by the fact that people *think* of their self-controlling capacities as limited (e.g., Martijn et al., 2002). Thus, people's expectations are the driving force behind ego depletion phenomena. In line with this, we proposed that self-control performance might not be a matter of energy alone, but also of expectancies about self-control. By now, we have repeatedly demonstrated that the activation of the expectation of "self-control as motivation" leads to significant improvements in self-control. These studies together strongly suggest that enactment of self-control does not inevitably lead to poorer performance on subsequent tasks. Ego depletion can be overcome when positive control expectancies are present.

It may be clear that *if* ego depletion and its negative effect on subsequent acts of self-control are inevitable, this is bad news for health education. After all, whether or not a person will engage in healthy behavior and will continue to do so often requires self-control. If people's limited capacity to manage health-related behavior explains why early ex-smokers light a cigarette the moment they experience stress, or why dieters can't resist the canteen's daily special, it is important to understand why self-control fails and whether it is possible to prevent negative effects of ego depletion. Interventions aiming at changing behavior that involve self-control should then account for people's limited strength. Possible ways to account for limited strength are to ensure that people change their behavior step by step instead of aiming at major changes all at once. Another strategy is to follow Baumeister's suggestion that training may enlarge self-controlling capacities. This means that people should be brought repeatedly into situations that appeal to their self-control. In the beginning, they will probably fail but they will gradually succeed more often in controlling unwanted thoughts, emotions or impulsive behavior.

However, if self-control success or failure can be explained in terms of differential expectations about self-control, interventions should start off differently. For example, interventions could start with an inventory and the explicit formulation of such expectations. If necessary, negative or inappropriate expectations should be changed for more positive and helpful expectations.

To summarize, an answer to the question why and how people lose or maintain their self-control is relevant both for theory and practice. Future research should focus on the question whether loss of control is an inevitable effect of "mental depletion" or whether changing expectations about self-control, and developing strategies to do so, enables people to maintain their control.

AUTHOR NOTE

Preparation of this chapter was supported by a grant of the Netherlands Organization for Scientific Research (NWO, Grant No. 402-01-049).

REFERENCES

Ajzen, I. & Madden, T.J. (1986). Prediction of goal-directed behavior: Attitudes, intentions, and perceived behavioral control. *Journal of Experimental Social Psychology, 22*, 453–474.

Alberts, H., Martijn, C. & de Vries, N.K. (2005). *Testing the Conservation Hypothesis: Do Strategies Aiming at Eliminating Ego Depletion Simply Delay its Effect?* Manuscript submitted for publication.

Alberts, H., Martijn, C., Greb, J., Merckelbach, H. & De Vries, N.K. (2005). *Carrying On or Giving In: The role of (implicit) cognition in overcoming ego depletion.* Manuscript submitted for publication.

Araya, T., Akrami, N., Ekehammar, B. & Hedlund, L.E. (2002). Reducing prejudice through priming of control-related words. *Experimental Psychology, 49*, 222–227.

Bandura, A. (1977). Self-efficacy: Toward a unifying theory of behavior change. *Psychological Review, 84*, 191–215.

Bargh, J.A., Chen, M. & Burrows, L. (1996). Automaticity of social behavior: Direct effects of trait construct and stereotype activation on action. *Journal of Personality and Social Psychology, 71*, 230–240.

Barkley, R.A. (1997). *ADHD and the Nature of Self-control*. New York: Guilford.

Baumeister, R.F. (2002). Yielding to temptation: Self-control failure, impulsive purchasing, and consumer behavior. *Journal of Consumer Research, 28*, 670–676.

Baumeister, R.F., Bratslavsky, E., Muraven, M. & Tice, D.M. (1998). Ego depletion: Is the active self a limited resource? *Journal of Personality and Social Psychology, 74*, 1252–1265.

Baumeister, R.F. & Exline, J.J. (2000). Self-control, morality, and human strength. *Journal of Social and Clinical Psychology, 19*, 29–42.

Baumeister, R.F. & Heatherton, T.F. (1996). Self-regulation failure: An overview. *Psychological Inquiry, 7*, 1–15.

Baumeister, R.F., Heatherton, T.F. & Tice, D.M. (1994). *Losing Control: How and why people fail at self-regulation*. San Diego, CA: Academic Press.

Baumeister, R.F., Muraven, M. & Tice, D.M. (2000). Ego depletion: A resource model of volition, self-regulation, and controlled processing. *Social Cognition, 18*, 130–150.

Bermant, G. (1976). Sexual behavior: Hard times with the Coolidge effect. In M.H. Siegel & H.P. Zeigler (Eds), *Psychological Research: The inside story*. New York: Harper & Row.

Carver, C.S. & Scheier, M.F. (1982). Control theory: A useful conceptual framework for personality-social, clinical and health psychology. *Psychological Bulletin, 92*, 111–135.

Dewsbury, D.A. (1981). Effects of novelty of copulatory behavior: The Coolidge effect and related phenomena. *Psychological Bulletin, 89*, 464–482.

Dijksterhuis, A., Van Knippenberg, A., Spears, R., Postmes, T., Stapel, D.A., Koomen, W. & Scheepers, D. (1998). Seeing one thing and doing another: Contrast effects in automatic behavior. *Journal of Personality and Social Psychology, 75*, 862–871.

Dweck, C.S., Chui, C. & Hong, Y. (1995). Implicit theories and their role in judgments and reactions: A world from two perspectives. *Journal of Personality and Social Psychology, 56*, 680–690.

Faber, R.J. & Vohs, K.D. (2004). To buy or not to buy? Self-control and self-regulatory failure in purchase behavior. In K.D. Vohs & R.F. Baumeister (Eds), *Handbook of Self-regulation* (pp. 509–524). New York: Guilford.

Furnham, A.F. (1988). *Lay Theories. Everyday understanding of problems in the social sciences*. Oxford, UK: Pergamon.

Langer, E.J. (1989). *Mindfulness*. Cambridge, MA: Perseus Books.

Lockwood, P. & Kunda, Z. (1997). Superstars and me: Predicting the impact of role models on the self. *Journal of Personality and Social Psychology, 73*, 91–103.

Martijn, C., Alberts, H. & Goedegebuure, F. (2005). *Positive Self-control Feedback Eliminates Ego Depletion*. Manuscript submitted for publication.

Martijn, C., Alberts, H., Merckelbach, H., Havermans, R., Huijts, A. & de Vries, N.K. (in press). If he can do it, then I can too: The influence of a role model on self-control and ego depletion. *European Journal of Social Psychology*.

Martijn, C., Tenbült, P., Merckelbach, H., Dreezens, E. & de Vries, N.K. (2002). Getting a grip on ourselves: Challenging expectancies about loss of energy after self-control. *Social Cognition, 20*, 441–460.

McConnell, A.R. (2001). Implicit theories: Consequences for social judgment of individuals. *Journal of Experimental Social Psychology, 37*, 215–227.

Metcalfe, J. & Mischel, W. (1999). A hot/cool-system analysis of delay of gratification: Dynamics of willpower. *Psychological Review, 106*, 3–19.

Mukhopadhyay, A. & Johar, G.V. (2005). Where there is a will, is there a way? Effects of lay theories of self-control on setting and keeping resolutions. *Journal of Consumer Research, 31*, 779–786.

Muraven, M. & Baumeister, R.F. (2000). Self-regulation and depletion of limited resources: Does self-control resemble a muscle? *Psychological Bulletin, 126*, 247–259.

Muraven, M., Baumeister, R.F. & Tice, D.M. (1999). Longitudinal improvement of self-regulation through practice: Building self-control strength through repeated exercise. *Journal of Social Psychology, 139*, 446–457.

Muraven, M., Collins, R.L. & Nienhaus, K. (2002). Self-control and alcohol restraint: an initial application of the self-control strength model. *Psychology of Addictive Behaviors, 16*, 113–120.

Muraven, M. & Slessareva, E. (2003). Mechanism of self-control failure: Motivation and limited resources. *Personality and Social Psychology Bulletin, 29*, 894–906.

Muraven, M., Tice, D.M. & Baumeister, R.F. (1998). Self-control as a limited resource: Regulatory depletion patterns. *Journal of Personality and Social Psychology, 74*, 774–789.

Schmeichel, B.J. & Baumeister, R.F. (2004). Self-regulatory strength. In R.F. Baumeister & K.D. Vohs (Eds), *Handbook of self-regulation: Research, theory, and applications* (pp. 84–98). New York: Guilford.

Schmeichel, B.J., Vohs, K.D. & Baumeister, R.F. (2003). Intellectual performance and ego depletion: Role of the self in logical reasoning and other information processing. *Journal of Personality and Social Psychology, 85*, 33–46.

Shallice, T. & Burgess, P. (1993). Supervisory control of action and thought selection. In A. Baddeley & L. Weiskrantz (Eds), *Attention: Selection, awareness, and control* (pp. 171–187). Oxford: Oxford University Press.

Srull, T.K. & Wyer, R.S. (1979). The role of category accessibility in the interpretation of information about persons: Some determinants and implications. *Journal of Personality and Social Psychology, 37*, 1660–1672.

Stapel, D. & Koomen, W. (2001). The impact of interpretation versus comparison mindsets on knowledge accessibility effects. *Journal of Experimental Social Psychology, 37*, 134–149.

Stapel, D.A. & Blanton, H. (2004). From seeing to being: Subliminal social comparisons affect implicit and explicit self-evaluations. *Journal of Personality and Social Psychology, 87*, 468–481.

Stapel, D.A., Koomen, W. & van der Pligt, J. (1996). The referents of trait inferences: The impact of trait concepts versus actor-trait links on subsequent judgments. *Journal of Personality and Social Psychology, 70*, 437–450.

Tangney, J.P., Baumeister, R.F. & Boone, A.L. (2004). High self-control predicts good adjustment, less pathology, better grades, and interpersonal success. *Journal of Personality, 72*, 271–322.

Tenbült, P., Dreezens, E. & Martijn, C. (2002). Over zelfcontrole en ego depletion: Is ego depletion het resultaat van energieverlies of schema-activatie? [On self-control and ego depletion: Is ego depletion the result of loss of energy or activation of a scheme?]. In D.A. Stapel, M. Hagedoorn & E. Van Dijk (Eds), *Jaarboek Sociale Psychologie 2001*. Delft, NL: Eburon.

Tice, D.M., Bratslavsky, E. & Baumeister, R.F. (2001). Emotional distress regulation takes precedence over impulse control: If you feel bad, do it! *Journal of Personality and Social Psychology, 80*, 53–67.

Vohs, K.D. & Heatherton, T.F. (2000). Self-regulatory failure: A resource-depletion approach. *Psychological Science, 11*, 249–254.

Vohs, K.D. & Schmeichel, B.J. (2003). Self-regulation and extended now: Controlling the self alters the subjective experience of time. *Journal of Personality and Social Psychology, 85*, 217–230.

Wallace, H.M. & Baumeister, R.F. (2002). The effects of success versus failure feedback on further self-control. *Self and Identity, 1*, 35–41.

Webb, T.L. & Sheeran, P. (2003). Can implementation intentions help to overcome ego-depletion? *Journal of Experimental Social Psychology, 39*, 279–286.

CHAPTER 9

Maintenance of Health Behavior Change: Additional Challenges for Self-regulation Theory, Research, and Practice

John B.F. de Wit

To fully profit from improvements in their personal health and quality of life, individuals who have managed to quit smoking, succeeded in taking up regular physical exercise, successfully improved their diet or effectively implemented changes in any other aspect of their lifestyle, need to maintain these behaviors over a wide range of contexts and extended periods of time, if not always and forever. Unfortunately but unsurprisingly, reviews of available research in a range of health behavior domains, such as weight loss (Jeffery et al., 2000), smoking cessation (Ockene et al., 2000), physical exercise (Marcus et al., 2000), and dietary behavior (Kumanyika et al., 2000), suggest that for most individuals long-term maintenance of health behavior change is difficult to achieve, and may be the exception rather than the rule. In this chapter I will argue that the prolonged maintenance of changes in health behavior presents major self-regulatory challenges, in addition to those inherent in mounting motivation to change and initiating action to attain a health goal, addressed in other chapters in this volume.

In a sense, the ubiquity of non-maintenance of health behaviors seems to suggest that at least in some behavioral domains individuals will never reach a point where they will be able to lay back comfortably and can entirely terminate efforts to self-regulate a given health behavior (cf. Brownell, Marlatt, Liechtenstein & Wilson, 1986). This is compellingly illustrated by the recovered alcoholic, former smoker, or earlier user of other addictive substances who perhaps for the rest of her or his life may need to retain a certain level of self-regulatory vigilance to effectively ensure long-term maintenance of the previously attained abstinence goal. Non-maintenance of health behaviors and relapse

Self-regulation in Health Behavior. Edited by Denise T.D. de Ridder and John B.F. de Wit.
© 2006 John Wiley & Sons Ltd.

into previously discarded behavioral patterns are notorious obstacles to successful long-term behavior change, although at times giving up may reflect adaptive disengagement from unattainable goals (see Rothermund, this volume). Unfortunately, maintenance and relapse have received only limited systematic attention in empirical tests of psychological theorizing of health behaviors, leaving largely unanswered the question of the (mal)adaptive nature of no longer sustaining behavior change. In addition, while substantial progress has been made in achieving short-term behavior change, much less attention has been devoted to important issues related to the successful promotion of maintenance of behavior change, which has proven far more difficult to instill (Wing, 2000a, 2000b).

In the remainder of this chapter I will first outline the challenges that the maintenance of health behavior change presents to achieving successful lifestyle modifications in a range of health-related domains. The chapter's central concern is with the influence of processes related to goal setting and goal striving on the successful outcome of self-regulated behavior change. The main part of the text therefore outlines the understanding of maintenance and relapse that is offered by contemporary theories of health behavior change, which generally were not devised to explain sustained health behavior change. In reviewing these theories' potential contributions, several self-regulation challenges will be considered in more detail, such as recovery from a lapse and the impact of such a slip on the long-term outcomes of the change process. Further self-regulation issues to be addressed include the influence of characteristics of the adopted health behavior goal on the successful maintenance of change, and the way sustained change is affected by resource demands that result from the shielding of protective health behavior goals over prolonged or indefinite periods of time.

To illustrate salient issues I will mostly draw on studies of sexual behavior change to prevent infection with sexually transmitted diseases and HIV, with an emphasis on work done by our own group among men who have sex with men. The non-maintenance of safer sex over time or context has become an established problem that has received quite some attention in behavioral epidemiology research among homosexual men. De Wit and Van Griensven (1994), for instance, used survival analysis to study the maintenance of safe sex among gay men in Amsterdam, and what they observed was as alarming as it was unexpected at the time. Almost all of about 400 participating men who had been practicing safer sex for at least one year reported some instance of risk-taking at a later point in time. After a maximum follow-up of almost eight years, 88% of respondents had failed to sustain safe sexual behaviors. Despite the apparent extent of non-maintenance, sustaining change of sexual behavior has only infrequently been addressed in health and social psychology.

MAINTENANCE OF HEALTH BEHAVIORS

The state of science related to achieving long-term behavior change across major health-related behaviors, notably smoking, physical exercise, and weight control, has been summarized in a series of comprehensive papers (see Wing 2000a). Overviews for disparate health behavior domains are similarly disconcerting, and if anything the papers show how difficult and unlikely prolonged maintenance of health behavior change is for most individuals. As Orleans (2000) put it: "Relapse remains the norm, regardless of the behavior in question (p. 77)." The overviews also testify to how little is known of the process of behavior change in general, and the factors promoting successful maintenance and recovery from lapse or relapse in particular. A detailed review of the literature on the maintenance of specific health behaviors is beyond the scope of this chapter, and the following is only intended to illustrate key maintenance issues in major domains.

Jeffery et al. (2000) note that over half of US adults have a weight level (corrected for height) that is of concern for their health. Moreover, historical trends in prevalence of overweight and obesity have generally been upward since the 1960s, in adults and children alike (National Center for Health Statistics, 2004). This increase in weight has been occurring despite high rates of dieting, suggesting that at the population level weight loss successes are being offset by ditto failures. The natural history of weight loss and regain among individuals who participate in behavioral treatments for obesity is remarkably consistent, and almost all fail to maintain change (Jeffery et al., 2000).

Decreasing cigarette smoking among adolescents and adults is also an important public health objective (e.g., United States Department of Health and Human Services, 2000), which has met with some success. However, in 2002 25% of adult men and 20% of adult women in the US were still current smokers (National Center for Health Statistics, 2004). The majority of smokers who managed to stop at a given time relapse (Ockene et al., 2000). About two thirds of relapse in smoking and other addictions occurs in the first three months (Hunt, Barnett, & Branch, 1971; cf. Ockene et al., 2000). Within one year more than three quarters of initial quitters may have relapsed, but relapse continues to occur thereafter (Centers for Disease Control and Prevention, 2005; Cohen et al., 1989).

Sexual behaviors, notably of men who have sex with men, changed dramatically in the 1980s, and researchers and practitioners were taken aback by an apparently sudden occurrence of relapse (e.g., Stall, Ekstrand, Pollack & Coates, 1990). For instance, de Wit, Van den Hoek, Sandfort and Van Griensven (1993) followed a cohort of HIV-negative and HIV-positive gay men, and a series of cross-sectional assessments showed that a decade into the HIV-epidemic, a significant increase had occurred in the proportion of men who engaged in risk-taking. Longitudinal data in addition illustrated substantial dynamics in individuals' safer and risky behaviors over time. Importantly, some men lapsed (24.9%), while an additional proportion had actually relapsed (31.0%).

Can Prolonged Behavior Change Be Achieved?

A substantial body of research illustrates that the prolonged maintenance of health behavior change presents major challenges for health promotion and disease prevention, and is difficult to attain. This is not to say, however, that sustained behavior change cannot be achieved at all, as the evidence reviewed thus far might have inadvertently suggested. Importantly, behavioral studies generally do not address individual behavioral dynamics over time, and hence do not allow any conclusions regarding the cumulative success, or lack thereof, of individuals' repeated change attempts. Exemplary of the typical approach to the study of maintenance of change are studies concerned with New Year's resolutions (e.g., Norcross, Mrykalo & Blagys 2002; Norcross, Ratzin & Payne, 1989; Norcross & Vangarelli, 1989). These studies show that some 40–50% of US adults make a New Year's resolution, mostly related to health behaviors (Norcross et al., 2002). Initial success in behavior change is substantial, but this declines rapidly over time.

Despite the difficulties involved in sustaining behavior change, Schachter (1982) has argued that individuals are capable of successfully maintaining change in their addictive-appetitive behaviors, notably smoking and obesity. However, sustained change may only come about after multiple attempts that individuals typically report. They make, for instance, the same resolutions year after year, illustrating that behavior change is a process rather than a discrete event (Cohen et al., 1989). Nevertheless, little is actually known of the dynamic aspects of behavior change, relapse, and eventual maintenance (Jeffery, 2000; Wing, 2000b).

UNDERSTANDING HEALTH BEHAVIOR MAINTENANCE

A host of factors affect maintenance of health behavior change at least to some extent, including personal/demographic, physiological, psychological, cognitive, and environmental/social context characteristics (Marcus, Bock & Pinto, 1997; Ockene et al., 2000). A typical list mostly encompasses barriers to sustained change, and relapse is better understood than successful maintenance (Orleans, 2000; see also Bandura, 1999). However, successful change reflects more than the mere absence of barriers, and understanding maintenance of health behavior change presumes a comprehensive conceptualization of barriers as well as enabling factors, and advances testable theories. Such theories, it has been suggested, should in particular answer the question how the processes involved in initiation of change differ from those involved in its maintenance (Jeffery et al., 2000). While Rothman and colleagues (King, Rothman & Jeffery, 2002; Rothman, 2000; Rothman, Baldwin & Hertel, 2004) contend that current models cannot adequately answer this question, I will first discuss the potential contributions of these health behavior theories that have been criticized for other reasons as well (see Conner & Norman, 2005).

Social-cognitive Theories of Motivation and Behavior

This category encompasses what are considered dominant health behavior theories (for overviews see De Wit & Stroebe, 2004; Conner & Norman, 2005). Social-cognitive models focus on the variables underlying behavioral decision-making (Fishbein et al., 2001), and in particular capture some of the more important motivational factors that underpin adoption of (health) behavior (cf. Armitage & Conner, 2000). Primarily these theories specify predictive models of proximal variables that determine the (non)performance of a behavior at a given point in time (Fishbein et al., 2001). This conceptual and empirical emphasis on the static prediction of behavior undoubtedly has promoted the view that social-cognitive theories are unsuited to understand and promote the maintenance of health behavior change (cf. Rothman, 2000; Rothman et al., 2004; also see Sheeran, Conner & Norman, 2001).

There are, however, at least two reasons why this conclusion is incorrect or premature at best. Social-cognitive theories are concerned with *ongoing* behavior, and assume that people will continue to behave as they have until something interrupts the normal flow of events (Fishbein et al., 2001). Behavioral outcomes to be predicted can therefore involve sustained patterns of behavior or even habits (for a consideration of habits, see Ajzen, 2002). Furthermore, according to the principle of compatibility, a behavior can be best predicted from measures of behavioral determinants that are equally general or specific in terms of target, action, context, and time as the outcome under consideration (Ajzen & Fishbein, 1977). This does not preclude the prediction of sustained change from any social-cognitive theory.

An early study demonstrating this point prospectively assessed predictors of relapse into unprotected intercourse with casual partners among gay men (De Wit, Van Griensven, Kok & Sandfort, 1993). The study was not explicitly framed as a test of the Theory of Planned Behavior, but a stronger intention to avoid intercourse with casual partners, higher condom use self-efficacy and a more favorable attitude regarding condom use with these partners promoted maintenance of safer sex over one year. More recently, my colleagues and I tested the prospective impact of beliefs regarding changes in HIV-related health threat on the risk of HIV-infection among homosexual men (Stolte, Dukers, Geskus, Coutinho & De Wit, 2004; Van der Snoek, De Wit, Mulder & Van der Meijden, 2005). Perceptions of health threat are one key component of the Health Belief Model and related conceptualizations, and we observed that men who did not believe that the threat of HIV-infection was reduced as a result of the availability of effective antiretroviral therapy were more likely to have maintained safer receptive intercourse with casual partners (Stolte et al., 2004), and were less likely to have acquired a sexually transmitted disease (Van der Snoek et al., 2005).

Researchers have also started to explicitly test the utility of the Theory of Planned Behavior in explaining health behavior maintenance (Armitage, 2005; Drossaert, Boer & Seydel, 2003; Sheeran at al., 2001). Sheeran and colleagues (2001) assessed participation in annual health screening in two consecutive years, but Theory of Planned Behavior variables failed to distinguish between consistent, initial, and delayed attendance groups, and only refused attendance could be discriminated. Drossaert et al. (2003) further conclude that Theory of Planned Behavior variables are more related to the initiation than the repeat participation in breast cancer screening. However, this seems mostly based on differences in proportions of variance explained since theoretically relevant variables could in fact predict consistent participation in a second or third round of screening.

Unfortunately, as Sheeran et al. (2001) acknowledge, the compatibility of their measures of behavioral determinants and outcomes was not optimal, and also involved differences in the action component (i.e., attending versus repeatedly or consistently attending), in addition to the noted time aspect (i.e., the one year delay). Indeed, in their conceptual replication Drossaert et al. (2003) included a more compatible measure of intention that did predict their indicators of maintenance. Armitage (2005) further noted that maintenance of behavior usually involves repeated performance. He assessed maintenance of physical activity weekly over a three-month interval and found that sustained behavior change was related to higher perceived behavioral control. Hence, while data are inconclusive, these studies do suggest that, when adequately operationalized, the Theory of Planned Behavior can explain behavioral maintenance. However, major findings are also compatible with Social Cognitive Theory.

Social Cognitive Theory

This model (Bandura, 1986) originated from a social-learning analysis of behavior, and was proposed as an integrative framework to explain and predict changes achieved by different modes of treatment (Bandura, 1977). As much a theory of behavior as a perspective on human functioning, the theory assumes a pivotal role for the exercise of human agency (e.g., Bandura, 1999), and advanced a self-regulation perspective psychological functioning (e.g., Bandura, 1991, 1998). Social Cognitive Theory considers most human behavior as purposively guided by goals that reflect the expected outcomes of prospective actions and provide the motivation to initiate behavior. Self-evaluative reactions to goal progress affect individuals' self-inducements to persist (e.g., Bandura, 1977).

The theory's single most important contribution is the proposition that expectations of personal or self-efficacy are central to effective self-regulation and affect the initiation as well as persistence of behavior change (e.g., Bandura, 1977). Self-efficacy beliefs reflect a person's conviction that he or she can successfully organize and execute the courses of action required to produce the desired outcomes. They exert their influence on behavior change by affecting the choice of behavioral alternatives or goal challenges, because people tend to avoid situations they believe exceed their capabilities, and instead prefer activities for which they judge themselves able. Through expectations of eventual success, self-efficacy also affects behaviors once they are initiated. Efficacy expectations determine the effort people expend and how long they persist in the face of obstacles, but self-efficacy only results in the desired performance if the person possesses the relevant capabilities.

The notion of self-efficacy has become incorporated in most health behavior theories (cf. Luszczynska & Schwarzer, 2005), and has been applied to a wide range of health-related problems and actions (for overviews see Bandura, 1998; Luszczynska & Schwarzer, 2005; Schwarzer & Fuchs, 1995). Marlatt, Baer and Quigley (1995) conceptualize self-efficacy beliefs according to their functional role in the health behavior change process, and suggest that successful maintenance is facilitated by coping self-efficacy and recovery self-efficacy, which involves restorative actions to get an individual back on track (Haaga & Stewart, 1992). Coping self-efficacy refers to a person's anticipatory efficacy to deal with relapse crises or his or her sense of capability to overcome barriers that may arise, and a recent prospective study of weekly levels of physical activity provided some direct support for the influence of maintenance self-efficacy as it has been relabeled (Luszczynska and Schwarzer, 2003), on sustained health behavior change (Sniehotta, Scholz & Schwarzer, 2005).

Relapse Prevention Approach

Marlatt's original (Marlatt & Gordon, 1985) and revised (Witkiewitz & Marlatt, 2004) cognitive-behavioral approach to relapse is one of only few health behavior models that explicitly address the maintenance phase of behavior change. Originally developed in the domain of addictions, the model can be applied to a wider range of health-related behaviors and other psychological issues (see Collier & Marlatt, 1995; Witkiewitz & Marlatt, 2004), and thus far has received moderate empirical support (Larimer, Palmer & Marlatt, 1999).

Reminiscent of its roots in social-learning and Social Cognitive Theory, the Relapse Prevention Approach assumes that an individual who has successfully adopted behavior change should increasingly experience self-efficacy or mastery over his or her behavior. Nevertheless, certain situations may exceed a person's capabilities for control. Such high-risk situations typically involve negative emotional states, interpersonal conflict, and social pressure (e.g., Marlatt, 1996). If a person can enact an effective cognitive or behavioral coping response, self-efficacy and sense of mastery increase and the likelihood of health-impairing behavior decreases. If, however, a person cannot perform a coping response, sense of self-efficacy and control diminish. The likelihood of a lapse is further increased if he or she expects positive effects of the abandoned behavior or substance.

The Relapse Prevention Approach proposes that whether a lapse results in relapse depends on a person's cognitive-affective reaction to the initial slip: the abstinence violation effect. This effect that is sometimes referred to as goal violation effect to signal applicability to non-abstinence rules (Collier & Marlatt, 1995), is comprised of two factors: a causal attribution of responsibility for transgressing a self-imposed rule, and an affective reaction to this attribution (Curry, Marlatt & Gordon, 1987). Marlatt (1985) proposed that cognitive dissonance is the key affective element of the abstinence violation effect, which results from the disparity between the individual's cognitions or beliefs about the self (e.g., as an abstainer) and the occurrence of a behavior that is at odds with this self-image (e.g., having smoked a cigarette). A reformulation of Festinger's (1957) Cognitive Dissonance Theory maintains that dissonance results from personal responsibility for aversive outcomes (J. Cooper & Fazio, 1984), and I propose that the abstinence/goal violation effect is a negative affective reaction to a self-attributed lapse.

This cognitive dissonance is experienced as psychological discomfort (Elliot & Devine, 1994), and can be reduced through a variety of strategies (cf. Stone, Wiegand, Cooper & Aronson, 1997). Most research studied attitude change as the preferred mode of dissonance reduction, and in keeping with the field's emphasis on this cognitive change, relapsed smokers who were high in self-esteem and hence experienced most dissonance, have been noted to reduce their risk perception (Gibbons, Eggleston & Benthin, 1997). An early study equally found that smokers reduced dissonance by minimizing personal danger (Pervin & Yatko, 1965), but smokers who intended to quit seemed less likely to endorse ideas that could reduce cognitive dissonance (Johnson, 1968). This suggests that changes in beliefs and behavior are mutually exclusive, and it is important to know when individuals engage in one rather than the other.

The way in which dissonance is reduced and the strategy's effectiveness should depend on the ease with which cognitions can be changed or added (Simon, Greenberg & Brehm, 1995; cf. Festinger, 1957), and this will typically result in the well-known attitude change effect. Only a few studies have addressed behavior change to resolve dissonance (e.g., Sherman & Gorkin, 1980; Stone, Aronson, Crain, Winslow & Fried, 1994), which was expected and found to occur when attitudes involved in the dissonant relationship were particularly central or important to the person, and resistant to change (Stone et al., 1997; Sherman & Gorkin, 1980). Walster, Berscheid and Barclay (1967) proposed that individuals select a dissonance reduction strategy that results in a stable solution, preferring one that is not challenged by present events or information, and is unlikely to come under future attack.

An important but potentially unstable strategy to alleviate cognitive dissonance in the health domain is to attempt to minimize the health threat. While such trivialization most likely is undermined by current and future evidence, it does seem part of individual's tool kit. Furthermore, it has been found to operate as an alternative for attitude change (Simon et al., 1995), although contemporary theory assumes that attitudes reflect beliefs. A study that helps to shed some light on this apparent incongruity, found support for the prediction that when beliefs and behavior are inconsistent, attitudes change in the direction of the beliefs, at least when it concerns condom use (Albarracín & McNatt, 2005, study 3). Further emphasizing the synergistic relation between beliefs and attitudes in resolving cognitive dissonance, De Wit and Stroebe (2005) propose that attitude change in the direction of the behavior only occurs when individuals can effectively trivialize potential health consequences. In their view this is most probable when serious negative health consequences for the individual are unlikely in the short term. Trivialization is unlikely to work when serious health consequences are highly probable in the near future, and no attitude change should then occur. Instead, in this situation dissonance will be resolved by motivational bolstering. Such bolstering of motivation and behavior has been established experimentally in the domain of weight control, and occurred as a result of priming restrained eaters with temptations, which automatically activated competing higher priority goals (Fishbach, Friedman & Kruglanski, 2003, study 5). Activated goals in turn inhibit these temptations, in particular when the goal of weight control is high in importance (Fishbach et al., 2003, study 4).

To test part of their reasoning, De Wit and Stroebe (2006) conducted a prospective field study of homosexual men and expected that men who were committed to safer sex but failed to do so, would experience cognitive dissonance. This should be greater for HIV-negative men, because their personal health threat arguably is higher. HIV-negative men were also expected to be less successful in trivializing the potential aversive outcomes, and show less attitude change. Outcomes supported these hypotheses. Also, negative affect and self-attribution of responsibility were significantly higher in HIV-negative men, and (partially) mediated the effect of serostatus on attitude change following risk behavior.

Polivy and Herman (2002) have noted that the repeated failures at change attempts make it difficult to understand why individuals persist, and they offer an explanation that conceptualizes the cycle of failure and renewed effort as a "false hope syndrome." Behavior change is thought to be motivated by unrealistic expectations about the amount, speed, and ease of the change, and its effects on other aspects of one's life. People, in other words, strive for unattainable goals and are likely to fail in their attempts to achieve them. However, instead of giving up people persist in their efforts if the desire to change remains. Explanations of the failure are thought to form the bridge to new hope. Notably, biased attributions of failure to unstable characteristics, such as lack of effort, make it correctable. Individuals subsequently try again because they continue to desire the same hoped-for consequences.

Stage Models of Behavior Change

Maintenance of change is specifically considered in a category of health behavior theories that propose that health behavior change involves the ordered transition through qualitatively different phases or stages. These stage models hold that individuals in the same stage face common barriers that differ from those in other stages, and may profit most from interventions that match specific barriers (see Weinstein, Rothman & Sutton, 1998). Stage models are popular, and several of them have been proposed for health behavior (see Sutton, 2005). One of these is the Precaution Adoption Process Model (e.g., Weinstein & Sandman, 1992), which distinguishes seven stages of change.

The dominant stage model in health psychology, Prochaska and colleagues' Transtheoretical Model (e.g., Prochaska, DiClemente & Norcross, 1992), was initially developed to understand smoking cessation, but has been applied to a wide range of health behaviors (e.g., Prochaska et al., 1994). The model distinguishes five stages: precontemplation (no intention to change in the next six months), contemplation (intention to take action in the next six months, but not the next 30 days), preparation (intends to take action in the next month, and has taken some steps), action (behavior change for less than six months), and maintenance (behavior change for more than six months). People can relapse and cycle through these stages several times before reaching maintenance, and progress through the stages is affected by the decisional balance of the pros and cons of changing (i.e., outcome expectations), confidence and temptation (i.e., self-efficacy), and cognitive-behavioral self-regulation strategies.

Some recent applications of the Transtheoretical Model were concerned with maintenance of behavior change, and in particular assessed the role of self-regulation processes of change (Norcross et al., 1994, 2002). For instance, via telephone interviews Norcross and colleagues (2002) followed New Year's resolvers and comparable nonresolvers over a period of six months. Resolutions mostly concerned health behaviors that require sustained change (i.e., weight loss, physical exercise, and smoking cessation), and the researchers found that resolvers who were still successful at six months follow-up were higher on self-efficacy, skills to change, and readiness to change (i.e., stage of change), as assessed before January 1. Into the New Year, successful and unsuccessful resolvers significantly differed in their self-regulation of change. Successful resolvers in particular were more likely to use cognitive-behavioral coping strategies (for similar findings, see Norcross et al., 1994).

The Transtheoretical Model has been extensively criticized on a number of grounds (e.g., Sutton, 2000), and the body of research offers little supportive evidence for the major tenets of the model, notably the superiority of matched interventions (cf. Sutton, 2005). With respect to the maintenance of behavior change, the Transtheoretical Model has been specifically criticized for solely distinguishing between the action and maintenance stages on the basis of the arbitrary length of time the behavior has been adopted, and for not distinguishing between self-regulation processes that promote initiating or sustaining change (Rothman, 2000; Rothman et al., 2004).

Satisfaction with Behavior Change

Rothman and colleagues (Rothman, 2000; Rothman et al., 2004) argue that current theories of health behavior either fail to consider maintenance of behavior altogether, or only distinguish between different phases but do not complement this with an understanding of factors that regulate transitions. They therefore propose a novel framework that offers both a description of features to assess what phase a person is in, as well as a series of hypotheses on the influence of specific factors throughout the behavior change process. To disentangle the concerns that guide initiation from those that figure in the maintenance of behavior change, Rothman et al. (2004) structure the process of behavior change into four phases that occur after people have decided to initiate a new pattern of behavior. These involve further distinctions in the broad initiation and maintenance phase, and include initial response, continued response, maintenance, and habit. Predictors of initiating action are outcome expectancies and, in particular, self-efficacy beliefs.

In the (novel) continued response phase individuals face challenges and unpleasant experiences, and risk lapse and relapse. Commitment and confidence are weakened to the extent that the new behavior is unpleasant or requires considerable mental or physical energy (Rothman et al., 2004). Successful completion of this phase is seen as a sign of recovery, and people who consistently engage in a new behavior acquire a sense of control over their actions. The struggle against relapse subsides, and in the maintenance phase the decision to continue the behavior is thought to become less a function of a person's ability to perform the behavior and more a function of the behavior's perceived value (Rothman et al., 2004). People are expected to begin to form an integrated assessment of the relative costs and benefits, and recent research suggests that the resulting satisfaction with the change does not only reflect a comparison of actual and expected outcomes, but also signals a consideration of the costs and other negative experiences related to the behavior change process (Jeffery, Kelly, Rothman, Sherwood & Boutelle, 2004). Transition to the habit phase only occurs when people are no longer actively concerned with their ability to engage in the behavior or their evaluation of the outcomes the behavior affords (Rothman et al., 2004), which may be difficult to attain for most individuals who attempt to change their unhealthy behavior.

The framework advanced by Rothman and colleagues (King et al., 2000; Rothman, 2000; Rothman et al., 2004) offers a promising new conceptualization of the health behavior change process that elegantly integrates social-cognitive theorizing and stage model assumptions, and substantially elaborates both types of accounts. In particular, Rothman and colleagues offer more precise predictions of the factors involved in the decision to initiate the behavior and those featuring in the decision to sustain behavior (cf. Brownell et al., 1986). These include the hypothesis that satisfaction with experienced outcomes should be the major determinant in the maintenance phase rather than outcome expectancies (also see Bandura, 1977; Gollwitzer, 1996; Locke & Latham, 2002; Strecher et al., 1995). Furthermore, they suggest that self-efficacy beliefs are most important when initiating and continuing the new behavioral pattern, and should become less influential in the maintenance and habit phases. Rothman's framework thus stresses the importance of volitional self-regulation processes in the earlier phases of the change process, and assumes that sustained motivation will be more important later on. However, some other approaches that equally invoke a notion of stages of change suggest that sustaining change may continue to involve self-efficacy beliefs and volitional strategies, as discussed below. In part this apparent contradiction may result from differences in the way action phases are conceived, which mostly does not include the distinction between continued response and maintenance proposed by Rothman et al. (2004).

Models of Behavioral Enaction

This class of health behavior theories includes models that elaborate the volitional processes that follow the formation of an intention to act (Armitage & Conner, 2000), the best known example of which probably is Gollwitzer's (e.g., 1999) theorizing on implementation intentions. Schwarzer's (e.g., 2001) Health Action Process Approach generally also is included in this category (cf. Armitage & Conner, 2000), although it may not qualify as a stage model (Sutton, 2005). Gollwitzer's well-known distinction between goal intentions ("I intend to reach Z"!; Gollwitzer, Fujita & Oettingen, 2004, p. 211) and implementation intentions ("If situation X is encountered, then I will perform the goal directed response Y!"; Gollwitzer et al., 2004, p. 212) grew out of the Model of Action Phases (e.g., Gollwitzer, 1996). This model proposes a distinction between the motivational issue of goal setting and the volitional issue of goal striving, which entail distinct tasks that promote the activation of specific cognitive procedures (i.e., mindsets) to facilitate their completion.

In the predecisional phase individuals consider wishes and set preferences, which is facilitated by a deliberative mindset in which the person analyses information in an impartial manner to arrive at the best decision. Progress to the next phase demands a decision to act or goal intention (i.e., a behavioral intention), and in the postdecisional but pre-actional phase the objective is to get started. This is promoted via effective planning in an implemental mindset, which is characterized by the selective processing of information favoring the adopted goal. This is the point where implementation intentions come into play, and the action phase involves bringing the goal pursuit to a successful end. In the evaluative or postactional phase the individual compares what has been achieved with what was desired, and decides whether further efforts are worthwhile and needed. This suggestion is revisited in Rothman's (e.g., 2000) proposition that maintenance of change depends on perceived satisfaction with the change. A comprehensive treatment of implementation intentions in health behaviors can be found elsewhere in this volume (also see Sheeran, Milne, Webb & Gollwitzer, 2005). Here I wish to note that the formation of implementation intentions has been shown to shield ongoing activities from unwanted influences and helps individuals stay on track, in addition to facilitating getting started (see Gollwitzer et al., 2004; Sheeran et al., this volume).

Furthermore, Sheeran et al. (2005) suggest a framework that distinguishes a range of volitional issues for which implementation intentions have been successfully used. These include maintaining wanted responses (such as continued participation in an exercise program) by mobilizing effort or a specific task orientation, preventing getting derailed by contextual threats (including attractive alternatives) or overcoming such threats, and controlling habitual responses. Some direct evidence for the beneficial effect on maintenance of behavior change is provided by Milne and Sheeran (2002; as cited in Sheeran et al., this volume) who showed that implementation intentions increased the sustained monthly performance of testicular self-examination over the course of one year. In addition, Luszczynska (in press) observed that patients who had suffered from myocardial infarction and were involved in an implementation intention intervention were more likely to maintain the number of physical activity sessions than patients in the control condition.

Health Action Process Approach

This health behavior model elaborated by Schwarzer (e.g., 2001), invokes the classic distinction between motivation and volition in behavior change (for an overview, see Gollwitzer, 1996), and explains "the mechanisms that operate whenever individuals become motivated to change their habits, adopt and maintain new behaviors, and attempt to resist temptations and recover from setbacks" (Sniehotta, Scholz et al., 2005, p. 145). While the model continues to be developed and different versions of the theory have been proposed (Sutton, 2005), the Health Action Process Approach is noteworthy because it is a rare attempt to integrate ideas from different theoretical traditions and bring some coherence to the otherwise fragmented health behavior theory landscape.

The Health Action Process Approach assumes that before individuals change their behavior they first develop an intention to change or adopt a goal, mainly based on their beliefs. Three variables are important in this motivational phase of goal setting: risk perception, outcome expectancies and perceived self-efficacy. These three predictors of intention are assumed to operate in concert, and the model proposes that risk awareness sets the stage for a further elaboration of thoughts about consequences and competences (Schwarzer, 2001; see also Sutton, 2005). The subsequent volitional phase in which a goal of behavior change is pursued, is further subdivided into a sequence of activities that, however, are not clearly distinct categories (Schwarzer, 2001), and include planning, initiation, maintenance, lapse management, and disengagement. These activities involve active self-regulation by planning the details of goal pursuit, trying to act, investing effort and persistence, and restarting when setbacks occur. At each point there are two predictors of success: the successful completion of the previous sub-stage, and an optimistic sense of control over the next one (Schwarzer, 2001). Perceived self-efficacy thus is the only predictor that operates in all phases, and the Health Action Process Approach proposes that corresponding, phase specific self-efficacy beliefs affect intention formation, planning processes, initiation and maintenance of behavior, and from lapse and relapse.

In the model, planning precedes the initiation of behavior change and involves developing a mental representation of a suitable future situation to enact a given behavior, as proposed by Gollwitzer (e.g., 1999). To further develop the concept of planning, a distinction has been made between action planning (i.e., implementation intentions), and coping planning (Sniehotta, Schwarzer, Scholz & Schüz, 2005). The latter refers to the mental simulation of overcoming anticipated barriers to action, and resulting coping plans were found important in later phases of the behavior change process of cardiac rehabilitation patients encouraged to exercise regularly (Sniehotta, Schwarzer et al., 2005).

Sutton (2005) gives an overview of research that has tested the Health Action Process Approach, and confirms that empirical applications of the model only recently have started to include measures of the proposed volitional processes. Some published studies assessed phase-specific self-efficacy (Luszczynska & Schwarzer, 2003; Schwarzer & Renner, 2000; Sniehotta, Schwarzer et al., 2005), and reported findings that support the expected relationships with planning and behavior change. Equally few studies directly tested (some of) the pathways the Health Action Process Approach specifies. In particular, planning was found to mediate the effect of intention on breast self-examination

(Luszczynska & Schwarzer, 2003), and physical exercise (Sniehotta, Scholz et al., 2005). Thus far, only one study assessed action control strategies as mediator of sustained behavior change (Sniehotta, Scholz et al., 2005), and findings generally are consistent with assumptions of the Health Action Process Approach. More such tests that address the proposed self-regulation processes will further establish the model's validity and applicability.

Models of Goal Setting and Goal Striving

Self-regulation can be considered a goal-guidance process that is directed at the attainment and maintenance of specific outcomes, and involves the setting of personal goals, steering behavior towards their achievement, and sustaining changes that have been brought about (Maes & Karoly, 2005). Goals are internal (mental) representations of desired states that have the potential to influence individuals' pursuits because of their content and process aspects (Gollwitzer & Moskowitz, 1996). Content pertains to the type of goal a person has selected, and in addition to a taxonomic classification includes properties of the adopted goal (e.g., specificity, difficulty) as well as its (hierarchical) relation to other goals (see also Austin & Vancouver, 1996). Goal processes refer to the striving towards the attainment of an adopted goal, and encompas the volitional processes broadly related to planning, initiation, and maintenance of behavior, as discussed above. In the remainder I will focus on the influence of goal content on the maintenance of (sexual) behavior change, and discuss the potential impact of repeated or prolonged self-control process on the successful maintenance of behavior change.

Goal Content Theories

Goal-Setting Theory (for an overview see Locke & Latham, 2002) is considered the prototype of a goal content theory (Gollwitzer & Moskowitz, 1996). The theory focuses primarily on motivation in work settings but is not limited to this domain (Locke & Latham, 2002), and the beneficial effects of setting goals for health behavior change have been discussed (e.g., Strecher et al., 1995). The core proposition of the theory is that challenging goals that are phrased in specific terms have a positive effect on performance, and more so than specific but moderate goals and challenging but vague goals (i.e., "do your best" goals). However, positive effects of goal setting only occur when individuals receive summary feedback on how they are doing in terms of progress towards the goal, when the task is not overly complex, and when the individual is committed to the goal (Locke & Latham, 2002). Performance should not be influenced by whether the goal is assigned, set participatively, or self-set, provided that individuals are committed to the goal. Nevertheless, other goal content theories, notably Self-Determination Theory (e.g. Ryan & Deci, 2000), note that self-motivation and external regulation result in functional and experiential differences. Autonomous motivation results in enhanced performance, persistence, and creativity, as well as heightened vitality, self-esteem and general well-being (Ryan & Deci, 2000), and such positive effects have also been obtained in the health behavior domain (for an overview, see Williams, 2002).

A health behavior goal that is unlikely to stimulate much personal commitment or reflect intrinsic motivation in most young persons is the promotion of sexual abstinence among adolescents to promote sexual health outcomes. Sex education that promoted abstinence has not resulted in any significant effect on behavior (Silva, 2002), and most success was observed in programs that promoted buying and using condoms (Jemmott & Jemmott, 2000). Nevertheless, risk-taking continues, and unprotected sex is more likely with "steady" than "casual" partners (for an overview see Misovich, Fisher & Fisher, 1997).

Sexual risk-taking can vary as a function of individuals' needs and goals (e.g., M.L. Cooper, Shapiro & Powers, 1998), and De Wit, Klep, and Beijk (2006) propose that initiating unprotected sex at some (early) point in the process of establishing a steady relationship operates as a signal of trust, which is important to normal relationship development. However, the goal to promote the relationship can be at odds with the protection of one's health, and this goal conflict is proposed to be resolved by motivated reasoning. A randomized vignette study provided support, and showed that college students intended to use condoms less with a steady than with a casual partner, although no risk-information was provided. As expected, the effect of partner type was mediated by the desire to trust the partner that resulted from relationship commitment, and promoted a more favorable construal of the partner. However, even when individuals are committed to health behavior they do not always initiate change, let alone maintain it.

Processes of Goal Striving

Having set a goal is an important first step in attaining it, but not one that guarantees success, because goal striving also calls upon volitional processes. As an illustration of this point, Koestner, Lekes, Powers and Chicoine (2002) documented in two separate meta-analyses that both goal self-concordance, reflecting the extent to which a goal reflects personal interests and values, and implementation intentions were significantly associated with goal progress. Moreover, in two original studies they obtained a significant interaction effect, indicating that goal self-concordance and implementation intentions combined synergistically to facilitate goal progress (Koestner, et al., 2002). Implementation intentions help individuals overcome self-regulation problems associated with getting started and persisting until the goal is reached (cf. Gollwitzer, 1999), the two problems that in particular plague successful striving for health goals (see Sheeran et al., this volume).

Once action has been initiated, self-regulation also involves protecting the ongoing goal pursuit from the intrusion of unwanted influences, such as distractions or situational priming of competing action tendencies, social pressures and habits (cf. Gollwitzer, 1999). In the language of Kuhl's (e.g., 2000) Personality Systems Interaction Theory, this volitional mode refers to a form of willing that is responsible for inhibiting impulsive actions and maintaining a focus on the activated goal. In his longstanding program of research, Mischel (e.g., Mischel & Ayduk, 2004) has documented that successful delay of gratification (i.e., not giving in to temptation and rejecting an immediate smaller reward for a delayed bigger reward) is related to the mental representation of the objects in a "cool" (i.e., informational) rather than "hot" (i.e., motivational) way, more than to whether or not attention is focused on the desirable temptations. According to Kuhl (e.g., 2000), individuals who are highly skilled at regulating their affect are referred to as "action-oriented," while their less proficient counterparts are considered "state-oriented" and assumed to be less successful at achieving health goals than action-oriented individuals (Fuhrmann & Kuhl, 1998), although findings are not supportive of such a moderation of health actions (Norman, Sheeran & Orbell, 2003).

In addition to views of self-control or "willpower" as acquired skill or individual difference, recent theorizing proposes that effective self-control depends on individuals' resources that can become depleted by a previous act of self-control (for overviews, see Muraven & Baumeister, 2000; Schmeichel & Baumeister, 2004; see also Martijn and colleagues, this volume). This "strength model" advanced by Baumeister and colleagues holds that overriding or inhibiting competing urges, behaviors or desires, can be difficult and effortful, and proposes that various acts of self-control draw on the same limited inner resource. As a result, self-control may become impaired and fail when recent demands have depleted the resource. This state of ego depletion is presumably not permanent and can be replenished by resting, much like a muscle that becomes fatigued by exertion (Muraven & Baumeister, 2000). Exercising self-control over time may increase the size of the reservoir, as when a muscle is trained. Furthermore, strategic automatization of goal pursuit seems to prevent ego depletion on a subsequent task (Webb & Sheeran, 2003).

The strength model of self-control predicts that circumstances that require continuous self-control may also lead to a breakdown in self-control (Muraven & Baumeister, 2000). Such demanding continuous self-control seems to be required when individuals attempt to sustain a health behavior change over time and repeatedly struggle to prevent lapse and relapse (e.g., resisting the urge to smoke; refusing a piece of delicious cake; forsaking condom use with a particularly attractive person). To the extent that prolonged self-control depletes the resource more quickly than it is replenished, a breakdown in self-control is likely. This should in particular be the case when maintaining behaviors that involve frequent or taxing self-control attempts, such as when attempting to maintain the long-term vigilance that is considered important for the success of interventions in the field of addictions (Brownell et al., 1986).

The notions of (physical) fatigue and acquiescence that are linked to ego depletion (Webb & Sheeran, 2005) closely resemble the proposition that gay men fail to maintain safer sexual behaviors because of safer sex fatigue or prevention burnout (Ostrow et al., 2002), referring to a decreased vigilance in maintaining safer sexual behaviors (Valdiserri, 2004). According to the Centers for Disease Control and Prevention (2001, as cited in Valdiserri, 2004), many older homosexual men find it difficult to maintain previously adopted safer sex practices over the course of their lifetime, and Ostrow et al. (2002) found that resulting safer sex fatigue predicted sexual risk-behavior, in particular among HIV-positive gay men.

In line with the limited strength-model of self-regulation, De Wit, Adam and Heijnen (2006) proposed that safer sex fatigue at least in part results from the prolonged self-control of sexual behaviors, and should be higher to the extent that men have self-restrained their sexual practices for a longer period of time. To test these hypotheses De Wit and colleagues developed a sexual restraint scale that correlated moderately and significantly with Ostrow et al.'s (2002) measure of fatigue. They also obtained a significant positive correlation with age, a proxy for the duration of restraint. Muraven and Slessareva (2003) propose that resources and motivation jointly predict self-control outcomes, and documented that ego depletion effects can be overcome by increasing individuals' motivation for self-control, referred to as the compensation hypothesis. Because the study by De Wit et al. (2006) did not directly test the limited resource assumption, safer sex fatigue may thus also reflect lowered motivation for condom use and reduced compensation. This alternative explanation is, however, unlikely because a positive correlation was obtained between sexual restraint and intention to use condoms: More restrained men were more likely to intend to use condoms, as expected.

Departing from the strength model, De Wit et al. (2006) propose that safer sex fatigue does not equal acquiescence but promotes a wish or desire to make up for missed experiences. This need for recovery is assumed to result in increased risky action tendencies, and present a motivational force that predicts intentions and risk-taking. In line with this hypothesis, higher need for recovery, for which a new measure was also developed, was related to a less favorable intention to use condoms. Furthermore, need for recovery was related to self-perceived risky changes in behavior, and prospectively predicted risk-taking. Need for recovery also correlated moderately with safer sex fatigue, and together these findings suggest that sexual risk-taking resulting from fatigue is an attempt to actively make up for missed opportunities, rather than merely passively going with the (risky) flow. Future research may establish if and under what conditions fatigue results in an active motivational state rather than a state of acquiescence, which needs this motivation can serve, and how the postulated active recovery contributes to an under-standing of ego depletion and resource substitution.

CONCLUSIONS

Studies of the behavior change process continue to document that sustained new health behavior patterns are an unlikely outcome of any one change attempt. Individuals may only achieve consistent change after giving it multiple tries, but why they repeatedly embark on missions that are likely to fail is not well known (Polivy & Herman, 2002). Understanding maintenance of health behavior change hence presents important chal-lenges to theory and research in fields dealing with health behaviors, notably health psychology and social psychology, and this is true as much to day as it was 20 years ago when major relapse theorists could note that interest in lapse and relapse was still relatively recent (Brownell et al., 1986). However, the large numbers of research needs they distinguished, ranging from the natural history of behavior change to effective coping strategies, are mostly unfulfilled.

Modern self-regulation research does not yet focus sufficiently on maintenance issues (Maes & Karoly, 2005), and the present chapter wants to underscore the important challenges health behavior maintenance poses for self-regulation theory, research, and practice. The relevance of the self-regulation approach for understanding and promoting maintenance of behavior change is evident from the myriad of processes that may be involved in attempting to sustain changes in health behavior and that can be derived from self-regulation theories. These involve issues related to goal setting and decision-making, planning action, and getting started, managing goal conflict and shielding against interference, evaluating change, and habituation of new behaviors. This wide range of processes reflect the respective stages of behavior change, and prevailing theories of health behavior differ in the stages they distinguish (if any), which may reflect differences in the types of health behaviors that are tacitly considered. As a result, theories also differ in the self-regulation issues they deem important and emphasize, further contributing to the overwhelming amount of themes and factors that can be found in the literature. Any advance in our understanding of health behavior maintenance should profit from establishing consensus regarding stages of change or the range of tasks involved in the process of behavior change (cf. Rothman et al., 2000).

A comparison of different models suggests that three basic stages can be distinguished, starting with a motivational phase in which individuals make a decision, establish commitment, and form an intention to change. Such a phase is inherent in all theories of health behavior (although not specified by Rothman et al., 2004), and is generally taken to involve deliberative goal setting that reflects the desired outcomes of a new behavior. However, a wealth of research now documents that goals that guide behavior are not always derived from active processing and suggests that self-regulation can equally start from automatically activated goals (e.g., Fitzsimons & Bargh, 2004; Shah, 2005). The goal guidance process, be it initiated deliberatively or automatically, terminates in a third phase when a new habit is created that puts further goal-directed behavior under automatic control (for an alternative view see Ajzen, 2002). This phase is thus far only distinguished by Rothman (2000; Rothman et al., 2004), but fits well with the increased attention for the role of habits in understanding social behavior (e.g., Wood, Quinn & Kashy, 2002). In the intermediary second phase individuals strive to attain their goals, and this more recently elaborated phase involves a diversity of volitional processes.

It is in their conceptualization of goal striving that current theories of behavior change differ most, and I propose that this volitional phase can be distinguished into two meaningful sub-phases: one involving preparing action and getting started, as advanced by behavioral enaction models (e.g., Gollwitzer, 1999; Schwarzer, 2001), and one referring to continuing or maintaining the change and evaluating process and outcomes (e.g., Rothman et al., 2004). Rothman et al. (2004) distinguish between continued engagement in the behavior and an evaluation of the results of behavior change (i.e., maintenance phase). Continued behavior is mostly considered to make up the main-tenance stage in other theories, while Rothman's maintenance stage seems to map on the evaluation phase proposed by Gollwitzer (e.g., 1996). I propose that continued response and evaluation together make up the maintenance sub-phase of goal striving. This phase was the main focus of this chapter, and the presented theories each offered a specific perspective on the deliberative processes that promote successful maintenance of behavior change.

Despite substantial theoretical diversity, however, only two main factors seem to be invoked in successful deliberative goal striving, although emphasis and labeling differ between theories: motivation and ability. Motivation for sustaining change involves a consideration of the expected outcomes of the new behavior that promotes commitment, as proposed by classic social-cognitive theories of behavior (cf. Fishbein et al., 2001) as well as goal content theories (e.g., Locke & Latham, 2002; Ryan & Deci, 2000). Motivation also reflects an evaluation of the change process and the outcomes that have actually been obtained (i.e., satisfaction), as stressed in more recent theorizing (e.g., Rothman et al., 2004). Ability encompasses individuals' beliefs regarding their competence (i.e., self-efficacy) that are now included in virtually any health behavior theory (cf. Bandura, 1998; Luszczynska & Schwarzer, 2005), as well as the skills and resources an individual possesses, and that are needed to overcome actual barriers to change (cf. Fishbein et al., 2001). A simple three-stage model of behavior change hence need invoke only two processes of change, albeit that they influence progress through phase-specific (Marlatt et al., 1995) or compatible (Ajzen & Fishbein, 1977) appraisals of self-efficacy (Schwarzer & Renner, 2000) and outcomes (Rothman et al., 2004). Motivation and ability may interact (e.g., De Wit & Stroebe, 1999), and synergistically contribute to the flexible strength individuals need to sustain behavior patterns over prolonged periods of time (cf. Muraven & Slessareva, 2003).

The above summary of self-regulation processes in behavior change obviously is incomplete and mainly serves to illustrate that the diverse theoretical approaches to health behavior can indeed be integrated in ways that may advance the field. It additionally serves to underscore the need for such theoretical integration and synthesis, as recently also noted by scholars who propose that the study of self-regulation is under construction (Karoly, Boekaerts & Maes, 2005). This is certainly true for the sub-field of self-regulation approaches that are concerned with the maintenance of behavior change, which can be characterized by a rapid proliferation of concepts and processes that for the most part remain to be tested. Such testing should be based on clear theorizing of the possible relations between different self-regulation processes (e.g., Sniehotta, Schwarzer et al., 2005), involve a direct comparison of the multitude of processes (e.g., Webb & Sheeran, 2005), assess the dynamics of behavior change (e.g., Armitage, 2005), and measure health outcomes (e.g., Van der Snoek et al., 2005). Most importantly, the issues presented here hopefully inspire future work.

REFERENCES

Ajzen, I. (2002). Residual effects of past on later behavior: Habituation and reasoned action perspectives. *Personality and Social Psychology Review, 6*, 107–122.

Ajzen, I. & Fishbein, M. (1977). Attitude-behavior relations: A theoretical analysis and review of empirical research. *Psychological Bulletin, 84*, 888–918.

Albarracín D. & McNatt, P.S. (2005). Maintenance and decay of past behavior influences: Anchoring attitudes on beliefs following inconsistent actions. *Personality and Social Psychology Bulletin, 31*, 719–733.

Armitage, C.J. (2005). Can the theory of planned behavior predict the maintenance of physical activity? *Health Psychology, 24*, 235–245.

Armitage, C.J. & Conner, M. (2000). Social cognition models and health behaviour: A structured review. *Psychology and Health, 15*, 173–189.

Austin, J.T. & Vancouver, J.B. (1996). Goal constructs in psychology: Structure, process and content. *Psychological Bulletin, 120*, 338–375.

Bandura, A. (1977). Self-efficacy: Toward a unifying theory of behavior change. *Psychological Review, 84*, 191–215.

Bandura, A. (1986). *Social Foundations of Thought and Action*. Englewood Cliffs, NJ: Prentice Hall.

Bandura, A. (1991). Social cognitive theory of self-regulation. *Organizational Behaviour and Human Decision Processes, 50*, 248–287.

Bandura, A. (1998). Health promotion from the perspective of social cognitive theory. *Psychology and Health, 13,* 623–649.

Bandura, A. (1999). A sociocognitive analysis of substance abuse: An agentic perspective. *Psychological Science, 10,* 214–217.

Bouton, M.E. (2000). A learning theory perspective on lapse, relapse, and the maintenance of behavior change. *Health Psychology, 19,* S57–S63.

Brownell, K.D., Marlatt, G.A., Lichtenstein, E. & Wilson, G.T. (1986). Understanding and prevention relapse. *American Psychologist, 41,* 765–782.

Centers for Disease Control and Prevention (2005). Cigarette smoking among adults—United States, 2003. *MMWR Morbidity and Mortality Weekly Report, 54,* 509–513.

Cohen, S., Lichtenstein, E., Prochaska, J.O., Rossi, J.S., Gritz, E.R., Carr, C.R., Orleans, C.T., Schoenbach, V.J., Biener, L., Abrams, D., DiClemente, C., Curry, S., Marlatt, G.A., Cummings, K.M., Emont, S.L., Giovino, G. & Ossip-Klein, D. (1989). Debunking myths about self-quitting: Evidence from 10 prospective studies of persons who attempt to quit smoking by themselves. *American Psychologist, 44,* 1355–1365.

Collier, C.W. & Marlatt, G.A. (1995). Relapse prevention. In A.J. Goreczny (Ed.), *Handbook of Health and Rehabilitation Psychology* (pp. 307–321). New York: Plenum.

Conner, M. & Norman, P. (2005). *Predicting Health Behaviour* (2nd edition). Maidenhead, UK: Open University Press.

Cooper, J. & Fazio, R.H. (1984). A new look at dissonance theory. In L. Berkowitz (Ed.), *Advances in Experimental Social Psychology* (Vol. 17, pp. 229–266). New York: Academic Press.

Cooper, M.L., Shapiro, C.M. & Powers, A.M. (1998). Motivations for sex and risky sexual behavior among adolescents and young adults: A functional perspective. *Journal of Personality and Social Psychology, 75,* 1528–1558.

Curry, S., Marlatt, G.A. & Gordon, J.R. (1987). Abstinence violation effect: Validation of an attributional construct with smoking cessation. *Journal of Consulting and Clinical Psychology, 55,* 145–149.

De Wit, J.B.F., Adam, P.C.G. & Heijnen, M.M. (2006). *Sexual Self-control as a Motivational Force Underlying Self-perceived, Intended and Actual Sexual Risk Behavior With Casual Partners Among Men Who Have Sex With Men.* Manuscript submitted for publication.

De Wit, J.B.F., Klep, A. & Beijk, C. (2006). *Motivated Reasoning Augments Health Risks in Intimate Relationships: The Case of Unprotected Sex as a Dangerous Signal of Trust.* Manuscript submitted for publication.

De Wit, J.B.F. & Stroebe, W. (1999). Social-cognitive modeling of sexual risk-taking in homosexual men. *Gedrag en Gezondheid, 27,* 48–55.

De Wit, J. & Stroebe, W. (2004). Social cognition models of health behaviour. In A. Kaptein & J. Weinman (Eds), *Health Psychology* (pp. 52–83). Oxford: BPS Blackwell.

De Wit, J.B.F. & Stroebe, W. (2006). *The Impact of Relapse on Condom Use Attitudes: Differences According to HIV-status.* Manuscript in preparation.

De Wit, J.B.F., Van den Hoek, J.A.R., Sandfort, Th.G.M. & Van Griensven, G.J.P. (1993). Increase in unprotected anogenital intercourse among homosexual men. *American Journal of Public Health, 83,* 1451–1453.

De Wit, J.B.F., Van Griensven, G.J.P., Kok, G.J., & Sandfort, Th.G.M. (1993). Why do homosexual men relapse into unsafe sex? Predictors of resumption of unprotected anogenital intercourse with casual partners. *AIDS, 7,* 1113–1118.

De Wit, J.B.F. & Van Griensven, G.J.P. (1994). Time from safer to unsafe sexual behaviour among homosexual men. *AIDS, 8,* 123–126.

Drossaert, C.H.C., Boer, H. & Seydel, E.R. (2003). Prospective study on the determinants of repeat attendance and attendance patterns in breast cancer screening using the theory of planned behaviour. *Psychology and Health, 18,* 551–565.

Elliot, A.J. & Devine, P.G. (1994). On the motivational nature of cognitive dissonance: Dissonance as psychological discomfort. *Journal of Personality and Social Psychology, 67,* 382–394.

Festinger, L. (1957). *A Theory of Cognitive Dissonance.* Oxford: Row, Peterson.

Fishbach, A., Friedman, R.S. & Kruglanski, A.W. (2003). Leading us not unto temptation: Momentary allurements elicit overriding goal activation. *Journal of Personality and Social Psychology, 84,* 296–309.

Fishbein, M., Triandis, H.C., Kanfer, F.H., Becker, M., Middlestadt, S.E. & Eichler, A. (2001). Factors influencing behavior and behavior change. In A. Baum, R.A. Revenson & J.E. Singer (Eds), *Handbook of Health Psychology* (pp. 3–17). Mahwah, NJ: Erlbaum.

Fitzsimons, G.M. & Bargh, J.A. (2004). Automatic self-regulation. In R.F. Baumeister and K.D. Vohs (Eds), *Handbook of Self-regulation. Research, Theory, and Applications* (pp. 151–170). New York: Guilford.

Fuhrmann, A. & Kuhl, J. (1998). Maintaining a healthy diet: Effect of personality and self-reward versus self-punishment on commitment to and enactment of self-chosen and assigned goals. *Psychology and Health, 13,* 651–686.

Gibbons, F.X., Eggleston, T.J. & Benthin, A.C. (1997). Cognitive reactions to smoking relapse: The reciprocal relation between dissonance and self-esteem. *Journal of Personality and Social Psychology, 72,* 184–195.

Gollwitzer, P.M. (1996). The volitional benefits of planning. In P.M. Gollwitzer & J.A. Bargh (Eds), *The Psychology of Action: Linking cognition and motivation to behavior* (pp. 287–312). New York: Guilford.

Gollwitzer, P.M. (1999). Implementation intentions: Strong effects of simple plans. *American Psychologist, 54,* 493–503.

Gollwitzer, P.M., Fujita, K. & Oettingen, G. (2004). Planning and the implementation of goals. In R.F. Baumeister & K.D. Vohs (Eds), *Handbook of Self-regulation. Research, Theory, and Applications* (pp. 211–228). New York: Guilford.

Gollwitzer, P.M. & Moskowitz, G.B. (1996). Goal effects on action and cognition. In E.T. Higgins & A.W. Kruglanski (Eds), *Social Psychology: Handbook of basic principles* (pp. 361–399). New York: Guilford.

Haaga, D.A.F. & Stewart, B.L. (1992). Self-efficacy for recovery from a lapse after smoking cessation. *Journal of Consulting and Clinical Psychology, 60,* 24–28.

Hunt, W.A., Barnett, L., & Branch, L. (1971). Relapse rates in addiction programs. *Journal of Clinical Psychology, 27,* 455–456.

Jeffery, R.W., Drewnowski, A., Epstein, L.H., Stunkard, A.J., Wilson, G.T. & Wing, R.R. (2000). Long-term maintenance of weight loss: Current status. *Health Psychology, 19 (Suppl.),* 5–16.

Jeffery, R.W., Kelly, K.M., Rothman, A.J., Sherwood, N.E. & Boutelle, K.N. (2004). The weight loss experience: A descriptive analysis. *Annals of Behavioral Medicine, 27,* 100–106.

Jemmott, J.B. 3rd, & Jemmott, L.S. (2000). HIV risk reduction behavioral interventions with heterosexual adolescents. *AIDS, 14 (Suppl. 2),* 40–52.

Johnson, R.E. (1965). Smoking and the reduction of cognitive dissonance. *Journal of Personality and Social Psychology, 9,* 260–265.

King, C.M., Rothman, A.J. & Jeffery, R.W. (2002). The Challenge Study: Theory-based interventions for smoking and weight loss. *Health Education Research, 17,* 522–530.

Koestner, R., Lekes, N., Powers, T.A. & Chicoine, E. (2002). Attaining personal goals: Self-concordance plus implementation intentions equals success. *Journal of Personality and Social Psychology, 83,* 231–244.

Kuhl, J. (2000). The volitional basis of personality systems interaction theory: Applications in learning and treatment contexts. *International Journal of Educational Research, 33,* 665–703.

Kumanyika, S.K., Van Horn, L., Bowen, D., Perri, M.G., Rolls, B.J., Czajkowski, S.M. & Schron, E. Maintenance of dietary behavior change. *Health Psychology, 19 (Suppl.),* 42–56.

Kunda, Z. (1990). The case for motivated reasoning. *Psychological Bulletin*, *108*, 480–498.

Larimer, M.E., Palmer, R.S. & Marlatt, G.A. (1999). Relapse prevention: An overview of Marlatt's cognitive-behavioral model. *Alcohol Research and Health*, *23*, 151–160.

Locke, E.A. & Latham, G.P. (2002). Building a practically useful theory of goal setting and task motivation. *American Psychologist*, *57*, 705–717.

Luszczynska, A. (in press). Effects of an implementation intention intervention on physical activity after MI mediated by the use of planning strategy. *Social Science and Medicine*.

Luszczynska, A. & Schwarzer, R. (2003). Planning and self-efficacy in the adoption and maintenance of breast self-examination: A longitudinal study on self-regulatory cognitions. *Psychology and Health*, *18*, 93–108.

Luszczynska, A. & Schwarzer, R. (2005). Social cognitive theory. In M. Conner & P. Norman (Eds), *Predicting Health Behaviour* (2nd edition; pp. 127–169). Maidenhead, UK: Open University Press.

Maes, S. & Karoly, P. (2005). Self-regulation assessment and intervention in physical health and illness: A review. *Applied Psychology: An International Review*, *54*, 267–299.

Marcus, B.H., Bock, B.C. & Pinto, B.M. (1997). Initiation and maintenance of exercise behavior. In D.S. Gochman (Ed.), *Handbook of Health Behavior Research II: Provider determinants* (pp. 335–352). New York: Plenum.

Marcus, B.H., Dubbert, P.M., Forsyth, L.H., McKenzie, T.L., Stone, E.J., Dunn, A.L. & Blair, S.N. (2000). Physical activity behavior change: Issues in adoption and maintenance. *Health Psychology*, *19*, (Suppl.), 32–41.

Marlatt, G.A. (1985). Relapse prevention: Theoretical rationale and overview of the model. In G.A. Marlatt & J.R. Gordon (Eds), *Relapse Prevention* (pp. 3–70). New York: Guilford.

Marlatt, G.A. (1996). Taxonomy of high-risk situations for alcohol relapse: Evolution and development of a cognitive behavioral model. *Addiction*, *91*, (Suppl.), 37–49.

Marlatt, G.A., Baer, J.S. & Quigley, L.A. (1995). Self-efficacy and addictive behavior. In A. Bandura (Ed.), *Self-efficacy in Changing Societies* (pp. 289–315). Cambridge: Cambridge University Press.

Marlatt, G.A. & Gordon, J.R. (1985). *Relapse Prevention*. New York: Guilford.

Mischel, W. & Ayduk, O. (2004). Willpower in a cognitive-affective processing system: The dynamics of delay of gratification. In R.F. Baumeister and K.D. Vohs (Eds), *Handbook of Self-regulation. Research, Theory, and Applications* (pp. 99–129). New York: Guilford.

Misovich, S.J., Fisher, J.D. & Fisher, W.A. (1997). Close relationships and elevated risk behavior: Evidence and possible underlying psychological processes. *Review of General Psychology*, *1*, 72–107.

Muraven, M. Baumeister, R.F. (2000). Self-regulation and depletion of limited resources: Does self-control resemble a muscle? *Psychological Bulletin*, *126*, 247–259.

Muraven, M. & Slessareva, E. (2003). Mechanisms of self-control failure: Motivation and limited resources. *Personality and Social Psychology Bulletin*, *29*, 894–906.

National Center for Health Statistics (2004). *Health, United States, 2004. With chart book on trends in the health of Americans*. Hyattsville, ML: National Center for Health Statistics.

Norcross, J.C., Mrykalo, M.S. & Blagys, M.D. (2002). *Auld Lang Syne*: Success predictors, change processes, and self-reported outcomes of New Year's resolvers and non-resolvers. *Journal of Clinical Psychology*, *58*, 397–405.

Norcross, J.C., Ratzin, A.C. & Payne, D. (1989). Ringing in the New Year: The change process and reported outcomes of resolutions. *Addictive Behaviors*, *14*, 205–212.

Norcross, J.C. & Vangarelli, D.J. (1989). The resolution solution: Longitudinal examination of New Year's change attempts. *Journal of Substance Abuse*, *1*, 127–134.

Ockene, J.K., Emmons, K.M., Mermelstein, R.J., Perkins, K.A., Bonollo, D.S. & Voorhees, C.C. (2000). Relapse and maintenance issues for smoking cessation. *Health Psychology*, *19*, (Suppl.), 17–31.

Orleans, C.T. (2000). Promoting the maintenance of health behavior change: Recommendations for the next generation of research and practice. *Health Psychology*, *19*, (Suppl.), 76–83.

Ostrow, D.E., Fox, K.J., Chmiel, J.S., Silvestre, A., Visscher, B.R., Vanable, P.A., Jacobson, L.P. & Strathdee, S.A. (2002). Attitudes towards highly active antiretroviral therapy are associated with sexual risk taking among HIV-infected and uninfected homosexual men. *AIDS, 16*, 775–780.

Pervin, L.A. & Yatko, R.J. (1965). Cigarette smoking and alternative methods of reducing dissonance. *Journal of Personality and Social Psychology, 2*, 30–36.

Polivy, J., & Herman, C.P. (2002). If at first you don't succeed. False hopes of self-change. *American Psychologist, 57*, 677–689.

Prochaska, J.O., DiClemente, C.C. & Norcross, J.C. (1992). In search of how people change: Applications to addictive behaviors. *American Psychologist, 47*, 1102–1114.

Prochaska, J.O., Velicer, W.F., Rossi, J.S., Goldstein, M.G., Marcus, B.H., Rakowski, W., Fiore, C., Harlow, L.L., Redding, C.A., Rosenbloom, D. & Rossi, S.R. (1994). Stages of change and decisional balance for 12 problem behaviors. *Health Psychology, 13*, 39–46.

Rothman, A.J. (2000). Toward a theory-based analysis of behavioral maintance. *Health Psychology, 19*, (Suppl.), 64–69.

Rothman, A.J., Baldwin, A.S. & Hertel, A.W. (2004). Self-regulation and behavior change. Disentangling behavioral initiation and behavioral maintenance. In R.F. Baumeister & K.D. Vohs (Eds), *Handbook of Self-regulation. Research, Theory, and Applications* (pp. 130–148). New York: Guilford.

Ryan, R.M. & Deci, E.L. (2000). Self-determination theory and the facilitation of intrinsic motivation, social development, and well-being. *American Psychologist, 55*, 68–78.

Schachter, S. (1982). Recidivism and self-cure of smoking and obesity. *American Psychologist, 37*, 436–444.

Schmeichel, B.J. & Baumeister, R.F. (2004). Self-regulatory strength. In R.F. Baumeister and K.D. Vohs (Eds), *Handbook of Self-regulation. Research, Theory, and Applications* (pp. 84–98). New York: Guilford.

Schwarzer, R. (1992). Self-efficacy in the adoption and maintenance of health behaviors: Theoretical approaches and a new model. In R. Schwarzer (Ed.), *Self-efficacy: Thought-control of action* (pp. 217–243). Washington, DC: Hemisphere.

Schwarzer, R. (2001). Social-cognitive factors in changing health-related behavior. *Current Directions in Psychological Science, 10*, 47–51.

Schwarzer, R. & Fuchs, R. (1995). Changing risk behaviors and adopting health behaviors: The role of self-efficacy beliefs. In A. Bandura (Ed.), *Self-efficacy in Changing Societies* (pp. 259–288). Cambridge: Cambridge University Press.

Schwarzer, R. & Renner, B. (2000). Social-cognitive predictors of health behavior: Action self-efficacy and coping self-efficacy. *Health Psychology, 19*, 487–495.

Silva, M. (2002). The effectiveness of school-based sex education programs in the promotion of abstinent behavior: A meta-analysis. *Health Education Research, 17*, 471–481.

Shah, J.Y. (2005). The automatic pursuit and management of goals. *Current Directions in Psychological Science, 14*, 10–13.

Sheeran, P., Conner, M. & Norman, P. (2001). Can the theory of planned behavior explain patterns of health behavior change? *Health Psychology, 20*, 12–19.

Sheeran, P., Milne, S.E., Webb, T.L. & Gollwitzer, P.M. (2005). Implementation intentions. In M. Conner & P. Norman (Eds), *Predicting Health Behaviour*, 2nd edition (pp. 276–323). Maidenhead, UK: Open University Press.

Sherman, S.J. & Gorkin, L. (1980). Attitude bolstering when behavior is inconsistent with central attitudes. *Journal of Experimental Social Psychology, 16*, 388–403.

Simon, L., Greenberg, J. & Brehm, J. (1995). Trivialization: The forgotten mode of dissonance reduction. *Journal of Personality and Social Psychology, 68*, 247–260.

Sniehotta, F.F., Scholz, U. & Schwarzer, R. (2005). Bridging the intention-behaviour gap: Planning, self-efficacy, and action control in the adoption and maintenance of physical exercise. *Psychology and Health, 20*, 143–160.

Sniehotta, F.F., Schwarzer, R., Scholz, U. & Schüz, B. (2005). Action planning and coping planning for long-term lifestyle change: Theory and assessment. *European Journal of Social Psychology*, *35*, 565–576.

Stall, R., Ekstrand, M., Pollack, L., McKusick, L. & Coates, T. (1990). Relapse from safer sex: The next challenge for AIDS prevention efforts. *Journal of AIDS*, *3*, 1181–1187.

Stolte, I.G., Dukers, N.H.T.M., Geskus, R.B., Coutinho, R.A. & De Wit, J.B.F. (2004). Homosexual men change to risky sex when perceiving less threat of HIV/AIDS since availability of highly active antiretroviral therapy: a longitudinal study. *AIDS*, *18*, 303–309.

Stone, J., Aronson, E., Crain, A.L., Winslow, M.P. & Fried, C.B. (1994). Inducing hypocrisy as a means of encouraging young adults to use condoms. *Personality and Social Psychology Bulletin*, *20*, 116–128.

Stone, J., Wiegand, A.W., Cooper, J. & Aronson, E. (1997). When exemplification fails: Hypocrisy and the motive for self-integrity. *Journal of Personality and Social Psychology*, *72*, 54–65.

Strecher, V.J., Seijts, G.H., Kok, G.J., Latham, G.P., Glasgow, R., DeVellis, B., Meertens, R.M. & Bulger, D.W. (1995). Goal setting as a strategy for health behavior change. *Health Education Quarterly*, *22*, 190–200.

Sutton, S. (2005). Stage theories of health behavior. In M. Conner & P. Norman (Eds), *Predicting Health Behaviour*, 2nd edition (pp. 223–275). Maidenhead; UK: Open University Press.

United States Department of Health and Human Services (2000). Healthy People 2010: Understanding and Improving Health (2nd edn). Washington, DC: US Government Printing Office.

Valdiserri, R.O. (2004). Mapping the roots of HIV/AIDS complacency: Implications for program and policy development. *AIDS Education and Prevention*, *16*, 426–439.

Van der Snoek, E.M., De Wit, J.B.F, Mulder, P.G.H & Van der Meijden, W.I. (2005). Incidence of sexually transmitted diseases and HIV infection related to perceived HIV/AIDS threat since highly active antiretroviral therapy availability in men who have sex with men. *Sexually Transmitted Diseases*, *32*, 170–175.

Walster, E., Berscheid, E. & Barclay, A.M. (1967). A determinant of preference among modes of dissonance reduction. *Journal of Personality and Social Psychology*, *7*, 211–216.

Webb, T.L. & Sheeran, P. (2003). Can implementation intentions help to overcome ego-depletion? *Journal of Experimental Social Psychology*, *39*, 279–286.

Webb, T.L. & Sheeran, P. (2005). Integrating concepts from goal theories to understand the achievement of personal goals. *European Journal of Social Psychology*, *35*, 69–96.

Weinstein, N.D., Rothman, A.J. & Sutton, S.R. (1998). Stage theories of health behavior: Conceptual and methodological issues. *Health Psychology*, *17*, 290–299.

Weinstein, N.D. & Sandman, P.M. (1992). A model of the precaution adoption process: Evidence from home radon testing. *Health Psychology*, *11*, 170–180.

Williams, G.C. (2002). Improving patients' health through supporting the autonomy of patients and providers. In E.L. Deci & R.M. Ryan (Eds), *Handbook of Self-determination Research* (pp. 233–254). Rochester, NY: University of Rochester Press.

Wing, R.R. (2000a). Maintenance of behavior change in cardiorespiratory risk reduction: Introduction to the proceedings from the National Heart, Lung and Blood Institute Conference. *Health Psychology*, *19*, (Suppl.), 3–4.

Wing, R.R. (2000b). Cross-cutting themes in maintenance of behavior change. *Health Psychology*, *19*, (Suppl.), 84–88.

Witkiewitz, K. & Marlatt, G.A. (2004). Relapse prevention for alcohol and drug problems: That was Zen, this is Tao. *American Psychologist*, *59*, 224–235.

Wood, W., Quinn, J.M. & Kashy, D.A. (2002). Habits in everyday life: Thought, emotion, and action. *Journal of Personality and Social Psychology*, *83*, 1281–1297.

CHAPTER 10

Hanging On and Letting Go in the Pursuit of Health Goals: Psychological Mechanisms to Cope with a Regulatory Dilemma

Klaus Rothermund

Health occupies a central place in personal and societal goal hierarchies (Brandtstädter, Renner & Baltes-Götz, 1989). Other things being equal, people have a strong tendency to foster personal health (e.g., stay in bed or take medicine to recover from illness) and to avoid health risks (e.g., avoid getting injured or eating foul food). There are many situations, however, in which health goals may stand in conflict with other goals and desires. To give just a few examples: A healthy diet is less tasty than chocolate or luxury dinners, regular physical exercise is less entertaining than reading a book or watching television, safe sex may be less pleasurable but reduces the risk of becoming infected with HIV, compliance with a medical treatment can be quite strenuous, high speed driving may give you a thrill but increases your accident hazard, smoking has a relaxing effect but increases the risk of developing cancer and cardiovascular diseases. In all these situations, pursuing health goals becomes difficult because other motivational forces tend to push persons away from the health-fostering behaviors and pull them toward other behavioral options that entail health threats.

CONFLICTS IN THE PURSUIT OF HEALTH GOALS

The Normative Stance: Trying to Make Health Behavior More Efficient

These conflict situations represent a major field of activity for health psychologists (Karoly, 1998). Health researchers are typically concerned with the question of how to secure commitment to health goals in the face of conflicting motivations and how to

Self-regulation in Health Behavior.   Edited by Denise T.D. de Ridder and John B.F. de Wit.

increase the persistence and efficiency of health-promoting behavior (Abraham, Sheeran & Johnston, 1998; Bandura, 1998; Maes & Gebhardt, 2000; Schwarzer, 1999). Ideally, research related to these questions will tell us how health goals can successfully be translated and implemented into efficient behaviors (Gollwitzer & Oettingen, 1998) and what factors and processes are necessary to shield health goals against competing alternatives (Fuhrmann & Kuhl, 1998). These are, of course, most interesting questions. In this chapter, however, I want to argue that these questions focus only on one side of an underlying regulatory dilemma in the pursuit of goals and will not always provide an adequate and comprehensive understanding of self-regulation in the domain of health goals and health behavior.

Attempting to improve the successful pursuit of health goals is rooted in the implicit normative conviction that—at least in the long run—health is always more important than other goals and desires. At first sight this view appears plausible because health is a central resource and is sometimes even a prerequisite for the successful pursuit of many other goals in life domains like family, work, or leisure activities (Brandtstädter, Meiniger & Gräser, 2003; Hobfoll, 1989). Seen from this perspective, choosing a health-promoting behavior always appears to be the rational choice whereas alternative desires and related behaviors represent mere temptations.

Focusing on examples like those listed above, it is hard to see what could be wrong with such an evaluative stance. A more comprehensive view of self-regulation processes, however, reveals that goal pursuit in the face of difficulties is often truly dilemmatic in nature. When difficulties arise during goal pursuit, there are two basic options: you can increase your effort and stay committed to the goal; alternatively, you can disengage from the goal. This situation can be characterized as a stability/flexibility dilemma (Bak & Brandtstädter, 1998; Rothermund, 1998; see also Goschke, 2002).

An Alternative Stance: Viewing the Pursuit of Health Goals as a Regulatory Dilemma

Characterizing the alternative between persistence and flexibility as a dilemma means that both options have their pros and cons; neither of which is by definition the more adaptive response. It can be adaptive to remain committed to a goal when difficulties arise and to increase efforts in order to overcome a problem. In fact, such a reactant increase of commitment and effort is necessary to achieve ambitious, long-range goals, for which difficulties inevitably will arise during goal pursuit. Almost by definition, such goals can never be achieved without persistence. On the negative side, however, stubborn persistence in the pursuit of a goal can also lead over to perseverance and the person may run the risk of becoming trapped in a losing course of action. Persistent effort amounts to a wasting of personal resources if a goal turns out to be unattainable or when the costs of pursuing it outweigh potential gains (entrapment or escalating commitment; see Brandtstädter & Wentura, 1995; Brockner & Rubin, 1985; Janoff-Bulman & Brickman, 1982).

The same ambiguity also holds for a disengagement response. Giving up or adjusting one's commitments helps to conserve scarce action resources and might neutralize emotional strain in a problematic situation (Brandtstädter & Rothermund, 1994; Rothermund & Brandtstädter, 1997a; Wrosch, Scheier, Miller, Schulz & Carver, 2003).

On the other hand, letting go of one's personal commitments in the face of difficulties can also be maladaptive. Giving up prematurely on a goal without exploiting available resources results in unnecessary failures and produces instability in goal orientations.

Benefits and Costs in the Pursuit of Health Goals

It is important to note that in many cases, this dilemma also applies to the pursuit of health goals. For example, there are lots of situations in which people are faced with large costs when they are trying to pursue their health goals and in which it is questionable whether these goals can be achieved at all. A paradigm case is the situation that is experienced by many elderly people. Old age is typically accompanied by age-related declines in physical fitness and health (Birren & Schaie, 2001; Schneider, Rowe, Johnson, Holbrook & Morrison, 1996). To maintain previous levels of functioning, older people can invest more time and energy in exercising or they might decide to abstain from all kinds of "unhealthy" nutrition. Maintaining youthful standards of fitness and doggedly trying to counteract age-related changes, however, is not necessarily the most adaptive response in this situation. Instead, personal health goals may be adjusted to the new situation to allow for a more realistic planning of health-promoting efforts that takes into account the reduced availability of action resources as well as the demands posed by other important goals (Rothermund & Brandtstädter, 2003a; Wrosch, Schulz, & Heckhausen, 2004). Old age, however, is by no means the only situation in which an active pursuit of health goals may reach its limits. For example, chronic diseases as well as chronic pain symptoms are often very difficult or even impossible to cure. A closer look at some of the examples mentioned above also shows that it is not entirely clear that a persistent commitment to ambitious health goals is always the best option. For example, medical treatments can have adverse physical side-effects that entail substantial restrictions of subjective life-quality or they may involve the investment of large amounts of private financial resources. In these cases, the decision to engage in or comply with such a treatment in the hope of improving one's health must be balanced against the potential costs. If the gains of an active pursuit of health goals are outweighed by their costs, acceptance of the status quo can be the better choice.

Limits of Personal Control over Health-related Outcomes

The previous examples highlight the fact that the potential to successfully pursue health goals by active attempts can be severely limited. We may not like to acknowledge this—after all, who would like to regard his or her health as being uncontrollable? One might even object that normally, we can achieve our health goals quite sufficiently. A closer look reveals, however, that this impression is not necessarily due to the overwhelming success of active attempts to improve health and fitness levels. Instead, we do not tend to waste much time reflecting about things we cannot change so that in everyday life, these limits and restrictions will typically not be apparent for very long. After some unsuccessful attempts to maintain the weight level we had as a 20-year-old person, we feel that after all, weight is not that important any more (and isn't that true?).

Or we might come to the conclusion that we can live quite well with the increasing level of high-pitch sounds in our ear that seemed quite unbearable and alarming when we noticed them for the first time. Another example: If the desire to have children is not fulfilled because of infertility, a married couple may become happy with an adopted child or may come to enjoy the positive sides of a life without children (e.g., having less constraints and obligations). As a result of these changes and adjustments, we tend to overlook that even health-related goals are constantly adjusted to the feasible range by the help of self-regulatory processes.

The previous arguments have emphasized that persistent commitment in the pursuit of given health goals is not always the most adaptive response in dealing with problems and difficulties. Health goals are like other goals with regard to the fact that difficulties and problems in the pursuit of these goals pose a self-regulatory dilemma. The tension between persistence and disengagement in difficult and demanding situations is one of the most fundamental problems in the regulation of health behavior. The central point is that neither stability nor flexibility is always adaptive. That is, our motivational system cannot use a simple default strategy that will always yield the best nor even a satisfying outcome. Both options involve the risk of massive negative consequences. What is needed for self-regulation to be truly adaptive is a subtle and delicately balanced combination of the two opposite options.

The remainder of this chapter is devoted to the question how the human motivational system handles the conflict between commitment and disengagement. As a theoretical framework, I draw on the dual-process model of assimilative and accommodative coping that was developed by Jochen Brandtstädter and colleagues (Brandtstädter, 1989; Brandtstädter & Renner, 1990; Brandtstädter & Rothermund, 2002a, 2002b).

THE DUAL-PROCESS MODEL OF ASSIMILATIVE PERSISTENCE AND ACCOMMODATIVE FLEXIBILITY

The dual-process model represents a conceptual framework for processes of action regulation and self-development (see Figure 10.1). According to the model, regulatory processes are activated by perceived or anticipated goal discrepancies. The model distinguishes between two fundamentally different ways to cope with these problems and difficulties; these are termed as *assimilative* and *accommodative* coping.[1] In this section, I will first present a brief general description of assimilative and accommodative coping and their determinants. A second part contains diverse applications of the dual process model to the domain of health. In a next section, I focus on the underlying cognitive processes that accompany assimilative and accommodative coping.

A first way of neutralizing discrepancies is to overcome the problem by investing more energy and effort. These active attempts are denoted as assimilative coping, because this form of coping aims at an assimilation of the current situation to the given goals and aspirations of a person. The assimilative mode largely corresponds to what has been

---

[1] Our usage of the terms assimilation and accommodation in the context of self-regulation processes should not be equated with the Piagetian (Piaget, 1970) terminology, which refers to basic processes in the development of cognitive or motoric schemas in interaction with their environment.

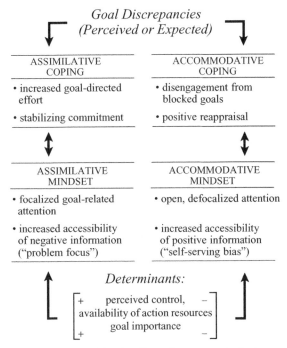

Figure 10.1   The dual-process model of self-regulation: Assimilative and accommodative coping, related cognitive mindsets, and determinants

described as persistent goal pursuit: It comprises processes aiming at effort mobilization and at stabilizing commitment to the goal.

A second, antagonistic mode of neutralizing perceived goal discrepancies is called accommodation. Accommodative coping consists in adjusting personal goals and aspirations to a given situation, which reduces discrepancies between goals and the personal situation. Accommodation can take the form of a positive reappraisal of a situation that was initially appraised as negative, which helps to alleviate the negative emotional impact of failures and losses. Another form of accommodation consists in reducing the importance of a blocked striving and/or in letting go of this goal. Disengaging from a commitment enables the person to withdraw action resources from a blocked goal and serves to avoid entrapment and escalation of commitment. Accommodative disengagement is also the basis for a reorientation toward other, more promising goals and projects (Brandtstädter & Rothermund, 2002a, 2002b; Rothermund, 1998; see also Wrosch, Scheier, Carver & Schulz, 2003).

Determinants of Assimilative and Accommodative Modes of Coping

A core element of the dual-process model consists in the specification of moderating conditions that determine whether an assimilative or accommodative mode of coping will prevail in dealing with a problematic situation. The specification of these determinants is of utmost importance for an understanding of how self-regulation tackles the stability/

flexibility dilemma because the nature of the self-regulation process in a specific situation depends on just these factors. According to the dual-process model, two factors stand out in this regard: first, perceived control over goal attainment, and second, the importance or centrality of the affected goal in the personal goal hierarchy.

Assimilative activities strongly depend on the perception of having high control over desired outcomes. For example, people differ with regard to self-efficacy beliefs, tenacity, or optimism, which predict active-assimilative coping with health problems (Luszczynska & Schwarzer, 2005; Scheier & Carver, 1992). Besides these global dispositional factors, more specific factors also have an influence on the tendency to actively influence goal achievement and to remain committed to a health goal, like controllability of a specific disease (Fournier, De Ridder & Bensing, 2002), availability of personal action resources (Rothermund & Brandtstädter, 2003a), or the knowledge how health goals can be promoted by specific activities. In case of low control-beliefs and in the absence of action resources or knowledge of relevant action strategies, assimilative activities typically decline, and an accommodative mode of coping becomes activated.

Besides control, goal centrality or substitutability is also of major importance for the regulation of coping modes. When a goal occupies a central place in a person's goal hierarchy, it cannot easily be substituted by alternative options. In this case, relinquishing the blocked goal is particularly difficult and painful because it involves a complete restructuring of the person's motivational structure. In such a situation, the assimilative mode of coping will dominate and tendencies to disengage from the goal will be inhibited. On the other hand, if a certain goal represents just one way to reach other, superordinate goals, or if the goal occupies only an isolated position in a person's goal hierarchy that is unrelated to other important goals and strivings, accommodative tendencies will become activated as soon as goal pursuit becomes difficult.

A final point is noteworthy with regard to the regulation of assimilative and accommodative coping. The activation (or inhibition) of these modes not only depends on external determinants like perceived control or importance. Over and above these influences, the two modes of coping are assumed to stand in an antagonistic, mutually inhibiting interrelation so that activation of one mode leads to the suppression of the other (Brandtstädter & Greve, 1994). For example, mobilizing additional energy and effort in order to achieve a goal when obstacles and problems arise during goal pursuit requires that the personal importance of the respective goal is maintained or even increased. Such a shielding of goal importance in the assimilative mode inhibits an accommodative tendency toward disengagement that would require a reduction of the subjective importance of the goal. It should be noted at this point, however, that although assimilation and accommodation cannot be activated simultaneously, both forms of self-regulation can become activated sequentially in the course of a coping episode (e.g., disengaging from a certain plan or strategy to reach a superordinate goal may set the stage for new, alternative forms of assimilative goal pursuit).

IMPLICATIONS OF THE DUAL-PROCESS MODEL FOR SELF-REGULATION IN THE DOMAIN OF HEALTH

The previous remarks have direct implications for the understanding of coping with health problems. A first point relates to the personal importance of health goals and to the adjustment of criteria that are used to define the concept of health. As was already stated in the introduction, health is an important resource for the pursuit of many other goals and strivings, and is in fact a prerequisite for living. In this sense, health can be considered to occupy a central place in personal goal systems. It therefore should be hard to disengage from the goal of being healthy. Stated the other way around, because illness interferes with the pursuit of most other goals, almost any possible attempt will be undertaken to become healthy again. However, absence of illness is just one of multiple meanings of the concept health, and it pays to take a closer look at possible variations and differentiations in the meaning of this term. Health is not just a simple binary dichotomy—either you have it or you don't—as the opposition of health and illness seems to suggest. Instead, there is substantial leeway in using specific personal criteria of what constitutes health and when a person feels justified to categorize him- or herself as healthy. These criteria can range from extraordinary fitness of an athlete (think of magazines like *Men's Health*) to still being able to live a life of one's own (out of hospital or out of a nursing home). In between these extremes, nearly all possible variations of criteria for being healthy exist. Subjective definitions of being healthy are not fixed, they can refer to given physical conditions, to the health status of same-aged people or any other reference group, or they may fluctuate depending on the nature of activities one wants to pursue. The conviction that health must always be of utmost personal importance, leaving no room for accommodation, may refer to only a very narrow meaning of the term health ("not being terminally ill"). Besides this truism, people can and apparently do adjust their subjective criteria of what constitutes health for them. In conclusion, it is important to acknowledge that the personal importance of health goals as well as criteria of being healthy differ within and between individuals. According to the dual-process model, these differences can result from accommodative processes.

Perceived Control Over Health

A second important aspect relates to the amount of perceived control over health-related outcomes and goals. Persistent commitment to health goals depends on the belief that behavioral efforts will improve one's health status. If this belief becomes frustrated by chronic failures to reach the intended goal, assimilative activities will also tend to decrease. It is important to note, however, that a reduction of assimilative activities does not necessarily imply disengagement or acceptance. If the blocked goal is very important for the person, chronic failure to reach the goal can result in a temporary (or permanent) deadlock. This combination of high importance with low control may lead to the development of degenerated intentions (i.e., the goal of being healthy is still of vital importance for the person although it has become a mere wish that is no longer linked with specific behaviours, plans, or strategies), which constitutes a major risk factor for depression (Kuhl & Helle, 1986).

SELF-REGULATORY PROCESSES IN COPING WITH HEALTH-RELATED PROBLEMS: EMPIRICAL ILLUSTRATIONS

In the following paragraphs, some empirical findings from the domain of coping with health-related problems are used to illustrate basic propositions of the dual-process model. These examples mostly emphasize the relevance of accommodative processes in coping with health problems and deficits. This is not meant to express that accommodation is always more important than assimilation. Instead, the focus on accommodative processes was chosen to complement the strong emphasis on active-assimilative coping processes that is typical for research on self-regulation in the health domain and is also well-documented in other chapters of this volume.

Emotional Buffering Effects of an Accommodative Coping Style

The core prediction of the dual-process model is that accommodative coping should help to reduce the negative impact of problems and losses on subjective well-being. Empirical support for this prediction was found in several studies investigating effects of accommodative coping with regard to goal discrepancies and critical life events in various life domains (Bak & Brandtstädter, 1998; Brandtstädter & Renner, 1990; Brandtstädter & Rothermund, 1994; Rothermund, Dillmann & Brandtstädter, 1994). The following overview describes studies that explicitly investigated emotional buffering effects of accommodative coping in the domain of health and disability.

Brandtstädter, Wentura and Greve (1993) assessed health problems with a checklist covering different categories of diseases. An overall index of health problems was computed by applying the *Seriousness of Illness Rating Scale* to these self-reported diseases (Wyler, Masuda & Holmes, 1968; modified after Bossé, Aldwin, Levenson & Ekerdt, 1987). Seriousness of Illness Rating scores were negatively related to measures of well-being and correlated positively with depression. The negative impact of diseases on measures of psychological adaptation, however, was dampened by an accommodative coping style (measured with the Flexible Goal Adjustment scale; Brandtstädter & Renner, 1990). For participants with low scores on Flexible Goal Adjustment, health problems were accompanied by depressive symptoms and low subjective well-being, whereas for participants scoring high on Flexible Goal Adjustment, well-being and depression were virtually unrelated to health problems and diseases.

Two other studies investigated effects of accommodative coping with regard to specific health problems and disabilities. Boerner (2004) investigated processes of adaptation to disability in a sample of people suffering from loss of vision. Accommodative coping, measured with the Flexible Goal Adjustment scale, had a beneficial effect on subjective well-being that was most pronounced for people who suffered from severe disabilities, indicating an emotional buffering effect. Schmitz, Saile and Nilges (1996) studied accommodative coping in a sample of chronic pain patients. In accordance with the previous findings, an accommodative coping style (high scores on the Flexible Goal Adjustment scale) reduced the negative impact of pain experience (pain intensity, pain-related disability) on depression. This result fits nicely with recent findings that acceptance is the strongest positive predictor of psychological adjustment in patients suffering from chronic pain or chronic illness (McCracken, 1998; McCracken, & Ecclestone, 2003; Schiaffino, Shawaryn & Blum, 1998). Another finding in the study by Schmitz and colleagues (1996) concerns the more immediate implications of accommodative coping for the reduction of pain symptoms. Active forms of coping with pain (e.g., action planning) had a positive effect on pain-related disability only when they were accompanied by an accommodative coping style. Apparently, being able to adjust one's goals to what can realistically be expected with regard to control over pain is an important requirement of choosing adequate forms of active coping (a similar finding has also been reported for coping with critical life events; see Rothermund & Brandt-städter, 1997a).

These findings illustrate the important role of accommodation for successful coping with health problems and disability. Accommodation is necessary if people are to accept losses and restraints in the domain of health and physical functioning. By enabling people to accept these deficits and losses as part of their personal situation, accommodation reduces the negative impact of these problems on life satisfaction and subjective well-being.

A Process Analysis of Accommodative Coping

The studies reviewed above investigated emotional buffering effects of a global accommodative coping style. In the following paragraph, I will take a closer look at the processes that are involved in accommodative coping and adjustment. The dual-process model identifies two major types of processes of accommodative coping: disengagement and positive reappraisal (see Figure 10.1).

The Process of Disengagement

Disengagement implies that the personal importance of a discrepant goal becomes downgraded so that it no longer occupies a central place in a person's goal hierarchy. Reducing the importance of a blocked goal is a prerequisite for withdrawing cognitive and action resources away from a problematic domain and for assigning them to other, more promising goals and projects.

Several studies have investigated processes of disengaging from blocked goals. Preliminary evidence for such a disengagement mechanism comes from findings that the perceived distance from a successful achievement of a certain goal typically shows a negative correlation with the subjective importance of the respective goal (i.e., perceiving a large distance to goal achievement is typically accompanied by low goal importance; Brandtstädter & Baltes-Götz, 1990; Brandtstädter & Renner, 1990; Brandtstädter, Rothermund & Schmitz, 1998). Due to the ambiguous nature of correlations, however, these findings do not provide unequivocal evidence for disengagement processes in response to perceived discrepancies; instead, the correlation might simply reflect that large goal discrepancies are more likely to emerge for unimportant goals because people are reluctant to invest effort and resources in domains that are not significant. To overcome these interpretational difficulties, Brandtstädter and Rothermund (2002a) analyzed longitudinal changes in goal importance. Their findings suggest a more complex picture of the process of adjusting the personal importance of goals. In this study, longitudinal changes in goal importance were regressed onto initial goal discrepancies but also on initially perceived control over goal achievement. In line with the previous findings, large initial discrepancies predicted a reduction of goal importance for goals that were perceived as being

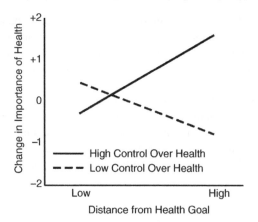

Figure 10.2 Longitudinal changes in the subjective importance of health as a function of initially perceived discrepancies in health goals and perceived control over health

uncontrollable, indicating a disengagement process. For controllable goals, however, initial discrepancies even led to a subsequent increase in goal importance, indicating reactant persistence that stabilizes goal commitment. Figure 10.2 illustrates this finding for the domain of health goals. This pattern of results indicates that discrepancies and perceived control interact in producing commitment to or disengagement from a goal. As predicted by the dual-process model, discrepancies trigger assimilative persistence if perceived control is high; on the other hand, encountering difficulties leads to an accommodative disengagement from the blocked goal if perceived control over goal achievement is low.

Reducing the importance of a certain goal is an obvious but also a somewhat blatant form of disengagement. In some cases, it might be difficult to completely disengage from a certain goal because this goal occupies a central place in a person's goal structure or because of external pressures to remain committed to the goal. In such cases, disengagement can take the form of adjusting previous aspirations or personal standards rather than abandoning the goal itself (in this case, the object of the disengagement process is a specific representation of a goal that is abandoned and replaced with a more feasible variant of the same goal). This adjustment of personal standards allows the person to remain committed to a certain abstract goal without becoming chronically frustrated.

Evidence for this more subtle form of disengagement was found in a recent study by Rothermund and Brandtstädter (2003a). Processes of coping with deficits in different domains of functioning (mental and physical health, everyday functioning) were assessed in a sample of middle aged and older adults. Functional deficits and losses in these domains were found to increase with age, particularly for old adults, who could no longer counteract functional declines by active-compensatory efforts. Interestingly, however, subjective contentment with personal levels of functioning was unrelated to age; satisfaction with personal performance remained stable even for the oldest cohorts of the sample. An explanation of this counterintuitive result can be found in processes of accommodative disengagement. In fact, older people employed a subtle form of disengagement to avoid potential frustration resulting from irreversible functional declines. Rothermund and Brandtstädter (2003a) found an age-related decrease in the importance to keep up with the performance levels of younger people in the respective domains. Additional analyses revealed that this lowering of personal standards buffered the negative relation between functional declines and contentment: increases in functional deficits no longer predicted dissatisfaction for participants who adjusted their personal standards during the longitudinal time interval of the study. This finding is particularly noteworthy because it also offers an explanation for the more general paradoxical finding that there is no age-related increase in depression nor decrease in subjective well-being despite a growing incidence of age-related problems with regard to health, mobility, fitness, or the loss of close relatives and friends (see Blazer, 1993; Diener & Suh, 1998; Rothermund & Brandtstädter, 2003b; Stock, Okun, Haring & Witter, 1983). Possibly, accommodative processes of adjusting personal standards to the feasible range play an important role in the prevention of frustration and depression in old age.

Positive Reappraisal

A second important form of accommodative coping with irreversible losses and deficits consists in adopting a new evaluation of a situation that was previously seen as being highly problematic. Finding a positive reappraisal of a negative situation may help to neutralize discrepancies without having to actively change the situation and also without having to disengage from the goals that are related to the problem. This second form of accommodative coping can take the form of seeing positive side-effects in a critical situation that are not obvious at first sight ("benefit finding," Affleck & Tennen, 1996; Tennen & Affleck, 2002). Alternatively, positive reappraisal may also result from viewing a stressful episode as an opportunity for developing maturity or personal growth, or as viewing it as an important experience that has helped to reveal what is of enduring importance in life and what is not (Aldwin & Sutton, 1998; Elliott, Kurylo & Rivera, 2002; Janoff-Bulman & Berger, 2000; Updegraff & Taylor, 2000).

Evidence for accommodative processes of constructing positive reappraisals in response to stressful situations or of experiencing gains as a result of critical life events has been found in several studies (Folkman, 1997; McFarland & Alvaro, 2000; Rothermund & Brandtstädter, 1997a; Rothermund & Meiniger, 2004; Taylor, 1983). These studies, however, typically did not investigate the functionality of these processes of meaning construction for psychological adjustment in a problematic situation. Evidence for the adaptive function of positive reappraisals in coping with health-related problems was reported by Wrosch, Heckhausen and Lachman (2000). In their study, positive reappraisal was found to buffer negative effects of perceived health stresses on subjective well-being. Importantly, these buffering effects were more pronounced for older people of the sample, indicating that accommodative processes are of increasing importance when efficient action resources to overcome health problems become scarce or are no longer available.

The research that was reviewed in the previous paragraphs has shown that reappraising negative situations in more positive terms or disengaging from barren goals and commitments are important ingredients of coping with health problems. Accommodation helps to accept irreversible losses and is of fundamental importance for understanding processes of psychological adjustment to intractable problems.

THE COGNITIVE MECHANISMS OF ASSIMILATION AND ACCOMMODATION

Assimilation and accommodation represent basic forms of self-regulation. The previous analyses have described these coping processes and their effects on commitment to and disengagement from health goals on a macro-level. It is important to emphasize, however, that neither assimilative persistence nor accommodative disengagement can be fully understood as the result of purely rational deliberation.

"Irrationality" of Assimilative Persistence

Maintaining or even increasing commitment to a goal when being confronted with difficulties provides the motivational basis for persistent and lasting goal pursuit (Kuhl, 1984, 2000). Although this can be a highly adaptive response in the long run, it cannot easily be explained in terms of a purely rational decision. Problems and difficulties in goal pursuit signal a reduced expectancy of achieving the goal and an increase in the expected costs that have to be invested to reach the goal. In a rational calculation of expectancies, costs, and benefits, problems and difficulties signal a lowering of the overall expected value of the respective goal and should thus reduce commitment to the goal or project (Atkinson & Feather, 1966; Feather & Newton, 1982). The reactant increase in goal importance that is in fact observed in the assimilative coping mode can only be understood in terms of a psychological mechanism that aims at *counteracting* this loss in value in order to prevent a destabilization of the goal commitment in the face of threat.

Emotional Attachment and Accommodative Disengagement

Seen from the outside, disengaging from a goal that has become unfeasible seems to be a most rational response. But again, although such a response can be highly adaptive for the conservation of action resources and for the emotional adjustment of a person, processes of an accommodative disengagement cannot be fully grasped in terms of rational calculation. Personal goals involve emotional attachments and are linked to self-definitions and cherished identities of a person (e.g., of being a successful athlete or of leading a life of one's own). Merely stating that it is no longer beneficial to pursue these goals because of an unfavorable cost/benefit ratio may perhaps help to suspend unsuccessful overt behavioral activities but is clearly not enough to neutralize deep emotional attachments. Disengagement is not complete without a real reduction of goal attractiveness that is not yet implicated by the insight that the goal is beyond one's reach (Wrosch et al., 2003). Similarly, just pointing out positive side-effects of a problematic situation—as it is sometimes done by relatives or close friends in order to console a person after a loss—does not suffice to convince the person that his or her situation is in fact desirable. Accepting a more positive view of one's situation, however, is not the result of a decision—otherwise, people would not suffer from rumination or depression (Brandtstädter & Rothermund, 2002a; Rothermund, 2003; Rothermund & Brandtstädter, 1997b).

Assimilative and Accommodative Mindsets

The main upshot of the previous arguments is that a full understanding of assimilative and accommodative coping requires an analysis of underlying psychological mechanisms that prepare our motivational system for assimilative persistence or for accommodative disengagement. It is a core assumption of the dual-process model that assimilative and accommodative coping are accompanied by corresponding modes of cognitive functioning, that is, by assimilative and accommodative *mindsets*[2] (Brandtstädter & Rothermund, 2002a, 2002b; Brandtstädter, Wentura & Rothermund, 1999; Rothermund, 1998). The basic idea is that parameters of automatic information processing are configured in such a way that either assimilation or accommodation is facilitated. In essence, the model specifies two main aspects of cognitive functioning that differentiate between assimilative and accommodative coping: selectivity of information processing and accessibility of valent information (see Figure 10.1).

Closed versus Open Modes of Information Processing

A first proposition of the dual-process model is that assimilative versus accommodative modes of coping are related to the selectivity or breadth of information processing (Rothermund, 1998). In a state of selective attention or vigilance, relevant or goal-related information has preferential access to processing resources whereas irrelevant information is inhibited (Tipper, 1992). A non-selective state of information processing, on the other hand, is characterized by intrusion effects of irrelevant, goal-unrelated information into the stream of processing (Kofta & Sedek, 1998).

According to the dual-process model, information processing is highly selective in the assimilative mindset. The focus of attention is directed at the current goal, which implies that goal-relevant information is processed with high priority, whereas goal-irrelevant or distracting information is blocked from accessing resource demanding processes. This kind of selectivity in the assimilative mode constitutes a goal-relevance principle of information processing (Rothermund, 1998). Focusing on goal-related information is essential for efficient goal pursuit and helps to shield the current goal against competing alternatives (Kuhl, 1984, 2000; Shah, Friedman & Kruglanski, 2002). A closed or focused mode of processing can thus be seen as an important prerequisite for persistent

---

[2] Psychologists of the Würzburg school introduced the concept of mindsets to denote different global configurations of the cognitive system (Marbe, 1915). More recently, the concept has been used by Heckhausen and Gollwitzer (1987; see also Gollwitzer & Kinney, 1989) to denote distinct modes of cognitive functioning during predecisional (deliberative mindset) and postdecisional (implemental mindset) states of the motivational/volitional process.

commitment to a goal, and is related to dispositional coping tendencies of tenacious goal pursuit (Shah et al., 2002).

In the accommodative mindset, the cognitive system is characterized by an open mode of information processing (Rothermund, 1998). Previously irrelevant or distracting information is no longer inhibited and regains access to cognitive resources. This neutralization of assimilative selectivity in the accommodative mindset is a prerequisite for withdrawing cognitive resources from a blocked goal and allocating them to other, more promising goal domains. The open mode of processing facilitates accommodative disengagement and paves the way for a reorienting toward new goals. This mode of processing constitutes another, more generalized relevance principle of information processing because cognitive resources are disengaged from content that is no longer relevant for the regulation of action and are transferred to potential new sources of relevance (Rothermund, 1998).

It should be noted that the influence between coping processes and cognitive mechanisms is assumed to be bidirectional (see Figure 10.1). Assimilative and accommodative coping are fostered by the corresponding cognitive mechanisms but macro-processes of coping, in turn, also entail closed or open modes of information processing (e.g., concentrating on a problem in an assimilative mode of coping can be both the effect and the cause of selective information processing).

Evidence for a corresponding switch between closed and open modes of information processing under assimilative and accommodative modes of coping has been gathered in a series of laboratory experiments. Activating an assimilative mindset, for instance by confronting participants with difficult but solvable tasks, led to an increased focusing on task-relevant information, whereas activating an accommodative mindset, for example by letting participants work on unsolvable tasks, was accompanied by an increase in distractibility and an intrusion of irrelevant information (Brandtstädter & Rothermund, 2002a; Lukas, 2003; Rothermund, 1998). Related evidence comes from experiments that were conducted in the tradition of learned helplessness research: Conforming to the predictions of the dual-process model, exposure to stress and problems that were uncontrollable led to an increased cognitive distractibility (Kofta & Sedek, 1998; Lee & Maier, 1988; Mikulincer, 1989; Mikulincer, Kedem & Zilkha-Segal, 1989; Rodd, Rosselini, Stock & Gallup, 1997).

In yet another experiment, closed versus open modes of processing were investigated with respect to pain sensitivity, which is of direct relevance to the health domain (Rothermund, Brandtstädter, Meiniger & Anton, 2002). In this study, participants were exposed to a series of painful pressure stimuli, the duration of which was either contingent on the performance in a simultaneous tracking task (controllable pain condition) or not (uncontrollable pain condition). Absolute durations of the pain stimuli were balanced between the two conditions by means of a yoked control design.[3] The aim of the study was to investigate effects of experiencing controllable versus uncontrollable pain on pain sensitivity. Changes in pain sensitivity were assessed by comparing pain sensitivity thresholds for heat stimuli before and after the application of the painful

---

[3] Pain durations for each participant in the uncontrollable pain condition were computed by averaging the pain durations of the preceding participant in the controllable condition across all trials of the tracking task.

pressure stimuli. In line with the predictions of the dual-process model, controllable pain led to an increase in pain sensitivity, that is, pain thresholds were lower after receiving painful stimuli that could be reduced in duration by personal effort. In this case, pain is a relevant signal for activating action resources in order to ward off the pain. An assimilative mode of coping is activated and attention is focused on goal-relevant information (i.e., pain), which in turn leads to an increase in pain sensitivity (*hyper-algesia*). Being exposed to uncontrollable painful stimuli, on the other hand, brought about a decrease in pain sensitivity (*hypoalgesia*), that is, pain thresholds were higher after receiving painful stimuli the duration of which could not be influenced by personal effort. In this case, pain is no longer relevant for the regulation of action because it cannot be controlled. An accommodative mode of coping is activated which neutralizes the dysfunctional focus on the pain and leads to a withdrawal of attentional resources away from the previously relevant source of information. Related findings of hyperalgesia after controllable pain and hypoalgesia after uncontrollable pain have also been reported in animal studies, which attests to the generality of the reported findings (Grau, Hyson, Maier, Madden & Barchas, 1981; Rodgers & Hendrie, 1983; for a review, see Maier, 1986).

Biases in the Cognitive Accessibility of Valent Information

The previous paragraph analyzed differences in the selectivity or breadth of information processing, regardless of valence. Another, albeit related proposition of the dual-process model is that assimilative versus accommodative modes of coping increase or decrease the accessibility of cognitions that have positive versus negative implications with regard to the current goal (Brandtstädter & Rothermund, 2002a; Brandtstädter et al., 1999).

Specifically, the dual-process model assumes that in the assimilative mindset, information processing is characterized by a problem focus: negative or threatening information should become highly accessible in the assimilative mode. Such a focus on problems and difficulties with regard to goal pursuit is functional for assimilative coping because problems and dangers are relevant for an efficient regulation of goal-related behavior. In the accommodative mode, on the other hand, processing is characterized by a focus on positive and self-assuring information. A high sensitivity for positive and relieving information paves the way for accommodative coping processes because it facilitates the construction of positive reappraisals and provides the basis for an acceptance of negative and goal-discrepant situations.

An increased sensitivity for problem-related versus positive information under assim-ilative versus accommodative modes of coping has been investigated in diverse research areas. A large number of studies have revealed that self-serving biases in the evaluation of personal attributes, feedback seeking, memory and attribution processes, or dissonance reduction are moderated by the controllability of the situation. Evidence for self-enhancing biases was found if the situation was perceived as being uncontrollable but not if a situation was perceived as being modifiable and open to personal control (Dunning, 1995; Duval & Silvia, 2002; Gilbert & Ebert, 2002; Green, Pinter & Sedikides, 2005; Pahl & Eiser, 2005; Trope, Gervey & Bolger, 2003). In a recent study by Rothermund, Bak and Brandtstädter (2005), students rated the degree to which they possessed attributes that were described as having either positive or negative implications for academic success. As predicted by the dual-process model, students showed a self-enhancement bias for self-evaluations regarding uncontrollable trait attributes, but showed an opposite bias for self-evaluations regarding attributes that were perceived as being modifiable and under the person's control. These findings indicate that controllability of attributes is critical for the activation of assimilative versus accommodative mindsets, leading to either a self-enhancement bias (low control, accommodation) or a problem-focus (high control, assimilation).

Wentura (1995; see also Wentura & Nüsing, 1999) conducted experiments that allowed a more direct assessment of changes in the cognitive accessibility of problematic information. Participants had to read text vignettes describing personally relevant situations (e.g., writing an exam, applying for a student scholarship abroad). After each scenario, a recognition test was conducted to assess the cognitive accessibility of the different pieces of information that were contained in the vignettes (short recognition latencies indicate high accessibility of the respective information). All scenarios contained information that could be used for a positive reappraisal of the situation if the story had a negative ending (most fellow students had considerable problems with the exam; most of your friends will remain at their home university). This potentially alleviating information was found to increase in accessibility after participants were informed that the episode had a frustrating outcome (failure, rejection), indicating an automatic tendency to focus on information that can be used for a positive reappraisal of the frustrating episode. This tendency was particularly strong for participants scoring high in Flexible Goal Adjustment (Wentura, Rothermund & Brandtstädter, 1995).

Another series of experiments investigated basic perceptual processes with regard to the detection of danger signals (Brandtstädter, Voss & Rothermund, 2004; Voss, Rothermund & Brandtstädter, in press). Multiple stimuli consisting of color-letter conjunctions were presented tachistoscopically in a visual search task. A certain combination (e.g., a yellow T) was randomly selected as a danger stimulus that signalled a possible loss of points. For one group of participants, loss of points was obligatory on the presentation of the danger stimulus (uncontrollable danger condition) whereas for another group, loss of points could be avoided by identifying the position of the danger stimulus in a subsequent location task (controllable danger condition). Signal detection analyses revealed that the perceptual sensitivity index 'd' was lower for danger stimuli compared to a neutral baseline in the uncontrollable condition, but was increased in the controllable danger condition. This pattern is in accordance with the predictions of the dual-process model: Perceptual defence was the default in the accommodative mode, whereas evidence of a heightened sensitivity for threatening stimuli that were relevant for action regulation (warding off the danger) was obtained in the assimilative mode.

Focusing on negative/problematic versus positive/alleviating information in an assimilative versus accommodative mindset is closely related to the regulation of health behavior. Increasing the accessibility of negative, threat-related information or focusing on the positive aspects of a situation should have a direct influence on processes of risk perception. Most models of health behavior identify personal risk estimates as one of the key predictors of health-related behavioral intentions and health-related behavior change (Maes & Gebhardt, 2000; Rippetoe & Rogers, 1987; Rogers & Prentice-Dunn, 1997;

Schwarzer, 1999; Weinstein, 1993). The dual-process model expands this perspective. Risk perceptions are not just seen as determinants of health behavior, but also reflect outcomes of self-regulation processes with control perceptions playing an important role in the formation of risk estimations. Specifically, the dual-process model predicts that high control triggers an assimilative mode of coping that sensitizes the person to possible risks and should increase risk estimations. In contrast, if health outcomes are seen as uncontrollable, risk-related information should become inhibited, because negative or threatening information is warded off in the accommodative mindset.

Many studies have revealed a tendency to underestimate personal health risks, a phenomenon that has been labelled as "unrealistic optimism" or as an "illusion of safety" (Thompson, Anderson, Freedman & Swan, 1996; Weinstein, 1980). Such a personal invulnerability bias, however, is not a ubiquitous phenomenon and seems to be subject to a number of moderating variables (see Renner & Schwarzer, 2003). Most important in the present context are effects of controllability on defensive tendencies of risk perception.

In early studies, Weinstein (1980, 1984) found that estimations of personal risks (i.e., probabilities of encountering negative events in the future) were lower in relation to "average" risk estimations for other people of the same age and gender. This optimistic bias was more pronounced for events that were controllable (see Alicke, 1985, for a similar finding in the domain of self-serving evaluative biases). The results of these studies, however, do not reflect pure biases with regard to probability estimates of personal risks because these estimates are confounded with evaluations of personal efforts (in the past, present or future) to prevent negative events. An underestimation of the likelihood to encounter controllable negative events in the future might therefore reflect a tendency to overestimate the personal potential to exert control over negative outcomes (i.e., an illusion of control, Alloy & Abramson, 1979; Gollwitzer & Kinney, 1989; Weinstein, 1984) rather than differences in risk estimations. These interpretational problems were avoided in other studies in which participants were randomly assigned to conditions of controllable and uncontrollable risks.

In an experimental study with a randomized assignment of participants to conditions, students were told that they tested either positively or negatively for a fictitious risk factor for a disease that typically emerges much later in life (Ditto, Jemmott & Darley, 1988). Students exposed to the positive test result reduced the personal relevance of the medical diagnosis by questioning the validity of the test compared to the participants that had received a favorable (i.e., negative) diagnosis. Importantly, the defensive bias following a threatening diagnosis was neutralized if participants were informed about a preventive treatment that would be effective in counteracting the negative effects of the risk factor that was diagnosed by the test. This reduction of defensiveness under conditions of control reflects the activation of an assimilative mindset, which directs the attentional focus to negative or problematic information and the way it can be counteracted. After receiving the threatening diagnosis, participants in the controllable condition might instantly have started to think about the treatment whereas participants in the uncontrollable condition might have thought about whether the test had been conducted properly or that a positive diagnosis was unlikely to be true because they had not observed any symptoms of the disease until then.

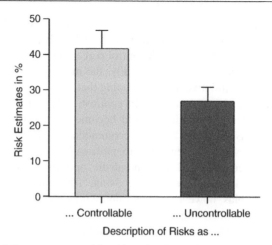

Figure 10.3 Probability estimates of health risks depending on the description of risks as controllable versus uncontrollable

A similar finding was obtained in a recent study by Rothermund and Voss (2005). Personal risk estimates were gathered for a number of fictitious situations, two of which were related to health problems. One of the scenarios assessed the probability of being infected with a dangerous virus after having spent a holiday in Africa, the other scenario concerned the probability of developing chronic problems with one's back due to working permanently in a sitting position. The scenarios were either presented in a standard version or in a controllable variant. In the standard version, risk estimates were assessed after a short description of the situation. The controllable variants were identical with regard to the description of health risks but contained additional information indicating that negative outcomes could be prevented by taking adequate measures (taking a vaccination that kills the virus even after infection, regular exercise to prevent the development of back problems). Each participant received both scenarios, one in the standard version and another in the controllable format (assignment of controllable and uncontrollable versions of the two scenarios to participants was counterbalanced). Risk estimates were significantly higher in the controllable condition (see Figure 10.3), indicating that perceived control goes along with an increased readiness to see a situation as threatening (similar findings have been reported with regard to dispositional optimism; Aspinwall & Brunhart, 1996, 2000). In a situation that does not contain any hints to counteract the emergence of health risks, on the other hand, an accommodative mindset is activated which leads to an inhibition of negative or problematic information.

The reported findings support the predictions of the dual-process model. Risk estimates apparently become adapted to personal control beliefs: Perceived influence or control over health-related outcomes sensitizes a person for negative and threatening information which facilitates efficient regulation of action to ward off dangers. Experiences of helplessness or perceptions of low control, on the other hand, shift the focus away from risks and dangers toward positive information that can be used for an alleviating or self-serving reappraisal of a problematic situation.

CONCLUSION

A theoretical analysis of self-regulation processes in the domain of health behavior has revealed two central components: assimilative persistence in the pursuit of health goals and flexible adjustment of goals and aspirations. I have argued that self-regulation in the health domain can be characterized as a regulatory dilemma, and that both forms of coping are necessary for an adaptive regulation of health behavior. Perceptions of personal control have been identified as a subtle psychological "switch" that activates either assimilative or accommodative forms of coping.

Current research in health psychology has typically emphasized processes of active goal-pursuit, problem-focused coping and stabilizing commitment to health goals (for a notable exception, see Brownlee, Leventhal & Leventhal, 2000). Analyzing the processes that underlie problem-focused coping is important for an understanding of what is necessary for a successful pursuit of health goals. These insights can be used to design interventions that aim at optimizing health behavior by increasing the range of personal control and influence.

In this chapter, emphasis has been put on a somewhat neglected aspect of self-regulation in the health domain. I have investigated processes that foster acceptance of health problems or disengagement from health goals. These processes are instigated if action resources are scarce and control over the achievement of health goals is low or nonexistent. Although we may not like to acknowledge this, there are many examples in the domain of health that can be characterized this way: unwanted infertility, terminal illness, incurable diseases, chronic pain, or age-related functional declines. It is important to note that even in these situations self-regulation does not come to a stop. Instead, processes of accommodation are of utmost importance to prepare the person for an adjustment to the problematic situation, to prevent that scarce resources are wasted in a futile attempt to change the unchangeable, and to reduce chronic emotional strain and prevent depression resulting from chronic failure.

The distinction between assimilative and accommodative forms of coping and of the conditions under which these different forms of self-regulation are adaptive also has important implications for practitioners in the domain of health psychology. Encouraging people to stay committed to ambitious health goals is advisable if there is a realistic chance that these goals will eventually be reached. If possible, such an encouragement should be accompanied with interventions aiming at an expansion of the personal control potential (Creer, 2000). It should not be overlooked that fostering active goal pursuit under conditions of low control or in a situation of low achievement probabilities does not come without costs. Action resources are invested that are no longer available for alternative options, experiences of failure can undermine control beliefs for future coping episodes, and commitment to goals that are in fact unfeasible represents a risk factor for the emergence of depression. Health psychologists might therefore try to initiate a process of reflecting about what may constitute an adequate and realistic goal in a specific situation and for a specific person. Such a counselling process can aim at sensitizing people to acknowledge negative future health consequences that are connected to certain risk behaviors like unsafe sex or drug consumption. Such a sensitizing process should always be accompanied by attempts to point out attractive alternative behaviors and to create a sense of confidence that these alternatives indeed represent a feasible option. On the other hand, if certain health goals should turn out as being unattainable or as extremely difficult to achieve, counselling should focus on how personal standards and habits can be adapted in order to make the given situation more acceptable (Gräser, 2005; Krause, 2003).

REFERENCES

Abraham, C., Sheeran, P. & Johnston, M. (1998). From health beliefs to self-regulation: Theoretical advances in the psychology of action control. *Psychology and Health, 13*, 569–591.

Affleck, G. & Tennen, H. (1996). Construing benefits from adversity: Adaptational significance and dispositional underpinnings. *Journal of Personality, 64*, 899–922.

Aldwin, C.M. & Sutton, K.J. (1998). A developmental perspective on posttraumatic growth. In R.G. Tedeschi, C.L. Park & L.G. Calhoun (Eds), *Posttraumatic Growth: Positive changes in the aftermath of crisis* (pp. 43–63). Mahwah, NJ: Erlbaum.

Alicke, M.D. (1985). Global self-evaluation as determined by the desirability and controllability of trait adjectives. *Journal of Personality and Social Psychology, 49*, 1621–1630.

Alloy, L.B. & Abramson, L.Y. (1979). Judgment of contingency in depressed and nondepressed students: Sadder but wiser? *Journal of Experimental Psychology: General, 108*, 441–485.

Aspinwall, L.G. & Brunhart, S.M. (1996). Distinguishing optimism from denial: Optimistic beliefs predict attention to health threats. *Personality and Social Psychology Bulletin, 22*, 993–1003.

Aspinwall, L.G. & Brunhart, S.M. (2000). What I do know won't hurt me: Optimism, attention to negative information, coping, and health. In J.E. Gillham (Ed.), *The Science of Optimism and Hope: Research essays in honor of Martin E.P. Seligman*, (pp. 163–200). Philadelphia, PA: Templeton Foundation Press.

Atkinson, J.W. & Feather, N.T. (1966). *A Theory of Achievement Motivation.* New York: John Wiley & Sons, Inc.

Bak, P.M. & Brandtstädter, J. (1998). Flexible Zielanpassung und hartnäckige Zielverfolgung als Bewältigungsressourcen: Hinweise auf ein Regulationsdilemma [Flexible goal adjustment and tenacious goal pursuit as coping resources: Hints to a regulatory dilemma]. *Zeitschrift für Psychologie, 206*, 235–249.

Bandura, A. (1998). Health promotion from the perspective of social cognitive theory. *Psychology and Health, 13*, 623–649.

Birren, J.E. & Schaie, K.W. (Eds). (2001). *Handbook of the Psychology of Aging* (5th edn). San Diego, CA: Academic Press.

Blazer, D. (1993). *Depression in late life* (2nd edn). St. Louis, MO: Mosby Year Book.

Boerner, K. (2004). Adaptation to disability among middle-aged and older adults: The role of assimilative and accommodative coping. *Journal of Gerontology: Psychological Sciences, 59B*, P35–P42.

Bossé, R., Aldwin, C.M., Levenson, M.R. & Ekerdt, D.J. (1987). Mental health differences among retirees and workers: Findings from the normative aging study. *Psychology and Aging, 2*, 383–389.

Brandtstädter, J. (1989). Personal self-regulation of development: Cross-sequential analyses of development-related control beliefs and emotions. *Developmental Psychology, 25*, 96–108.

Brandtstädter, J. & Baltes-Götz, B. (1990). Personal control over development and quality of life perspectives in adulthood. In P.B. Baltes & M.M. Baltes (Eds), *Successful Aging: Perspectives from the behavioral sciences* (pp. 197–224). Cambridge, MA: Cambridge University Press.

Brandtstädter, J. & Greve, W. (1994). The aging self: Stabilizing and protective processes. *Developmental Review, 14*, 52–80.

Brandtstädter, J., Meiniger, C. & Gräser, H. (2003). Handlungs- und Sinnressourcen: Entwick-lungsmuster und protektive Effekte [Action resources and meaning resources: Developmental patterns and protective effects]. *Zeitschrift für Entwicklungspsychologie und Pädagogische Psychologie*, *35*, 49–58.

Brandtstädter, J. & Renner, G. (1990). Tenacious goal pursuit and flexible goal adjustment: Explication and age-related analysis of assimilative and accommodative strategies of coping. *Psychology and Aging*, *5*, 58–67.

Brandtstädter, J., Renner, G. & Baltes-Götz, B. (1989). Entwicklung von Wertorientierungen im Erwachsenenalter: Quersequentielle Analysen [Development of values in adulthood: Cross-sequential analyses]. *Zeitschrift für Entwicklungspsychologie und Pädagogische Psychologie*, *21*, 3–23.

Brandtstädter, J. & Rothermund, K. (1994). Self-percepts of control in middle and later adulthood: Buffering losses by rescaling goals. *Psychology and Aging*, *9*, 265–273.

Brandtstädter, J. & Rothermund, K. (2002a). Intentional self-development: Exploring the interfaces between development, intentionality, and the self. In L. J. Crockett (Ed.), *Agency, Motivation, and the Life Course: Nebraska symposium on motivation*. (Vol. 48, pp. 31–75). Lincoln, NE: University of Nebraska Press.

Brandtstädter, J. & Rothermund, K. (2002b). The life-course dynamics of goal pursuit and goal adjustment: A two-process framework. *Developmental Review*, *22*, 117–150.

Brandtstädter, J., Rothermund, K. & Schmitz, U. (1998). Maintaining self-integrity and efficacy through adulthood and later life: The adaptive functions of assimilative persistence and accom-modative flexibility. In J. Heckhausen & C.S. Dweck (Eds), *Motivation and Self-regulation Across the Life Span* (pp. 365–388). New York: Cambridge University Press.

Brandtstädter, J., Voss, A. & Rothermund, K. (2004). Perception of danger signals: The role of control. *Experimental Psychology*, *51*, 24–32.

Brandtstädter, J. & Wentura, D. (1995). Adjustment to shifting possibility frontiers in later life: complementary adaptive modes. In R.A. Dixon & L. Bäckman (Eds), *Compensating for Psychological Deficits and Declines* (pp. 83–106). Mahwah, NJ: Erlbaum.

Brandtstädter, J., Wentura, D. & Greve, W. (1993). Adaptive resources of the aging self: Outlines of an emergent perspective. *International Journal of Behavioral Development*, *16*, 323–349.

Brandtstädter, J., Wentura, D. & Rothermund, K. (1999). Intentional self-development through adulthood and later life: Tenacious pursuit and flexible adjustment of goals. In J. Brandtstädter & R.M. Lerner (Eds), *Action and Self-development: Theory and research through the life span* (pp. 373–400). Thousand Oaks, CA: Sage.

Brockner, J. & Rubin, J.Z. (1985). *Entrapment in Escalating Conflicts: A social psychological analysis*. New York: Springer.

Brownlee, S., Leventhal, H. & Leventhal, E.A. (2000). Regulation, self-regulation, and construction of the self in the maintenance of physical health. In M. Boekaerts, P.R. Pintrich & M. Zeidner (Eds), *Handbook of Self-regulation* (pp. 369–416). San Diego, CA: Academic Press.

Creer, T.L. (2000). Self-management of chronic illness. In M. Boekaerts, P.R. Pintrich & M. Zeidner (Eds), *Handbook of Self-regulation*, (pp. 601–629). San Diego, CA: Academic Press.

Diener, E. & Suh, M. E. (1998). Subjective well-being and age: An international analysis. In K.W. Schaie, M.P. Lawton & M. Powell (Eds), *Annual Review of Gerontology and Geriatrics: Focus on emotion and adult development*. (Vol. 17, pp. 304–324). New York: Springer.

Ditto, P.H., Jemmott, J.B. & Darley, J. M. (1988). Appraising the threat of illness: A mental representational approach. *Health Psychology*, *7*, 183–201.

Dunning, D. (1995). Trait importance and modifiability as factors influencing self-assessment and self-enhancement motives. *Personality and Social Psychology Bulletin*, *21*, 1297–1306.

Duval, T.S. & Silvia, P.J. (2002). Self-awareness, probability of improvement, and the self-serving bias. *Journal of Personality and Social Psychology*, *82*, 49–61.

Elliott, T.R., Kurylo, M. & Rivera, P. (2002). Positive growth following acquired physical disability. In C.R. Snyder & S.J. Lopez (Eds), *Handbook of Positive Psychology* (pp. 687–699). New York: Oxford University Press.

Feather, N.T. & Newton, J.W. (1982). Values, expectations, and the prediction of social action: An expectancy-valence analysis. *Motivation and Emotion, 6*, 217–244.

Folkman, S. (1997). Positive psychological states and coping with severe stress. *Social Science and Medicine, 45*, 1207–1221.

Fournier, M., De Ridder, D. & Bensing, J. (2002). How optimism contributes to the adaptation of chronic illness. A prospective study into the enduring effects of optimism on adaptation moderated by the controllability of chronic illness. *Personality and Individual Differences, 33*, 1163–1183.

Fuhrmann, A. & Kuhl, J. (1998). Maintaining a healthy diet: Effects of personality and self-reward versus self-punishment on commitment to and enactment of self-chosen and assigned goals. *Psychology and Health, 13*, 651–686.

Gilbert, D.T. & Ebert, J.E. (2002). Decisions and revisions: The affective forecasting of changeable outcomes. *Journal of Personality and Social Psychology, 82*, 503–514.

Gollwitzer, P.M. & Kinney, R.F. (1989). Effects of deliberative and implemental mindsets on illusion of control. *Journal of Personality and Social Psychology, 56*, 531–542.

Gollwitzer, P.M. & Oettingen, G. (1998). The emergence and implementation of health goals. *Psychology and Health, 13*, 687–715.

Goschke, T. (2002). Volition und kognitive Kontrolle [Volition and cognitive control]. In J. Müsseler & W. Prinz (Eds), *Allgemeine Psychologie* (pp. 271–335). Heidelberg: Spektrum.

Gräser, H. (2005). Developmental counseling. In W. Greve, K. Rothermund & D. Wentura (Eds), *The Adaptive Self: Personal continuity and intentional self-development*, (pp. 299–321). Göttingen: Hogrefe & Huber.

Grau, J.W., Hyson, R.L., Maier, S.F., Madden, J. & Barchas, J.D. (1981). Long-term stress-induced analgesia and activation of the opiate system. *Science, 213*, 1409–1411.

Green, J., Pinter, B. & Sedikides, C. (2005). Mnemic neglect and self-threat: Trait modifiability moderates self-protection. *European Journal of Social Psychology, 35*, 225–235.

Heckhausen, H. & Gollwitzer, P.M. (1987). Thought contents and cognitive functioning in motivational versus volitional states of mind. *Motivation and Emotion, 11*, 101–120.

Hobfoll, S.E. (1989). Conservation of resources: A new attempt at conceptualizing stress. *American Psychologist, 44*, 513–524.

Janoff-Bulman, R. & Berger, A.R. (2000). The other side of trauma: Towards a psychology of appreciation. In J.H. Harvey & E.D. Miller (Eds), *Loss and Trauma: general and close relationship perspectives* (pp. 29–44). Philadelphia, PA: Brunner-Routledge.

Janoff-Bulman, R. & Brickman, P. (1982). Expectations and what people learn from failure. In N.T. Feather (Ed.), *Expectations and Actions*, (pp. 207–237). Hillsdale, NJ: Erlbaum.

Karoly, P. (1998). Expanding the conceptual range of health self-regulation research: A commentary. *Psychology and Health, 13*, 741–746.

Kofta, M. & Sedek, G. (1998). Uncontrollability as a source of cognitive exhaustion. In M. Kofta, G. Weary & G. Sedek (Eds), *Personal Control in Action: Cognitive and motivational mechanisms* (pp. 391–418). New York: Plenum Press.

Krause, M. (2003). The transformation of social representations of chronic disease in a self-help group. *Journal of Health Psychology, 8*, 599–615.

Kuhl, J. (1984). Volitional aspects of achievement motivation and learned helplessness: Toward a comprehensive theory of action control. In B.A. Maher (Ed.), *Progress in Experimental Personality Research* (Vol. 13, pp. 99–171). New York: Academic Press.

Kuhl, J. (2000). A functional-design approach to motivation and self-regulation: the dynamics of personality systems interactions. In M. Boekaerts, P.R. Pintrich & M. Zeidner (Eds), *Handbook of Self-regulation* (pp. 111–169). San Diego, CA: Academic Press.

Kuhl, J. & Helle, P. (1986). Motivational and volitional determinants of depression: The degenerated-intention hypothesis. *Journal of Abnormal Psychology, 95*, 247–251.

Lee, R.K. & Maier, S.F. (1988). Inescapable shock and attention to internal versus external cues in a water discrimination escape task. *Journal of Experimental Psychology: Animal Behavior Processes, 14*, 302–310.

Lukas, C. (2003). Handlungsregulation bei Misserfolg. Eine empirische Studie zur Aufmerksamkeitslenkung bei hartnäckiger Zielverfolgung und flexibler Zielanpassung [Action regulation after failure: Effects of tenacious goal pursuit and accommodative goal adjustment on attention allocation]. *Trier: Universität Trier.* Unpublished Master's Thesis.

Luszczynska, A. & Schwarzer, R. (2005). The role of self-efficacy in health self-regulation. In W. Greve, K. Rothermund & D. Wentura (Eds), *The Adaptive Self: Personal continuity and intentional self-development* (pp. 137–152). Göttingen: Hogrefe & Huber.

Maes, S. & Gebhardt, W. (2000). Self-regulation and health behavior: The health behavior goal model. In M. Boekaerts, P.R. Pintrich & M. Zeidner (Eds), *Handbook of Self-regulation* (pp. 343–368). San Diego, CA: Academic Press.

Maier, S.F. (1986). Stressor controllability and stress-induced analgesia. In D.D. Kelly (Ed.), *Stress-induced Analgesia* (Vol. 467, pp. 55–72). New York: New York Academy of Sciences.

Marbe, K. (1915). Der Begriff der Bewußtseinslage [The concept of mindset]. *Fortschritte der Psychologie und ihrer Anwendungen, 3*, 27–39.

McCracken, L.M. (1998). Learning to live with pain: Acceptance of pain predicts adjustment in persons with chronic pain. *Pain, 74*, 21–27.

McCracken, L. M. & Eccleston, C. (2003). Coping or acceptance: What to do about chronic pain? *Pain, 105*, 197–204.

McFarland, C. & Alvaro, C. (2000). The impact of motivation on temporal comparisons: Coping with traumatic events by perceiving personal growth. *Journal of Personality and Social Psychology, 79*, 327–343.

Mikulincer, M. (1989). Cognitive interference and learned helplessness: The effects of off-task cognitions on performance following unsolvable problems. *Journal of Personality and Social Psychology, 57*, 129–135.

Mikulincer, M., Kedem, P. & Zilkha-Segal, H. (1989). Learned helplessness, reactance, and cue utilization. *Journal of Research in Personality, 23*, 235–247.

Pahl, S. & Eiser, J.R. (2005). Valence, comparison focus and self-positivity biases: Does it matter whether people judge positive or negative traits? *Experimental Psychology, 52*, 303–310.

Piaget, J. (1970). Piaget's theory. In P.H. Mussen (Ed.), *Carmichael's Manual of Child Psychology* (Vol. 1, pp. 703–732). New York: John Wiley & Sons, Inc.

Renner, B. & Schwarzer, R. (2003). Social-cognitive factors in health behavior change. In K.A. Wallston & J. Suls (Eds), *Social Psychological Foundations of Health and Illness* (pp. 169–196). Malden, MA: Blackwell.

Rippetoe, P.A. & Rogers, R.W. (1987). Effects of components of protection-motivation theory on adaptive and maladaptive coping with a health threat. *Journal of Personality and Social Psychology, 52*, 596–604.

Rodd, Z.A., Rosellini, R.A., Stock, H.S. & Gallup, G.G., Jr. (1997). Learned helplessness in chickens (Gallus gallus): Evidence for attentional bias. *Learning and Motivation, 28*, 43–55.

Rodgers, R.J. & Hendrie, C.A. (1983). Social conflict activates status-dependent endogenous analgesic or hyperalgesic mechanisms in male mice: Effects of naloxone on nociception and behaviour. *Physiology and Behavior, 30*, 775–780.

Rogers, R.W. & Prentice-Dunn, S. (1997). Protection motivation theory. In D.S. Gochman (Ed.), *Handbook of Health Behavior Research: Personal and social determinants* (Vol. 1, pp. 113–132). New York: Plenum Press.

Rothermund, K. (1998). Persistenz und Neuorientierung: Mechanismen der Aufrechterhaltung und Auflösung zielbezogener kognitiver Einstellungen [Persistence and reorientation: Maintaining and dissolving goal-related cognitive sets]. Trier: University of Trier: Unpublished doctoral dissertation. Internet document: http://ub-dok.uni-trier.de/diss/diss11/19990701/19990701.htm.

Rothermund, K. (2003). Automatic vigilance for task-related information: Perseverance after failure and inhibition after success. *Memory and Cognition, 31,* 343–352.

Rothermund, K., Bak, P.M. & Brandtstädter, J. (2005). Biases in self-evaluation: Effects of attribute controllability. *European Journal of Social Psychology, 35,* 281–290.

Rothermund, K. & Brandtstädter, J. (1997a). Entwicklung und Bewältigung: Festhalten und Preisgeben von Zielen als Formen der Bewältigung von Entwicklungsproblemen [Development and coping: Holding on to and letting go of goals as forms of coping with developmental problems]. In C. Tesch-Römer, C. Salewski & G. Schwarz (Eds), *Psychologie der Bewältigung* (pp. 120–133). Weinheim: Psychologie Verlags Union.

Rothermund, K. & Brandtstädter, J. (1997b). Zum Verständnis der Assimilations-Akkommodations-Theorie [Understanding the assimilation-accommodation theory]. In C. Tesch-Römer, C. Salewski & G. Schwarz (Eds), *Psychologie der Bewältigung* (pp. 162–171). Weinheim: Psychologie Verlags Union.

Rothermund, K. & Brandtstädter, J. (2003a). Coping with deficits and losses in later life: From compensatory action to accommodation. *Psychology and Aging, 18,* 896–905.

Rothermund, K. & Brandtstädter, J. (2003b). Depression in later life: Cross-sequential patterns and possible determinants. *Psychology and Aging, 18,* 80–90.

Rothermund, K., Brandtstädter, J., Meiniger, C. & Anton, F. (2002). Nociceptive sensitivity and control: Hypo- and hyperalgesia under two different modes of coping. *Experimental Psychology, 49,* 57–66.

Rothermund, K., Dillmann, U. & Brandtstädter, J. (1994). Belastende Lebenssituationen im mittleren und höheren Erwachsenenalter: zur differentiellen Wirksamkeit assimilativer und akkommodativer Bewältigung [Differential efficiency of assimilative and accommodative coping with stressful life situations in middle and late adulthood]. *Zeitschrift für Gesundheitspsychologie, 4,* 245–268.

Rothermund, K. & Meiniger, C. (2004). Stress-buffering effects of self-complexity: Reduced affective spill-over or self-regulatory processes? *Self and Identity, 3,* 263–281.

Rothermund, K. & Voss, A. (2005). Probability estimates of health risks depend on controllability. Unpublished data.

Scheier, M.F. & Carver, C.S. (1992). Effects of optimism on psychological and physical well-being: Theoretical overview and empirical update. *Cognitive Therapy and Research, 16,* 201–228.

Schiaffino, K.M., Shawaryn, M.A. & Blum, D. (1998). Examining the impact of illness representations on psychological adjustment to chronic illnesses. *Health Psychology, 17,* 262–268.

Schmitz, U., Saile, H. & Nilges, P. (1996). Coping with chronic pain: Flexible goal adjustment as an interactive buffer against pain-related distress. *Pain, 67,* 41–51.

Schneider, E.L., Rowe, J.W., Johnson, T.E., Holbrook, N.J. & Morrison, J.H. (Eds). (1996). *Handbook of the Biology of Aging* (4th edn). San Diego, CA: Academic Press.

Schwarzer, R. (1999). Self-regulatory processes in the adoption and maintenance of health behaviors: The role of optimism, goals, and threats. *Journal of Health Psychology, 4,* 115–127.

Shah, J.Y., Friedman, R. & Kruglanski, A.W. (2002). Forgetting all else: On the antecedents and consequences of goal shielding. *Journal of Personality and Social Psychology, 83,* 1261–1280.

Stock, W.A., Okun, M.A., Haring, M.J. & Witter, R.A. (1983). Age and subjective well-being: A meta-analysis. In R.J. Light (Ed.), *Evaluation studies: Review annual,* (Vol. 8, pp. 279–302). Beverly Hills, CA: Sage.

Taylor, S.E. (1983). Adjustment to threatening events: A theory of cognitive adaptation. *American Psychologist, 38,* 1161–1173.

Tennen, H. & Affleck, G. (2002). Benefit-finding and benefit-reminding. In C.R. Snyder & S.J. Lopez (Eds), *Handbook of Positive Psychology* (pp. 584–597). New York: Oxford University Press.

Thompson, S.C., Anderson, K., Freedman, D. & Swan, J. (1996). Illusions of safety in a risky world: A study of college students' condom use. *Journal of Applied Social Psychology, 26*, 189–210.

Tipper, S.P. (1992). Selection for action: The role of inhibitory mechanisms. *Current Directions in Psychological Science, 1*, 105–109.

Trope, Y., Gervey, B. & Bolger, N. (2003). The role of perceived control in overcoming defensive self-evaluation. *Journal of Experimental Social Psychology, 39*, 407–419.

Updegraff, J.A. & Taylor, S.E. (2000). From vulnerability to growth: Positive and negative effects of stressful life events. In J.H. Harvey & E.D. Miller (Eds), *Loss and Trauma: general and close relationship perspectives* (pp. 3–28). Philadelphia, PA: Brunner-Routledge.

Voss, A., Rothermund, K. & Brandtstädter, J. (in press). Motivated binding: Top-down influences in a conjunction search task. In H. D. Zimmer, A. Mecklinger & U. Lindenberger (Eds), *Handbook of Binding and Memory: Perspectives from cognitive neuroscience*. Oxford: Oxford University Press (to appear in April, 2006).

Weinstein, N.D. (1980). Unrealistic optimism about future life events. *Journal of Personality and Social Psychology, 39*, 806–820.

Weinstein, N.D. (1984). Why it won't happen to me: Perceptions of risk factors and susceptibility. *Health Psychology, 3*, 431–457.

Weinstein, N.D. (1993). Testing four competing theories of health-protective behavior. *Health Psychology, 12*, 324–333.

Wentura, D. (1995). *Verfügbarkeit entlastender Kognitionen [Accessibility of palliative cognitions]*. Weinheim: Psychologie Verlags Union.

Wentura, D. & Nüsing, J. (1999). Situationsmodelle in der Textverarbeitung: Werden emotional entlastende Informationen automatisch aktiviert? [Situation models in text comprehension: Will emotionally relieving information be automatically activated?] *Zeitschrift für Experimentelle Psychologie, 46*, 193–203.

Wentura, D., Rothermund, K. & Brandtstädter, J. (1995). Experimentelle Analysen zur Verarbeitung belastender Informationen: differential- und alternspsychologische Aspekte [Experimental studies on the processing of negative information: Differential and age-related aspects]. *Zeitschrift für Experimentelle Psychologie, 42*, 152–175.

Wrosch, C., Heckhausen, J. & Lachman, M.E. (2000). Primary and secondary control strategies for managing health and financial stress across adulthood. *Psychology and Aging, 15*, 387–399.

Wrosch, C., Scheier, M.F., Carver, C.S. & Schulz, R. (2003). The importance of goal disengagement in adaptive self-regulation: When giving up is beneficial. *Self and Identity, 2*, 1–20.

Wrosch, C., Scheier, M.F., Miller, G.E., Schulz, R. & Carver, C.S. (2003). Adaptive self-regulation of unattainable goals: Goal disengagement, goal reengagement, and subjective well-being. *Personality and Social Psychology Bulletin, 29*, 1494–1508.

Wrosch, C., Schulz, R. & Heckhausen, J. (2004). Health stresses and depressive symptomatology in the elderly: A control-process approach. *Current Directions in Psychological Science, 13*, 17–20.

Wyler, A.R., Masuda, M. & Holmes, T.H. (1968). Seriousness of illness rating scale. *Journal of Psychosomatic Research, 11*, 363–374.

Index

Printed and bound by CPI Group (UK) Ltd, Croydon, CR0 4YY

27/10/2024

14580152-0002

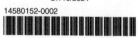